Diagnostic Imaging of the Premature Infant

Diagnostic Imaging of the
Premature Infant

Edited by

Rodrigo Dominguez, M.D.

Associate Professor
Departments of Radiology and Pediatrics
University of Texas Medical School at Houston
Radiologist
Hermann Hospital, Lyndon B. Johnson General Hospital,
  and Shriners Hospital for Crippled Children, Houston Unit
Houston, Texas

Churchill Livingstone
New York, Edinburgh, London, Melbourne, Tokyo

Library of Congress Cataloging-in-Publication Data

Diagnostic imaging of the premature infant / edited by Rodrigo
  Dominguez.
         p.   cm.
    Includes bibliographical references and index.
    ISBN 0-443-08740-7
    1.   Infants (Premature)—Diseases—Diagnosis. 2. Pediatric
diagnostic imaging.   I. Dominguez, Rodrigo.
    [DNLM: 1. Diagnostic Imaging—in infancy & childhood. 2. Infant,
  Premature. 3. Infant, Premature, Diseases—diagnosis. WS 410
  D536]
  RJ255.6.D52D53 1992
  618.92'011—dc20
  DNLM/DLC
  for Library of Congress   91-36199
                                                          CIP

Distributed in the United Kingdom by Churchill Livingstone, Robert Stevenson House, 1–3 Baxter's Place, Leith Walk, Edinburgh EH1 3AF, and by associated companies, branches, and representatives throughout the world.

Accurate indications, adverse reactions, and dosage schedules for drugs are provided in this book, but it is possible that they may change. The reader is urged to review the package information data of the manufacturers of the medications mentioned.

The Publishers have made every effort to trace the copyright holders for borrowed material. If they have inadvertently overlooked any, they will be pleased to make the necessary arrangements at the first opportunity.

Acquisitions Editor: *Nancy Mullins*
Copy Editor: *David Terry*
Production Designer: *Jill Little*
Production Supervisor: *Sharon Tuder*
Production services provided by Bermedica Production, Ltd.
Cover design by Paul Moran

Printed in the United States of America

First published in 1992   7 6 5 4 3 2 1

Contributors

Mauricio Castillo, M.D.
Assistant Professor, Department of Radiology, University of Texas Medical School at Houston; Neuroradiologist, Lyndon B. Johnson Hospital, Houston, Texas

Rodrigo Dominguez, M.D.
Associate Professor, Departments of Radiology and Pediatrics, University of Texas Medical School at Houston; Radiologist, Hermann Hospital, Lyndon B. Johnson General Hospital, and Shriners Hospital for Crippled Children, Houston Unit, Houston, Texas

Roma Ilkiw, M.D.
Assistant Professor, Division of Pediatric Cardiology, Department of Pediatrics, University of Texas Medical School at Houston; Attending Physician, Department of Pediatrics, Hermann Hospital, Houston, Texas

Seiji Kitagawa, M.D.
Assistant Professor, Department of Pediatrics, University of Texas Medical School at Houston; Attending Physician, Division of Pediatric Gastroenterology, Department of Pediatrics, Hermann Hospital, Houston, Texas

Lamk M. Lamki, M.D., F.R.C.P.C.
Professor, Department of Radiology, University of Texas Medical School at Houston; Radiologist, Hermann Hospital and Lyndon B. Johnson General Hospital, Houston, Texas

David G. Oelberg, M.D.
Associate Professor, Division of Neonatal/Perinatal Medicine, Department of Pediatrics, University of Texas Medical School at Houston; Attending Physician, Department of Pediatrics, Herman Hospital, Houston, Texas

Ignacio Pastor, M.D.
Associate Professor, Department of Radiology, Autonomous University of Madrid Medical School; Radiologist, La Paz Childrens Hospital, Madrid, Spain

Lawrence Robinson, M.D.
Associate Professor, Departments of Radiology and Pediatrics, University of Texas Medical School at Houston; Radiologist, Hermann Hospital, Lyndon B. Johnson General Hospital, and Shriners Hospital for Crippled Children, Houston Unit, Houston, Texas

A. Aguirre Vila-Coro, M.D.

Adjunct Assistant Professor, Department of Ophthalmology, University of Texas Medical School at Houston, Houston, Texas; Medical Director, Omega Eye Care Center, Jackson, Tennessee

Louis K. Wagner, Ph.D.

Associate Professor, Department of Radiology, University of Texas Medical School at Houston; Adjunct Associate Professor, University of Texas Graduate School of Biomedical Sciences; Medical Physicist, Department of Radiology, Lyndon B. Johnson General Hospital, Houston, Texas

Foreword

Late in the 1960s the advent of special care nurseries for newborn and premature infants led to a great surge of activity and knowledge in this area, and this continued throughout the 1970s and into the early 1980s. Much of what was learned in this group of patients eventually was transferred to the care of older children, and indeed, even adults. To be sure, the intensive care nursery was the precursor of intensive care medicine, and all the while, diagnostic imaging grew hand in hand with this clinical discipline. Beginning with simple chest and abdominal radiographs and then progressing to ultrasonography, computed tomography, and magnetic resonance imaging, diagnostic imaging remains a most important clinical tool in the investigation of these infants.

With all of this occurring, it was inevitable that lower and lower birthweight infants would be accepted to these nurseries. Eventually, a subdiscipline related primarily to the premature and low-birthweight infant developed. The care and treatment of these infants usually is delegated to a small, special group of closely knit physicians who understand the peculiarities of the disease processes in this early stage of life. Dr. Dominguez is one of these physicians and has had a long-standing interest in the field. Out of this interest and in conjunction with a number of equally devoted colleagues, he has produced this volume on the subject. This book is designed not only to provide information regarding the various disease entities encountered but also as an approach to the investigation, treatment, and final disposition of these patients.

Dr. Dominguez is a thorough and dedicated physician and I believe this book will be very useful for all disciplines involved in the care of these infants. It is a pleasure as well for me to note that this endeavor also comes from Texas, where the industrious, innovative, and bold can flourish. I wish Dr. Dominguez and his colleagues the best of luck with this book.

Leonard E. Swischuk, M.D.
Professor, Departments of Radiology and Pediatrics
University of Texas Medical Branch at Galveston
Director, Division of Pediatric Radiology
Department of Radiology, Child Health Center
Galveston, Texas

Preface

Presently, the most significant problems in perinatal medicine are those associated with an infant that is born prematurely or has a low birthweight (LBW). LBW infants represent over 200,000 live births each year in the United States. Although their absolute number has declined (due in part to the decreasing birth rate), our infant mortality rate, closely related to the number of LBW infants, remains high and well above the levels found in other developed countries. Its causes are controversial and not all that clear: poverty, accompanied by inadequate access to health care and proper alimentation; failure to uphold personal responsibilities (negative parental behaviors and attitudes, especially in cases of illegitimate or out-of-wedlock infants); high numbers of teenage pregnancies; smoking and drug and alcohol consumption rising among pregnant women. Very recent statistics have shown a moderate drop in the infant mortality rate due primarily to medical advances, for which we are paying a high price.

LBW infants (those weighing under 2,500 g) born prematurely or retarded in intrauterine growth are 40 times more likely to die in the neonatal period than are infants of normal birthweight. LBW survivors have an increased incidence of disability from a broad range of conditions, including neurodevelopmental handicaps, congenital anomalies, respiratory illnesses, and complications acquired during neonatal intensive care.

While many scientific medical advances were made during the first half of this century, there was little understanding of the diseases that affected premature infants. It was not until the late 1940s that the pathophysiology of respiratory distress syndrome (RDS) or hyaline membrane disease (HMD) was partially understood, and oftentimes well-intentioned treatment caused harmful side effects.

Awareness of the increased morbidity in surviving LBW infants, coupled with a greater understanding of fetal and infant nutrition, pharmacology, and pathophysiology, has advanced the development of perinatal care in the last two decades.

During the 1960s, neonatologists identified two "new" diseases that are major problems in the newborn intensive care unit (NICU): necrotizing enterocolitis (NEC) and bronchopulmonary dysplasia (BPD). Furthermore, since the survival of 1,500-g (4-lb) infants is now routine, difficult questions are now being asked about the 750-g (1 ½-lb) or 500-g (1-lb) infants. Since yesterday's miracle has become today's standard expectation, it is hard to define what constitutes a heroic measure and what should be the limits of our efforts. Most neonatologists agree that the salvage of an infant born at 25 to 26 weeks' gestation represents the limit of contemporary medical practice.

There have been other breakthroughs in the care of preterm infants, in part because of the space race and because of the rapid development of computers. New technology has changed the care-taking policies and the appearance of the NICU. Now older treatment techniques can be monitored more carefully and used more effectively with much less risk of complications. There have been almost unbelievable advances in respirator design and in monitoring technology, with a substantial reduction in the volume of blood necessary for diagnostic tests. Pediatric ventilators did not exist 25 years ago; now there are many specialized types. Infants who could not be fed in past years can now be maintained on intravenous hyperalimentation. New drugs can be used to control premature labor, often preventing delivery for crucial days or weeks. Various types of steroid drugs, such as betamethasone or dexamethasone, can be given to the mother in an attempt to prevent HMD; this disorder is now curable by the instillation of artificial surfactant.

Along with other medical advances, sophisticated imaging techniques are providing more accurate diagnoses and are making possible preventive measures and better treatments; in doing so they are decreasing the morbidity and mortality of the LBW infant. Prenatal factors contributing to high risk in neonates and LBW for premature infants are now being detected by ultrasound and magnetic resonance imaging (MRI); even though no definitive treatment exists for congenital malformations, a better understanding of their pathophysiology is emerging from these diagnostic studies.

The portable capability of real-time ultrasound has tremendously facilitated the diagnosis of acute abdominal problems and the monitoring of cerebral hemorrhagic and ischemic lesions at cribside. Computed tomography along with the development of new NICUs have contributed substantially to the decrease in perinatal morbidity from neurologic causes, while duplex Doppler ultrasound and MRI are providing insights into the physiology of blood flow of the labile premature brain and permitting clearer anatomic descriptions of cerebral and spinal congenital anomalies.

An understanding of new advances in perinatal medicine requires a comprehensive update of diagnostic imaging and its different applications in this field, which overrides obstetrics, pediatrics, and intensive care medicine. Providing such an update is our goal in the present book

I have assembled a team of pediatricians and radiologists specialized in neonatal diagnostic imaging, cardiology, gastroenterology, and ophthalmology to update the reader in the field of diagnosis of the disease processes commonly encountered in the premature infant. It is not our intention to offer a comprehensive book on pediatric radiology, nor to write extensively about the pathologic processes imaged here, but to chart diagnostic guidelines in this relatively recent field of pediatrics. This manual is in-tended for medical students and pediatric residents on clinical rotation through the NICU and for specialized pediatric nurses and respiratory therapists so that they may understand, order, analyze, and screen diagnostic imaging procedures in a more rational and cost-efficient manner. Radiologists in training and general radiologists will probably find this book helpful and may use it as a consultative aid.

Suggestions and criticisms to improve and fulfill the aims of this book are welcomed, as this will help to accomplish our goal of serving best the medical community and its direct beneficiaries, these premature infants.

Rodrigo Dominguez, M.D.

Contents

Clinical Considerations of the Premature Infant

David G. Oelberg

1

Many advances have occurred in biotechnology over the past 40 years to foster the development of perinatal-neonatal medicine. Early progress in the administration of oxygen, maintenance of body temperature, treatment of infections with antibiotics, and provision of parenteral fluids have opened the pathway to such recent innovations as fetal surgery, intrauterine transfusions, extracorporeal membrane oxygenation (ECMO), and administration of exogenous surfactant. These and related improvements in diagnostic and therapeutic procedures have increased the limits of viability and reduced the mortality and morbidity of more developed premature newborns.

Delivery prior to 37 weeks' gestation defines prematurity. The subpopulation of premature or low-birthweight (LBW) newborns is further subdivided into moderately low-birthweight (MLBW), very low-birthweight (VLBW), and extremely low-birthweight (ELBW or "micropremie") newborns.[1] Delivery between 37 and 32 weeks' gestation and average birthweights between 2,500 and 1,500 g characterize the MLBW newborns. Delivery between 31 and 28 weeks' gestation and birthweights of 1,499 to 1,000 g define the VLBW newborns. Finally, "micropremies" are delivered at gestational ages less than 28 weeks with birthweights less than 1,000 g.

The characterization of newborns by both gestational age and birthweight is important for identification of relatively overweight and underweight newborns. While most newborns are appropriately sized for their gestational ages, some are born "large for gestational age" (LGA) and others "small for gestational age" (SGA) (the latter are also referred to as having intrauterine growth retardation, or IUGR).[2] Identification of LGA and SGA newborns is critical because certain underlying diseases are frequently associated with each size category.[3]

Approximately 7 percent of all births in the United States are premature.[4] Approximately 1 percent of the LBW newborns are of the VLBW or ELBW subpopulations.[4] It comes as no surprise that mortality increases as a direct function of decreasing gestational age. Prior to 20 years ago, death rates of VLBW and ELBW newborns remained high while survival of the MLBW neonate increased to about 95 percent.[5] Over the past two decades, however, the greatest increases in survival have occurred in the VLBW and ELBW populations. In general, declines in mortality rates for VLBW and ELBW newborns paralled one another for the past 20 years. However, as survival of all VLBW newborns approached that of the MLBW population at 95 percent, survival of ELBW newborns remained directly related to gestational age despite improvements.[5]

As survival increases in the ELBW population, the limit of viability fluctuates. Unfortunately, many decisions regarding management of very sick newborns today occur without knowledge of what impact these diagnostic or therapeutic interventions may have on future quality of survival. With this general limitation in mind, as well as individual considerations regarding local practices, available resources, and parental desires, the limit of viability in the United States approaches 23 weeks' gestation or 500 g birthweight.

Encouragingly, as mortality decreases for LBW and VLBW newborns, morbidity also decreases in both frequency and severity. Twenty-five years ago the incidence rates of major neurosensory handicaps such as cerebral palsy, mental retardation, and blindness were about 50 percent and 30 percent for VLBW

1

and MLBW newborns, respectively.[1] More recently, investigators cite incidence rates of major neurosensory handicaps of 4 to 10 percent, 10 to 15 percent, and 12 to 20 percent for MLBW, VLBW, and ELBW newborns, respectively.[6] On the other hand, minor disabilities, including learning disorders, developmental delays, or conditions requiring special education, remain of considerable concern in the ELBW and VLBW populations because as many as 30 to 70 percent of these infants are affected.

The remainder of this chapter provides an overview of the common diseases encountered by LBW newborns. To this end, the first sections introduce the reader to fetal and neonatal developmental physiology. These physiologic principles serve as a framework upon which subsequent chapter sections review fetal and neonatal diseases. Although diseases of the premature newborn cannot be addressed independently from those encountered by full-term newborns, emphasis is upon diseases of the premature infant. Like other general reviews of this type, the chapter should be regarded as a stimulus for in-depth study of selected topics rather than a thorough survey of fetal and neonatal diseases.

FETAL AND PREMATURE NEONATAL PHYSIOLOGY

Concepts of Development and Adaptation

Fetal and premature neonatal physiology are the direct consequence of development and adaptation.[7] Development is the process of structural and functional changes that transforms the fertilized egg from an embryo to a fetus. This process prepares the fetus for successful adaptation to the stresses of extrauterine life. Adaptation of organ systems occurs in harmony with development as both contribute to the structural and functional competency of the newborn. Adaptation is the relative capability of organ systems to respond to intrauterine or, more commonly, extrauterine stresses with accelerated structural or functional competency.

The developmental sequence is tightly controlled by the genetic template, identified maternal/fetal regulatory mechanisms (e.g., hormones, growth factors) and unknown factors that for lack of a better term are known as the "biological clock." It is relatively insensitive to outside influences such as radiation and maternal drugs except during "critical periods" of development, which tend to occur during the first trimester of pregnancy for the embryo and fetus in general, and which are restricted to narrow windows of time for individual organ systems. Like development, adaptation of individual organ systems also proceeds at different rates from one system to another. However, adaptation is a more dynamic process that promotes alteration of selected organ systems by intrauterine or extrauterine stresses, thus resulting in positive (lung maturation) or negative (IUGR) consequences.

The LBW newborn represents a unique situation requiring premature adaptation of fetal physiology to extrauterine stresses. Successful adaptation of this type becomes more likely as gestational age and postnatal age (age after birth) increase. Because humans are dependent upon respiration for life, the first organ systems to undergo relatively rapid transition from fetal to neonatal physiology are the cardiovascular and pulmonary systems. The gastrointestinal, renal, immunologic, and hematopoietic systems are capable of gradual transition while the central nervous and musculoskeletal systems are relatively incapable of accelerated transition.

Much of the morbidity and mortality of LBW newborns are attributable to accelerated attempts at premature adaptation. Premature adaptation results in higher incidence rates of selected diseases such as necrotizing enterocolitis, periventricular hemorrhage, bronchopulmonary dysplasia, and retinopathy of prematurity. Additional consideration of these diseases occurs later in the chapter.

Physiology of the Fetomaternal-Placental Unit

Functions of the placenta include protection of the fetus and pregnancy, provision of fetal nutrition and respiration, and excretion of toxic metabolites.[8] Most of these functions are accomplished by the shunting of maternal arterial blood into intervillous spaces. Chorionic villi containing fetal arteriovenous networks extend into intervillous spaces, placing villi in direct contact with maternal blood. Accordingly, exchange of molecules proceeds with only three layers of fetal tissue separating the maternal and fetal circulations. While the intimate relationship of these circulations fosters exchange of metabolites, the potential for intermixing of circulations and subsequent "immunization" of the mother by fetal antigens increases.

Toxic products of the fetus, such as carbon dioxide, urea, and uric acid, are carried to the placenta for excretion via the umbilical arteries, while nutrients such as oxygen, glucose, amino acids, minerals, free fatty acids, and vitamins are returned via the umbilical vein. Production of amniotic fluid provides mechanical protection of the fetus, and passage of maternal immunoglobulin G antibodies during the last trimester provides the fetus with protection from infection. In addition, maintenance of pregnancy and normal development depend upon the synthesis and secretion of selected protein and steroid hormones. Disruption of the above functions usually result in abnormal development, premature delivery, or fetal death.

Unique Aspects of Fetal and Premature Neonatal Physiology

Characteristic differences exist between fetal, premature neonatal, term neonatal, and adult physiology because of structural or functional differences resulting from limited development and adaptation. In the following sections an overview of the more significant differences is presented by organ system.

Central Nervous System

The presence of the periventricular germinal matrix prior to 34 to 36 weeks of gestation is a major anatomic difference between immature and mature brains. The germinal matrix is a poorly differentiated, highly vascularized body of tissue that gives rise to neuronal and glial components of the developing cerebral cortex.[9] The limited support of tortuous, thin-walled capillary networks by connective tissue, the susceptibility of capillary endothelium to ischemic injury, and retrograde transmission of elevated central venous pressure to the cerebral venous system are among the many factors considered important to the development of periventricular hemorrhage. The germinal matrix is particularly susceptible to ischemia because it is contained within the boundary zone of arterial circulations supplying the basal ganglia and the brain stem. In addition, impaired autoregulation of cerebral blood flow in the face of hypercapnia results in pressure-passive cerebral blood flood, and the autoregulatory plateau is shifted to the left in fetuses and newborns, thus magnifying the impact of even mild hyper- or hypotension upon the hemorrhage-prone germinal matrix.

Some other differences of the fetal–premature neonatal brain relate to decreased development of the cerebral cortex. The cortical pile and gyral pattern of the cortex are less complex, and synaptic interconnections between neurons are primitive. Synthesis and release of neurotransmitters are limited, and myelination is not promoted by premature delivery. In summary, the central nervous system (CNS) is relatively resistant to accelerated development and adaptation despite premature delivery, but it is susceptible to reversible or irreversible injury in the face of extrauterine stresses because of structural and functional immaturity.

Cardiovascular System

Major differences exist between the circulatory circuits of fetuses and neonates.[8,10] In utero, well-oxygenated blood returning from the placenta via the umbilical vein and ductus venosus mixes with poorly oxygenated blood of the superior and inferior venae cavae. At the right atrium about two-thirds of the blood flow is pumped to the right ventricle while one-quarter crosses the foramen ovale to the left atrium, where it is joined by about 10 percent returning from the pulmonary circulation. The right ventricular output is pumped into the pulmonary artery; however, because of elevated pulmonary vascular resistance, all but 10 percent of the flow shunts across the ductus arteriosus to join the left ventricular output in the aorta. About one-half of the arterial systemic flow circulates to the body while the other half travels to the placenta via the umbilical arteries. At birth, constriction of the ductus arteriosus, ductus venosus, and umbilical vessels, functional closure of the foramen ovale, and decrease of pulmonary vascular resistance upon aeration cause a transition from the fetal pattern of parallel systemic and placental circulations to the adult pattern of serial systemic and pulmonic circulations. In the LBW newborn completion of the transition may be prolonged, thus resulting in persistent shunting across an abnormally patent ductus arteriosus.

In addition to differences in the circulatory circuits, differences also exist between mature and immature myocardial tissue. Functionally, calcium adenosine triphosphatase (ATPase) activity, calcium uptake rate, responsiveness to sympathetic tone, and tension development capacity per cross section of myocardium are decreased in immature myocardium.[11] Structurally, the concentrations of sarcoplasmic reticulum and myofibrils are also reduced. As a result of these limitations, cardiac output of newborns, unlike that of adults, is very rate dependent.

Pulmonary

Immature anatomy, biochemistry, and respiratory control distinguish the pulmonary physiology of fetuses and premature newborns from that of full-term newborns. Proximally, abnormally increased compliance of upper airways results from reduced or inadequate support by connective tissues and cartilage, thus predisposing the airways to collapse during inspiration. Increased chest wall compliance resulting from underdeveloped costochondral and costosternal joints and undermineralized ribs limits effective ventilation to the point of respiratory failure. Obligate nose breathing—especially in the presence of nasal obstruction—and dependence upon diaphragmatic breathing with little intercostal breathing also limits ventilatory capacity. The number of terminal airways composed of respiratory saccules, alveolar ducts, and alveoli—the sites of gas exchange—are decreased. Moreover, limited differentiation of respiratory epithelia potentially limits optimal pulmonary functioning.

Much has been written about the biochemical immaturity of premature lungs, and the interested reader is referred to much more thorough reviews, of which there are many.[12-14] For the purpose of this chapter details of the biochemistry and regulatory pathways are excluded. The net result is deficient synthesis, release, and reuptake of disaturated phosphatidylcholine, specific apoproteins, and other phospholipids such as phosphatidylglycerol. Apoproteins are recently discovered components of surfactant that are likely to influence intra-alveolar activity and reuptake of phospholipids as well as other undefined functions. Accordingly, the functional activity of surfactant may be more dependent upon nonlipid components than previously believed.

Although control of respiration is also immature, the level(s) at which delays occur are not well delineated.[15] The blunted responsiveness of carotid bodies to hypoxia and of central chemoreceptors to carbon dioxide and acidosis are important but may be less important than blunted vagally mediated reflexes and chest wall stretch reflexes. Immaturity of the brain stem reticular activating system may figure even more importantly—particularly in accounting for differences that occur between different states of sleep or activity.

Gastrointestinal System

Premature delivery of the fetus limits the capacity of the gastrointestinal tract to adapt to the extrauterine environment at all levels.[16,17] Although gastrointestinal motility proceeds in a craniocaudal direction, suck and swallow are uncoordinated until 34 to 36 weeks of gestation. Concomitantly, impaired gastroesophageal sphincter function and delayed gastric emptying predispose to gastroesophageal reflux. Immature neuromuscular development proceeding in a craniocaudal direction, uncoordinated peristaltic waves, increased antiperistaltic activity, decreased gastrointestinal hormonal activities, and impaired gastrocolic and rectosphincteric reflexes collectively contribute to delayed small and large bowel transit times in the LBW newborn. In addition to delays in motility, absorption of selected nutrients is also affected. Limited digestion of starch, lactose, and protein and delayed glucose absorption have a direct impact upon carbohydrate and protein absorption. Similarly, reductions in lipase activity and the bile salt pool impair digestion of fat and absorption of fat and fat-soluble vitamins. Delayed "gut closure" resulting in increased absorption of antigenic macromolecules increases the potential for sensitizing the premature gut to foreign antigens. The effects of premature delivery are also apparent in the liver as evidenced by (1) decreased detoxification and clearance of endogenous or exogenous toxins or drugs and (2) decreased synthesis of bile salts and other products of hepatic metabolism.

Renal System

Increased susceptibility of the LBW newborn to extrarenal water losses magnifies the difficulty of maintaining salt and water balance in the presence of immature renal function. Increased extrarenal water losses occur because of immature epidermis, increased surface-to-volume ratio of the body, tachypnea and thermal instability resulting in hyperthermia. With regard to renal function, incomplete nephrogenesis reduces glomerular filtration rate.[18] Concentrating ability is decreased by reduced medullary tonicity, variable response to antidiuretic hormone (ADH), shortened loops of Henle, and inhibitory activities of endogenous compounds such as prostaglandin E_2. Redistribution of renal blood flow from inner to outer portions of the renal cortex also may influence glomerular and tubular functions. Fractional excretion of sodium is also elevated at birth, especially in the presence of an increased sodium load. Collectively, the above factors account for the limited adaptation of the kidneys to birth and the very high incidence of salt and water disturbances in VLBW and ELBW newborns.

Hematopoietic System

At delivery the hemoglobin/hematocrit and white blood cell count of LBW newborns are slightly lower than those of full-term newborns. Typically, as oxygen saturation of hemoglobin dramatically rises at birth, erythropoietin production drops, thus resulting in a fall in erythropoiesis. The fall in new red cell production is compounded by the shortened life span of fetal red cells, thus producing a physiologic anemia that is more severe for LBW infants than for full-term infants.

Immune System

The host defense mechanisms of the fetus and LBW newborn are deficient at multiple levels.[19] For the purpose of this chapter they are classified by factors relating to the body surface, primary immune or neutrophil response, secondary immune or lymphocyte response, and limited availability of maternal milk. Susceptibility of the fragile epidermis to breakdown from decreased epithelialization and percutaneous intra-arterial or intravenous catheters; skin colonization by pathogenic, bacterial hospital flora; compromised ciliary activity of the respiratory tract; and reduced antimicrobial activity in tears and saliva collectively limit the barrier function of body surfaces to invasion by infectious agents.

Neutrophil response to infection is initially limited by smaller pools of neutrophilic stem cells and reduced stem cell proliferative capacity during infection. These limitations restrict the bone marrow's capacity for releasing large neutrophil populations into the systemic circulation in the face of infectious challenge. Concentrations of specific and nonspecific opsonins are reduced, and activity of the alternate complement pathway is decreased. In addition, impaired chemotaxis by the neutrophils and reduced bactericidal activity occur.

The most specific immune responses are performed by cell-mediated (T cell) and humoral (B cell) systems. In fetuses and LBW newborns the percentage of T cells, in general, and the quantity of T-suppressor cells are decreased. Immunoglobulin G

(IgG), IgA, IgM, IgD, and IgE production are absent. The full-term newborn acquires maternal IgG antibodies via transport across the placenta during the last trimester of gestation. However, LBW infants are deprived of these antibodies because of delivery prior to completion of the third trimester. Enteral intake of fresh maternal milk provides secretory IgA, macrophages, and B and T cells to the gut, but the limited capacity of LBW newborns for acceptance of enteral feedings often precludes this opportunity.

Endocrine/Metabolic Systems

The fetal endocrine system is independent of the maternal system because neurohypophyseal, adrenal, thyroid, and parathyroid hormones and insulin do not cross the placenta. Nevertheless, maternal metabolites and drugs are capable of exerting influence upon fetal endocrine function in a stimulatory or inhibitory capacity. A particularly good example of this occurs in the infant of the diabetic mother. Overabundance of maternal nutrients results in increased placental transport of nutrients to the fetus, who responds with fetal and, subsequently, neonatal hyperinsulinemia. In addition to fetal and maternal production of hormones, placental production of selected peptide hormones and steroidal hormones also occurs.[20]

Endocrine system development is divided into three phases.[7] The first occurs in the first trimester and results in the rudimentary development of the glandular tissue. The second results in the differentiation of the different tissues, and the third involves increasing end-organ responsiveness to the different hormones. Although detailed consideration of developing individual endocrine organs is not appropriate for this chapter, these issues are discussed again in the section regarding diseases of the endocrine systems.

The fetus' most rapid weight gain occurs at 32 to 38 weeks' gestation.[21] Achievement of this weight gain requires about 100 to 110 cal/kg/day. Maintenance of the same rate of gain is seldom realized in LBW newborns in the first days to weeks of life because of decreased endogenous energy stores, inadequate caloric intake (<100 cal/kg/day), and extrauterine stresses (e.g., temperature instability, infection, lung disease) that divert metabolic requirements away from growth. Glucose provides about 50 percent of the energy requirements in the fetus.[22] Maternally derived amino acids and free fatty acids are also transported across the placenta. Energy stores increase five-fold between 32 and 38 weeks by fat and glycogen deposition. At birth, successful metabolic adaptation requires that glycogenolysis maintain glucose homeostasis until establishment of gluconeogenesis and provision of an external source of glucose. Hepatic glycogen stores are depleted within 24 hours in the full-term newborn and sooner in the LBW newborn. Metabolic adaptation also requires that lipolysis release fatty acids and glycerol from fat stores. Heat results from energy production and, accordingly, thermal stability of the newborn depends upon successful metabolic adaptation.[23]

Musculoskeletal System

By comparison with adults, the neonate's skull is disproportionately large but the face is small because of the small jaw, absence of paranasal sinuses, and small facial bones.[7] Sutures are not fused and fontanels are present. Rapid growth of the skull accompanies growth of the brain. Ossification of the long bones begins within the first trimester, and by 12 weeks primary centers of ossification develop in nearly all bones. Secondary centers appear after birth. Nevertheless, mineralization of the bones in LBW newborns is less than that in full-term newborns.

FETAL MONITORING

Prenatal Methods of Diagnosis

Perinatologists rely upon four diagnostic methods for assessing fetal maturity or detecting fetal anomalies, genetic abnormalities, errors of metabolism and other selected diseases in high-risk pregnancies: ultrasonography, amniocentesis, fetoscopy, and chorionic villus sampling.[24] The most common indications for these procedures in early pregnancy are advanced maternal age ($>$ 35 years); prior delivery of an affected newborn; and couples with prior history of one or more pregnancy losses or balanced chromosomal translocation in one of the members. In later stages of pregnancy these procedures are employed to assess maturation, monitor disease progress, and screen for unsuspected fetal anomalies.

Ultrasonography

Ultrasonography is the most commonly employed procedure for screening for fetal and placental anomalies, determining the number of fetuses, monitoring progress of known fetal disease, and assessing fetal growth and maturation.[25] Although some have questioned its safety, most consider the procedure as safe to mother and fetus.

Amniocentesis

Amniocentesis is an outpatient procedure during which a needle is passed percutaneously into the amniotic sac under ultrasonographic guidance.[26] Fetal cells sloughed from the skin and the respiratory, gastrointestinal, and urogenital tracts are available for analysis in the amniotic fluid, as are selected biochemical markers of disease or maturation. Tissue culture of fetal cells permits analysis of the karyotype, thus providing prenatal diagnosis of chromosomal abnormalities. Elevated α-fetoprotein concentrations support the diagnosis and serve as a screen for open neural tube anomalies. Lecithin-to-sphingomyelin (L/S) ratios predict biochemical maturation of fetal lungs. Bilirubin concentrations facilitate management of fetuses with Rh isoimmune disease. Despite the usefulness of amniocentesis however, its benefits must be considered relative to risks that may be as high as 1 spontaneous abortion per 200 to 300 procedures.

Fetoscopy

Fetoscopy resembles amniocentesis except that a large-bore fiberoptic scope is passed into the amniotic cavity through a surgical incision.[27] Samples of fetal skin or fetal venous blood become available for diagnostic purposes by this procedure. The risk of fetal loss is 5 to 10 percent.

Chorionic Villus Sampling

Chorionic villus sampling requires transabdominal or transcervical aspiration of chorionic villi into tissue culture medium.[27] Culture of the tissue permits diagnosis of chromosomal abnormalities and inborn errors of metabolism as early as 8 weeks of gestation — the primary advantage of this procedure. The risk of pregnancy loss is about 2 percent.

Fetal Surveillance during High-Risk Pregnancy

The purpose of fetal surveillance during pregnancy is to prevent intrauterine death and minimize intrauterine asphyxia. To achieve this purpose, markers have been developed individually and markers have been combined as scores in an attempt to maximize sensitivity without sacrificing specificity. Of historic interest, the measurement and interpretation of estriol assays met with limited success, and the assays disappeared for the most part from clinical practice as electronic fetal heart rate monitoring and ultrasonography developed. Performance of antenatal fetal heart rate monitoring generally proceeds by one of two protocols.[28] In the nonstress test baseline heart rate and variability are evaluated in relation to fetal movements. Based on sensitivity, specificity, and predictive value, a normal nonstress test indicates a healthy fetus. By contrast, an abnormal nonstress test lacks predictive value and sensitivity. In selected cases an abnormal nonstress test provides an indication for an oxytocin challenge test or contraction stress test. Under these conditions oxytocin-induced contractions of the uterus test placental reserve.

In addition to screening for congenital anomalies, ultrasonography is particularly useful for assessing gestational age, detecting intrauterine growth retardation, determining placental placement, and combining pulsed Doppler ultrasound with real-time linear array ultrasonography to provide fetal blood flow measurements. Ultrasonographic determinations of fetal tone, movements, breathing activity, and amniotic fluid volume and electronic determination of heart rate reactivity comprise the biophysical profile.[29] The biophysical profile is another score developed for early determination of fetal compromise and possible need for early delivery.

Fetal Monitoring during Labor

Electronic fetal monitoring provides the most common method of fetal supervision during labor.[30] This technique monitors changes in fetal heart rate relative to intrauterine pressure or extrauterine tone. Changes in fetal heart rate occur as early, late, and variable decelerations. Implications of these decelerations are outside the scope of this discussion, but it is noteworthy that not all patterns indicate impending fetal compromise. Under occasional circumstances withdrawal of capillary fetal blood gas samples from a presenting part (e.g., the scalp) aids in the assessment of fetal status. Of course, performance of this technique requires ruptured amniotic membranes and concomitant cervical dilatation.

DISEASES OF AND DAMAGE TO THE FETUS

Intrauterine Growth Retardation

Low birthweight results from prematurity or abnormal fetal growth rate. Abnormal fetal growth rate gives rise to the syndrome of intrauterine growth retardation (IUGR). IUGR is subdivided into symmetric IUGR, wherein weight, length, and head circumference are small for gestational age, and asymmetric IUGR, wherein weight is affected with sparing of the head circumference and variable sparing of length. Symmetric IUGR results from fetal insults occurring very early in gestation, whereas asymmetric IUGR results from later insults. In general, IUGR occurs under circumstances of inadequate maternal supply of fetal nutrients, ineffective placental transport systems, or abnormal fetal utilization of supplied nutrients.

During pregnancy, clinical markers and ultrasound examinations provide indicators of IUGR. Decreased growth of uterine fundal height on clinical examination or decreased estimated fetal weight based on biparietal diameter of the head, head circumference, abdominal circumference, and femur length on ultrasound examination support the prenatal diagnosis of IUGR. Following delivery, newborns with birthweights less than tenth percentile for gestational age are victims of IUGR. Additionally, physical signs of decreased subcutaneous fat and hypothermia and laboratory findings of hypoglycemia, hypocalcemia, and polycythemia increase suspicion of IUGR. Prepartum management, possibly including premature delivery of the fetus, depends upon the etiology of IUGR and the gestational age of the fetus. Postpartum management is directed at treatment of neonatal diseases directly responsible for IUGR, if present, and of the metabolic or hematologic consequences of IUGR. Long-term prognoses for catch-up growth and development depend upon etiology.

Rh/ABO Isoimmune Hemolytic Anemia

Isoimmune hemolytic anemias in the fetus and newborn result from maternal sensitization to antigens on fetal and newborn red cells, production of antigen-specific IgG antibodies, and passage of antibodies across the placenta into fetal circulation. In the case of Rh sensitization, antibody production is stimulated by entrance of Rh+ red cells into the circulation of Rh− mothers. Because anti-A and anti-B antibodies occur naturally in 0− mothers, entrance of red cells into the maternal circulation is unnecessary for sensitization to the A and B antigens. Prior to the development of Rh immune globulin for prevention of sensitization in Rh− mothers, approximately 1 to 2 percent of pregnancies were affected. Successful programs of prophylaxis reduce sensitization to about 0.1 percent.[31] The incidence of ABO incompatibility is about 15 percent.[32]

The condition associated with intrauterine hemolytic anemia resulting from binding of anti-Rh antibodies to fetal red cells defines erythroblastosis fetalis. In its mildest form the newborn develops hyperbilirubinemia with variable degrees of anemia. The severest manifestation occurs as hydrops fetalis, characterized by congestive heart failure, severe anemia, generalized edema, hypoproteinemia, and pleural, pericardial, or peritoneal effusions. Mortality is as high as 5 to 10 percent.[31] By contrast, the most common manifestation of ABO incompatibility is hyperbilirubinemia, which, if recognized and treated, is associated with minimal morbidity.

Prevention of maternal sensitization to Rh antigen with the immune globulin provides the mainstay of management in mothers at risk. If erythroblastosis fetalis develops, then frequent assessment of amniotic fluid bilirubin pigment employing amniocentesis may indicate the need for ultrasound-directed intrauterine transfusion or early delivery.[33] Ultrasonography also detects early development of hydrops fetalis. Postpartum management is directed at treatment of hydrops fetalis and, in all cases of isoimmune hemolytic anemia, treatment of hyperbilirubinemia with phototherapy or exchange transfusion.

Spontaneous Abortions and Late Fetal Death

For the purpose of this chapter spontaneous abortions and late fetal death are defined as fetal death occurring prior to 20 weeks' and after 20 weeks' gestation, respectively. Etiologies include chromosomal abnormalities, congenital malformations, maternal disease, infection, immunologic factors, and obstetric complications. Lethal chromosomal abnormalities account for the single greatest percentage of spontaneous abortions.[34] Among late fetal deaths, 25 percent are associated with congenital malformations — half of which are associated with chromosomal abnormalities.[35] Maternal illnesses such as systemic lupus erythematosus, diabetes mellitus, renal disease, and congenital heart disease contribute another significant percentage of fetal wastage in early and late gestation. In addition to the TORCH agents, an increasing number of bacterial and viral agents have been implicated as contributing to fetal wastage. Immunologic rejection of fetal or placental antigens by maternal antibodies also contributes to early or late loss of pregnancy. Finally, structural abnormalities of the uterus, cervix, or placenta also cause early and late fetal death.

Umbilical Cord Accidents

Cord accidents result from structural anomalies of the cord, abnormal cord insertion in the placenta, nuchal cord entanglement, or prolapse of the cord. Among the structural anomalies that predispose to cord rupture, unusually short cords and velamentous cord insertion are the most common. In velamentous umbilical cords membranous cord vessels pass over the internal os of the uterus, thus predisposing them to rupture or thrombosis. Abnormally long cords predispose to knot formation and nuchal cord entanglement — the longer the cord the greater the number of nuchal loops. However, if nuchal entanglement occurs, the tightest loops occur with the shortest cords. Prolapse of the cord arises when a segment of the umbilical cord precedes the fetal presenting part. Associated and, presumably, predisposing conditions include prematurity, IUGR, oligohydramnios, and fetal malpresentations.

Pregnancy-Induced Hypertension and Eclampsia

In general, hypertensive disease associated with pregnancy refers to a group of hypertensive disorders requiring further division into chronic hypertension, when hypertension precedes pregnancy or 20 weeks' gestation, and pregnancy-induced hypertension, when hypertension occurs after 20 weeks' gestation.[36] Pre-eclampsia implies superimposed proteinuria and edema associated with chronic hypertension or pregnancy-induced hypertension. Associated seizures define eclampsia. The pathophysiology remains unknown but altered vascular reactivity and increased vasospasm of vascular beds predominate. Management of pregnancy-induced hypertension includes early recognition and screening of mothers at risk, frequent assessment of fetal well-being, bed rest, and reduction of blood pressure with antihypertensive and diuretic medications in mild to moderately affected mothers, and hospitalization, sedation, seizure prevention, and early delivery in severely affected mothers.

Placenta Previa

Central placenta previa occurs when the placenta completely covers the internal os of the uterus. Partial placenta previa describes placental localization at the edge of the os. Morbidity and mortality results from abortion, hemorrhage, and IUGR. Management is guided by aggressive blood volume replacement, hospitalization of symptomatic mothers, and tocolysis of preterm delivery in the presence of immature fetal lungs. Upon determination of mature lungs or at term gestation, elective delivery ensues.

Intrauterine TORCH Infections

The acronym "TORCH" serves as a reminder of the most common intrauterine infections: *t*oxoplasmosis, *o*ther (syphilis), *r*ubella, *c*ytomegalovirus, and *h*erpes simplex. Although this acronym recalls the best characterized intrauterine infections, it is recognized that many other transplacentally acquired infections exist. These include human immunodeficiency virus (HIV)—acquired immunodeficiency syndrome (AIDS), hepatitis B virus, coxsackievirus, and rubeola. Despite inclusion of herpes simplex in this group of transplacentally acquired infections, the vast majority of these infections develop during passage through the birth canal.

Clinical manifestations of these infections are grouped into the following presentations: (1) asymptomatic, (2) early or late fetal death, (3) prematurity, (4) IUGR, (5) congenital malformations, (6) disseminated sepsis, and (7) localized infection. Asymptomatic infections are typically cytomegalovirus, hepatitis A or B, enteroviruses, and toxoplasmosis, Intrauterine death occurs most frequently with syphilis and rubella. Different investigators associate rubella, toxoplasmosis, syphilis, cytomegalovirus, hepatitis B, and poliovirus with prematurity. IUGR occurs with toxoplasmosis, rubella, cytomegalovirus, syphilis, and rubeola. Congenital malformations result from rubella and cytomegalovirus infections occurring early in gestation. Disseminated infection indicative of sepsis suggests herpes simplex or syphilis, whereas localized infection with focal inflammation and destruction of tissue results from any of the agents. Long-term consequences of the infections relate directly to the clinical manifestations, but psychomotor retardation, growth retardation, and sensory impairments are common in severely affected infants.

Birth Injuries

With modern obstetric practice birth injuries are reduced to a minimum. Fetal scalp electrodes and fetal blood sampling occasionally result in scalp abscesses. On occasion, vacuum extraction gives rise to scalp lacerations, cephalohematomas, and rare intracranial hemorrhage. Complications of forceps extraction include cephalohematomas and rare facial nerve palsies. Fractures of the clavicle, humerus, or femur occur most frequently during rapid delivery of large fetuses in breech position or in fetal distress. Similarly, brachial plexus injuries usually result from lateral flexion of the neck and concomitant traction of cervical roots and plexus during delivery of LGA fetuses with abnormal presentations. Erb's palsy resulting in the "waiter's tip" posture is the most common palsy associated with birth injury.

Multiple Pregnancy

The incidences of twinning, triplets, and quadruplets are approximately 1:80, 1:8,000, and 1:512,000 pregnancies, respectively.[37] Approximately 25 percent of twins are monozygous or "identical." The perinatal death rate of twins is about four times that of singleton pregnancies. Among the fetal complications associated with multiple pregnancy, the most common include prematurity, IUGR, abnormal presentations, congenital malformations, polyhydramnios, and twin-twin transfusions.

Prior to the past decade, as many as 50 percent of multiple pregnancies escaped antepartum detection. Current figures suggest that detection now occurs in 90 percent of such pregnancies prior to delivery. Careful antepartum surveillance of fetal well-being is necessary to minimize fetal morbidity and mortality. In most cases aggressive management prevents preterm delivery prior to lung maturation. Protocols for optimal methods of delivery depend upon presentation of the fetuses and fetal size. Although long-term follow-up studies of growth and intellectual development in twins are small in number, most investigators regard observed delays in growth and intellect as consequences of prematurity rather than twinning.

Oligohydramnios and Polyhydramnios

Diminished and excessive collections of amniotic fluid define oligohydramnios and polyhydramnios, respectively. Fetal urine output, rate of fetal swallowing, pulmonary secretions, and presence of chronic amniotic fluid leakage are important factors contributing to the dynamics of amniotic fluid balance. In oligohydramnios, the two most common causes relate to reduced fetal urine output or chronic amniotic fluid leakage. Renal hypoplasia, dysplasia, and obstructive lesions most commonly account for reduced urine output. Reduced fetal swallowing from obstruction of the upper gastrointestinal tract or neurologic impairment, as in central and peripheral nervous system diseases, commonly account for fetal causes of polyhydramnios. Common maternal causes include diabetes mellitus, multiple pregnancy, and erythroblastosis fetalis. In a third of cases no maternal or fetal etiology is attributable to the disorder.

Products of pregnancies complicated by oligohydramnios or polyhydramnios do better if detected during pregnancy. Detection is initiated by clinical suspicion during prenatal care and confirmed by ultrasound examination. Management may include early delivery, particularly in the presence of mature lung indices. Oligohydramnios predisposes to fetal compression syndrome, whereby lung hypoplasia develops, facial anomalies occur, extremities are contracted, and IUGR occurs—in addition to renal defects that may be present. It is worth emphasizing that the pulmonary hypoplasia and associated pulmonary hypertension are frequently lethal. The major complications of polyhydramnios result from abnormal presentations and the primary maternal or fetal conditions giving rise to polyhydramnios. Morbidity and mortality of the fetus/newborn depend upon the primary maternal/fetal diseases.

Congenital Malformations

For the purpose of this chapter considerations of most congenital malformations appear later during review of individual organ systems. However, a few general concepts are reviewed at this time. Major malformations are defined as those that are life threatening or that require prompt surgical attention. By contrast, minor malformations are regarded as variations of normal that, in general, are not surgically corrected except for cosmetic purposes. Major malformations occur in about 2 percent of newborns while minor malformations occur in about 12 percent.[38] Malformations present as localized (most commonly) or multiple anomalies depending upon whether one or several defects occur, respectively. Known etiologies of malformations, in order of decreasing frequency, are multifactorial inheritance, mendelian inheritance, chromosomal abnormalities, and teratogenic influence.[38] Chromosomal abnormalities result from nondisjunction, translocation, and deletion. Of the localized malformations, multifactorial inheritance accounts for the majority of cases, but for multiple malformations chromosomal abnormalities predominate. Detection of most congenital malformations occurs upon physical examination after birth, but as ultrasound examinations of the fetus become more common, earlier intrauterine detection results.

DISEASES OF THE PREMATURE NEWBORN

As suggested in prior discussions, newborns deliver prematurely for different reasons—some directly attributable to disorders of the mother, fetus, or placenta and others related to uncontrollable premature onset of labor. In addition to the problems associated with intrauterine or fetal conditions, the premature newborn copes with an additional group of problems associated with premature adaptation to the extrauterine environment. Among the most common diseases observed in premature newborns during the first week are hypothermia, hypoglycemia, hypocalcemia, hyperbilirubinemia, respiratory distress syndrome, sepsis, patent ductus arteriosus, intraventricular hemorrhage, apnea, and acid-base, salt, or fluid imbalances. The remainder of this chapter considers the diseases affecting premature newborns. After initial discussions of asphyxia, sepsis neonatorum, and retinopathy of prematurity, review of the remaining diseases are organized by organ systems. Where appropriate, epidemiology, pathophysiology, clinical presentation, treatment, and prognosis are considered. It is worth emphasizing at this point that newborns often present with nonspecific clinical pictures.

The newborn's inability to provide historic information and describe symptoms often limits the diagnostic process to impressions derived from the physical examination, laboratory test results (often of limited sensitivity and/or specificity), and one's knowledge of the most likely diseases.

Asphyxia

The incidence of asphyxia increases in the presence of prematurity. Asphyxia results from conditions occurring before or during delivery that interrupt gas exchange between the placenta and fetus. Thus, conditions that reduce placental blood flow to the fetus (placenta abruptio, placenta previa, IUGR, or cord accidents), reduce maternal blood flow to the placenta (maternal hypotension or pre-eclampsia), or decrease maternal arterial oxygen saturation predispose to asphyxia. With interruption of gas exchange fetal pCO_2 and base deficit rise and pO_2 and pH fall. Without prompt resuscitation of asphyxiated newborns heart rate, systemic blood pressure, and blood flow to vital organ systems (brain, heart, lungs, kidneys, and gut) fall, causing irreversible tissue damage. Clinical presentation at birth reflects involvement of the affected organ systems. Hence, newborns may present with hypotonia, seizures, apnea, congestive heart failure, hypotension, acidosis, respiratory failure, oliguria, hypoglycemia, hypothermia, or hypocalcemia. Following initial cardiopulmonary and metabolic stabilization, treatment is directed at management of the involved organ systems.

Sepsis Neonatorum

The overall incidence of sepsis in newborns is approximately 10:1,000.[39] In premature newborns that figure jumps to about 160:1,000. In the United States group B β-hemolytic streptococci account for the majority of infections acquired within the first few days of life. Pneumonia associated with respiratory distress is the most common focus of infection. Other relatively common organisms include *Staphylococcus aureus, Staphylococcus epidermidis, Escherichia coli, Klebsiella pneumoniae, Enterobacter cloacae, Listeria monocytogenes,* and group D streptococci. Following prolonged hospitalization, particularly in patients who are receiving parenteral alimentation via a central venous catheter or are chronically ventilated, gram-negative bacilli, methicillin- resistant *S. aureus* or *S. epidermidis,* and *Candida albicans* assume greater importance.

In a majority of infants the precise portal of infection remains obscure. It is clear that neonatal sepsis is associated with prolonged rupture of amniotic membranes, maternal fever, and chorioamnionitis. While it is tempting to speculate that bacteria enter the fetal circulation via infected placental membranes or that fetuses are colonized with pathogenic bacteria during passage through the birth canal, it is also known that only a fraction of newborns delivered under these circumstances develop sepsis. Accordingly, it is suggested that other factors such as transplacental passage of protective antibodies play a role in the prevention of neonatal sepsis. In instances in which the normal integrity of the skin is violated by puncture wounds or foreign bodies are inserted into blood vessels or the trachea, the portal of infection is more clear.

The clinical presentation of sepsis neonatorum may be subtle or obvious. Vague signs include temperature instability, hypoglycemia, feeding intolerance, hypotonia, and apnea or tachypnea. Alternatively, it may present with respiratory failure, seizures, septic shock, or disseminated intravascular coagulation. Laboratory findings commonly include leukocytosis or leukopenia with an increased immature-to-total neutrophil ratio and positive cultures of blood, cerebrospinal fluid, or urine. Treatment is directed at the infection and includes antibiotics, and in the case of associated complications, assisted ventilation, blood and platelet replacement, anticonvulsants, and vasopressors. Despite the disappointing experience with leukocyte transfusions, recent evidence suggests that immunoglobulin therapy is of value. Mortality is variable but probably ranges from 10 to 30 percent in modern neonatal intensive care units.[40]

Retinopathy of Prematurity

With the advent of continuous electronic oxygen monitoring and efforts to maintain pO_2 below 100 mmHg, the incidence of retinopathy of prematurity (ROP) has decreased from epidemic proportions— particularly in infants with birthweights greater than 1,000 g. ROP is rare in infants with birthweights greater than 1,8000 g and uncommon for birthweights between 1,500 and 1,800 g. ROP results from abnormal proliferation of small retinal vessels. Normal retinal vascularization begins at 16 weeks of gestation. In contrast to normal vascularization resulting in otherwise normal vision, proliferation of the abnormal vessels subsequently may result in (1) rapid regression with visual defects that are correctable by lenses; (2) delayed regression causing scarring of the retina that is correctable by lenses but carries a risk of eventual retinal detachment; or (3) minimal regression, exudation from vessels, inflammation of the vitreous, and severe scarring of the retina that produces retinal detachment and subsequent blindness.

The pathogenesis of ROP is not fully elucidated but relates to cytopathic effects of excess oxygen on immature retinal vessels. Oxidant-induced injury of the immature endothelium has prompted the use of antioxidant therapy with limited efficacy. Early detection of ROP depends upon screening ophthalmic examinations of infants at risk by 6 to 8 weeks of age. The most promising therapy for infants with the severest forms of disease is cryotherapy, which attempts to prevent retinal detachment. The long-term prognosis for infants with birthweights less than 1,000 g is a 5 percent incidence of blindness.[41]

Diseases of the Central Nervous System

Periventricular Hemorrhage

Periventricular hemorrhage (PVH) is a disease of LBW newborns. Evolving from rupture of the subependymal germinal matrix, which normally disappears at about 35 to 36 weeks of gestation, PVH usually occurs in newborns delivered prior to this gestational age. Overall, the incidence of PVH in premature newborns is 40 to 50 percent.[42] In VLBW newborns the published incidence ranges between 30 and 70 percent. Severity of PVH varies from those hemorrhages isolated to the subependymal region to those that rupture into the ventricular system and those that extend into cerebral tissue.

In addition to prematurity, several other conditions predispose to PVH, thus providing clues as to its pathogenesis. Respiratory distress syndrome, asphyxia, pneumothorax, apnea, patent ductus arteriosus, hypervolemia, hyperosmolality, and hypotension predispose to PVH. The germinal matrix is a weakly supported network of thin-walled capillaries that rupture in the presence of increased intracapillary pressure, decreased endothelial integrity, or decreased external support. Loss of autoregulation of cerebral blood flow predisposes to endothelial injury and acute increases in intracapillary pressure.

Although victims of PVH may present with seizures, anemia, bulging fontanels, hypotonia, or apnea, the majority are asymptomatic. Screening ultrasound examinations of the brain in infants at risk are the cornerstone of diagnosis. Computed tomography (CT) or magnetic resonance (MR) imaging exams are useful but less practical in sick newborns because of high cost and nonportability. There is no specific treatment for PVH. Anticonvulsants control seizure activity; other symptoms are treated expectantly.

The primary complications of PVH are posthemorrhagic hydrocephalus (PHH), cerebral palsy, and mental retardation. PHH occurs in moderate to severe cases of PVH, with incidence rates of 15 to 25 percent in moderate and 65 to 100 percent in severe cases.[43] PHH results from inflammation and scarring caused by blood in the intraventricular space. Scarring disrupts normal patterns of cerebrospinal fluid flow and reabsorption, thus producing hydrocephalus. Initially, PHH is treated with serial lumbar or ventricular punctures to remove excess accumulation of cerebrospinal fluid. Medications are used in an attempt to reduce fluid production with variable efficacy. However, in cases that fail to respond to these initial therapies placement of a ventriculoperitoneal shunt provides continuous drainage of excessive fluid into the peritoneum. Multiple etiologies, including PVH and PHH, contribute to the development of cerebral palsy and mental retardation. These two neurologic deficits are of sufficient importance to merit separate consideration later in the chapter.

Other Types of Intracranial Hemorrhage

In addition to PVH, three other types of intracranial hemorrhage occur in neonates. Subdural hemorrhages are uncommon in premature newborns because pathogenesis usually relates to delivery of a relatively large head through a relatively small or rigid birth canal. By contrast, subarachnoid hemorrhages occur in both preterm and term newborns in association with asphyxia. Because the source of bleeding is venous, the consequences are usually mild. The most common presentation, particularly in premature newborns, is asymptomatic. Other presentations occur with seizures or, rarely, with massive hemorrhage and death. The prognosis for infants presenting with seizures, as for those who are asymptomatic, is very good. Intracerebellar hemorrhages, like PVH, are unique to preterm newborns. The pathogenesis is generally unknown, but there is an association with severe PVH and with occipital molding. Clinically, the infants often demonstrate a catastrophic course resulting in death.

Periventricular Leukomalacia

Periventricular leukomalacia (PVL) results from reduced cerebral blood flow to border zones of the middle, anterior, and posterior cerebral arteries. Ischemia of the border zones produces coagulation necrosis, followed by proliferation of astrocytes, endothelia, and macrophages and eventual cavitation or thinning of periventricular white matter. Clinically, PVL occasionally contributes to death, but more commonly it gives rise to the spastic diplegia form of cerebral palsy.

Seizures

PVH and severe asphyxia are the most common causes of seizures in the preterm newborn. The next most frequent causes are metabolic in nature and include hypoglycemia, hypocalcemia, hypomagnesemia, hyperphosphatemia, and hypo- or hypernatremia. Another frequent cause is infection of the central nervous system, as in meningitis or encephalitis. Occasionally, withdrawal from narcotics or barbiturates or inadvertent injection of local anesthetics accounts for seizure activity. Clinical presentations of seizures usually differ from those typical of older children and adults. The most common presentation is subtle because it is easily overlooked by the untrained eye. Its manifestations include apnea, sucking activity, tongue thrusting, deviation of the eyes, or "rowing" or "pedaling" activity of the limbs. Other seizure types include clonic, tonic, or myoclonic forms. Treatment of seizures caused by metabolic disturbances or CNS infection is directed at treatment of the metabolic disorder or infection. Seizures resulting from infection, PVH, and asphyxia are treated with anticonvulsants such as phenobarbital. The prognosis for normal development depends upon the etiology of seizure. In general, PVH and CNS infections carry the worst prognoses.

Spina Bifida

Spina bifida refers to a group of disorders resulting from incomplete dorsal closure of the neural tube or surrounding vertebral column. The most common and most benign of the lesions is spina bifida occulta, which occurs as a defect in the posterior lumbosacral vertebral arch. Clinically, it is usually asymptomatic and presents as a sacral dimple, tuft of hair, or angioma. Occasionally subcutaneous benign tumors such as lipomas or dermoid cysts are associated, causing symptoms from pressure on the cord or tethering of the cord. The next most common disorder is meningomyelocele. This presents as a dorsal outpouching of meninges and neural elements beyond the vertebral arch. The Arnold-Chiari malformation, consisting of a complex brain stem malformation, small posterior fossa, herniation of the cerebellar vermis through the foramen magnum, and hydrocephalus from aqueductal forking is often associated with meningomyeloceles. Etiology is unknown but a familial component is present in some cases. Diagnosis is obvious from physical examination and frequently made prepartum by ultrasound examination. Treatment consists of surgical closure of the meningomyelocele sac within 24 hours of delivery, eventual treatment of hydrocephalus with a ventriculoperitoneal shunt, and evaluation of neurologic, orthopaedic, and urologic functions. Prognoses vary with the size and location of the lesion, and, in general, only a minority of patients achieve normal intelligence. Meningoceles resemble meningomyeloceles except that neural tissue is absent from the sac. Overall, prognosis is much better than that of meningomyeloceles. Finally, myeloschisis and craniorachischisis totalis represent lethal conditions in which newborns present with splayed exposure of the neural plate, thus resulting in profound neurologic deficit and death from sepsis.

Meningitis and Encephalitis

Bacterial meningitis occurs with frequencies as high as 1:1,000 births and with a prevalence for premature newborns.[44] The most common organisms are the same as those observed in sepsis neonatorum, with group B β-hemolytic streptococci and *E. coli* accounting for 65 percent of infections. Clinical presentations are similar to those of sepsis neonatorum, and seizures are often present. Cerebrospinal fluid findings of bacterial growth in culture, bacterial organisms on smear, increased white blood cells, decreased glucose, and increased protein confirm the diagnosis of meningitis. Antibiotic therapy and supportive therapy constitute the cornerstones of treatment. Mortality from neonatal bacterial meningitis is as high as 20 to 40 percent, and 30 to 50 percent of survivors suffer permanent neurologic damage.[44] Aseptic meningitis in the neonatal period, although known to occur, is relatively uncommon except in association with encephalitis occurring with cytomegalovirus, varicella, herpes simplex type 2, and rubella infections. Of newborns with disseminated or localized herpes simplex type 2 infection or symptomatic rubella and cytomegalovirus, encephalitis is common. Diagnosis is usually based on confirmation of the disease at other body sites, abnormal cerebrospinal fluid findings, viral isolation from brain tissue or cerebrospinal fluid, seizures, coma, or an abnormal electroencephalogram. With the exception of herpes, for which a specific anti-viral agent is available, treatment is supportive. Prognosis is poor, with both mortality and morbidity approaching 75 percent.[44]

Mental Retardation and Cerebral Palsy

Mental retardation refers to impaired intellectual abilities measured by learning ability, abstract thinking, sensory memory, verbal expression, and social adjustment. Operationally, it is defined by formal intelligence testing, which measures intelligence in terms of intelligence quotient (IQ) or ratio of mental age to chronologic age. Despite identified problems with this measure, persons with IQs less than 75 are considered mentally retarded. Over 100 identified factors are associated with mental retardation, and the incidence in premature newborns is two to three times greater than that in the population at large. Other investigators find the average IQ of preterm infants at school age to be about 10 points less than that of otherwise normal classmates. The specific factors contributing to decreased intellectual abilities in LBW newborns probably include placental insufficiency, PVH, hypoxic injury of the CNS, suboptimal nutrition, and CNS infections.

Cerebral palsy refers to a nonprogressive motor deficit resulting from injury to the CNS during the pre- or perinatal period. Spastic diplegia is the most common type associated with prematurity, and 50 percent of those infants with spastic diplegia are premature newborns.[45] It is characterized by spasticity, rigidity, and contractures of the lower extremities with secondary involvement of upper limbs. Intelligence is usually normal or borderline low. PVH, PVL, and hydrocephalus constitute the most common causes of spastic diplegia in the premature newborn. Treatment is directed at maximizing mobility and normal motor development with stretching exercises and orthopaedic appliances and procedures.

Diseases of the Cardiovascular System

Persistent Patent Ductus Arteriosus

Persistent patency of the ductus arteriosus is most common in premature infants, females, and newborns surviving respiratory distress syndrome.[46] It is the most common cause of heart diseases presenting in preterm infants, accounting for approximately 40 percent of cases. It is commonly associated with other congenital heart diseases. The ductus arteriosus conducts blood flow between the aorta and the left pulmonary artery. It usually constricts to functional closure during the first day of life in term infants. In preterm infants, closure is commonly delayed secondary to decreased pO_2 and ductal muscle mass and increased levels of circulating prostaglandins. With increased pulmonary vascular resistance (e.g., during respiratory distress syndrome), blood flow through the ductus is from the pulmonary artery to the aorta, thus promoting hypoxemia. With a fall in pulmonary vascular resistance (e.g., as respiratory distress syndrome resolves) blood flow reverses, causing increased pulmonary blood flow, left ventricular volume overload, and congestive heart failure. The clinically significant patent ductus arteriosus presents with a systolic murmur, increased pulse pressures, and signs of mild to severe congestive heart failure such as poor feeding, tachycardia, pulmonary edema, hepatosplenomegaly, and peripheral edema. Diagnosis is supported by cardiomegaly and pulmonary edema on chest radiograph and confirmed by echocardiography. Closure is effected by administration of the prostaglandin inhibitor indomethacin or by surgical ligation of the ductus. Prior to closure supportive therapy such as diuretics, fluid restriction, and respiratory support is directed at treatment of congestive heart failure.

Other Congenital Heart Diseases

Of other congenital heart diseases presenting during the neonatal period and associated with preterm infants, the most common are ventricular septal defect and coarctation of the aorta.[47] Ventricular septal defects often present initially in the nursery as systolic murmurs without associated symptoms. However, as pulmonary vascular resistance falls a large blood flow from the left to the right ventricle may develop depending upon the size of the defect. In the presence of large left-to-right shunts, pulmonary edema and congestive heart failure result. Diagnosis is confirmed by echocardiography, and treatment is directed at management of congestive heart failure until palliative or corrective surgery is performed. Discussion of coarctation of the aorta is beyond the scope of this chapter because of its frequent occurrence as a complex cardiac malformation rather than an isolated lesion. Finally, in the newborn with cyanosis it is useful to remember the "five Ts" causing cyanotic heart disease—transposition of the great vessels, tetralogy of Fallot, truncus arteriosus, tricuspid atresia, and total anomalous pulmonary venous drainage.

Persistent Fetal Circulation

Persistent fetal circulation, or persistent pulmonary hypertension, most commonly occurs in premature newborns in association with respiratory distress syndrome. Less frequently associated conditions include sepsis neonatorum, asphyxia, and polycythemia. Clinically, persistent fetal circulation presents as severe hypoxemia resembling congenital cyanotic heart disease. Hypoxemia results from shunting of poorly oxygenated blood from the left pulmonary artery to the aorta through a patent ductus arteriosus or from the right to the left atrium through a patent foramen ovale secondary to increased pressures in pulmonary arteries and the right atrium. In respiratory distress syndrome, persistent fetal cirulation contributes to but is not the major cause of associated hypoxemia. Generally speaking, persistent fetal circulation is primarily a disease of term newborns.

Diseases of the Pulmonary System

Respiratory Distress Syndrome

Prior to the availability of exogenous surfactant, which appears to have dramatically reduced the mortality directly resulting from respiratory distress syndrome (RDS), 50 to 70 percent of deaths in preterm newborns were associated with RDS.[48] Incidence is inversely related to gestational age, and in LBW infants the incidence is 10 to 15 percent while in VLBW infants it is greater than 70 percent. Intrauterine stress, IUGR, maternal administration of steroids 24 to 48 hours prior to delivery, and female sex of the newborn constitute factors that reduce the incidence of RDS.

RDS results from insufficient availability of surfactant produced by type II pneumocytes lining the alveolar spaces and, in the most immature newborns, insufficient alveolar surface area necessary for the available capillary beds to provide adequate gas exchange. Surfactant availability depends upon adequate synthesis, release, and turnover to ensure sufficient quantities of the phospholipid material. Prematurity and perinatal insults such as asphyxia reduce availability. In the absence of sufficient quantities, alveolar surface tension increases; atelectasis occurs; hypoventilation and intrapulmonary shunts develop producing hypoxemia, hypercarbia, and acidosis; capillary damage occurs; and plasma proteins leak into the alveolar spaces. This cascade of events further compromises availability or surfactant.

Clinically, infants with RDS usually present within 6 hours of delivery with tachypnea, expiratory grunting, nasal flaring, intercostal retractions, and variable degrees of cyanosis. Management includes support of metabolic parameters and nutrition, oxygen supplementation, and continuous positive airway pressure (CPAP) or assisted ventilation. In addition, evaluation for bacterial pneumonia with initiation of antibiotic therapy is usually indicated because pneumonia and RDS are clinically indistinguishable. More recently, administration of exogenous surfactant via endotracheal instillation is proving efficacious by occurrence of clinical improvement within minutes to hours.

Transient Tachypnea of the Newborn

By comparison with RDS, transient tachypnea of the newborn (TTN) is a relatively benign disease. As many as a third of premature newborns present with this disease, but mortality is rare. Etiology is related to delayed absorption of fetal fluid from the lung. Although resolution commonly occurs within 24 to 72 hours of delivery, severity is variable and appears directly related to gestational age. In VLBW newborns initial respiratory support may require assisted ventilation, whereas in near-term newborns oxygen supplementation is usually sufficient. Clinical presentation is similar to those of RDS and pneumonia. The disease is self-limited, and prognosis is excellent. However, as for RDS, evaluation for pneumonia and administration of antibiotics are often initiated.

Wilson-Mikity Syndrome and Chronic Pulmonary Insufficiency of the Premature Infant

Diagnoses of Wilson-Mikity syndrome and chromic pulmonary insufficiency of the premature infant (CPIP) are reserved for VLBW infants who do not require assisted ventilation in the first days of life but who subsequently develop respiratory distress of undetermined etiology. Respiratory distress is secondary to atelectasis and overly distended areas of lung, and it may progress to eventual need for assisted ventilation. Radiographic examinations vary from normal radiographs to others that are indistinguishable from bronchopulmonary dysplasia. Most likely, CPIP and Wilson-Mikity syndrome represent extremes of the same disease process wherein CPIP is the milder of the two forms. Both the inability to radiographically distinguish between Wilson-Mikity syndrome and bronchopulmonary dysplasia and the aggressive use of assisted ventilation in VLBW newborns during the first hours of life have markedly restricted the diagnosis of Wilson-Mikity syndrome in nurseries today.

Pneumonia

Pneumonia is associated with as many as 20 percent of neonatal deaths. Etiologies may be divided into those acquired transplacentally, those acquired by aspiration, and those acquired during delivery or postpartum. Transplacental agents include the TORCH agents and *Listeria monocytogenes*. Aspiration of amniotic fluid or meconium may give rise to infections by streptococci, pneumococcus, or *E. coli*. Intrapartum or postpartum pneumonias result from any of the agents causing sepsis neonatorum as well as respiratory syncytial virus, other respiratory viral pathogens, *Chlamydia trachomatis*, and *Candida albicans*. The clinical presentation may be similar to that of sepsis neonatorum or more specific, with cyanosis, tachypnea, grunting, nasal flaring, intercostal retractions, rales, wheezes, and an abnormal chest radiograph. Treatment is directed at specific antibiotic therapy of the infection and support of respiratory distress.

Air Leak Syndromes

In most nurseries, the incidence of air leak syndromes in premature newborns receiving assisted ventilation is 10 to 30 percent. Air leak results from rupture of alveoli followed by extravasation of air into lung interstitial tissue. This event gives rise to pulmonary interstitial emphysema. Subsequently, air may dissect proximally along the bronchoalveolar tree to the mediastinum, thus resulting in pneumomediastinum. From the mediastinum air may cause a pneumothorax by dissecting into the pleural space or pneumopericardium by dissecting into the pericardium. Either event represents a medical emergency requiring immediate evacuation of air from the pleural space or pericardium. Although pneumopericardia are relatively uncommon, mortality is high secondary to cardiac tamponade. Rarely, air dissects beyond the thorax into the peritoneum (pneumoperitoneum) or into subcutaneous tissues of the head or neck. Diagnosis of these conditions is made by radiographic examination and clinical suspicion based on rapid deterioration of infants at risk. Treatment of pneumothorax begins with the placement of a chest tube in the pleural space and subsequent application of negative pressure. If tolerated by the infant, attempts are made to reduce applied ventilatory pressures.

Congenital Malformations

Although congenital malformations of the lung occur in premature newborns, they do not occur with increased frequency except for one entity. Laryngotracheomalacia occurs as a developmental delay that improves with time. It results from inadequate cartilaginous development of the larynx or trachea and reduced intraluminal diameter of the newborn airway, thus permitting collapse of the airways during respiration. Characteristically, if involvement occurs proximal to the vocal cords, stridor is inspiratory; if it occurs distal to the cords, then stridor is expiratory. Specific treatment is usually unnecessary, but if edema of the upper airway occurs or respiratory secretions increase, then assisted ventilation may be required.

Although congenital laryngotracheal stenosis is rare, acquired laryngotracheal stenosis secondary to prolonged intubation is observed in premature newborns requiring prolonged assisted ventilation. Symptoms are similar to those of laryngotracheomalacia, and treatment consists of racemic epinephrine, tracheotomy, or surgical split of the cricoid cartilage depending upon the type and severity of stenosis.

Pulmonary Hemorrhage

Pulmonary hemorrhage most commonly occurs in VLBW newborns receiving assisted ventilation. Although the etiology is somewhat elusive, patent ductus arteriosus with a large intrapulmonary shunt, sepsis neonatorum, pneumonia, or congenital heart disease is commonly associated. Most commonly infants present with rapid deterioration, and blood is suctioned from the endotracheal tube. Treatment is supportive, with continued assisted ventilation and transfusion of red blood cells and clotting factors.

Apnea of Prematurity

Apnea of prematurity occurs in as many as 25 percent of premature newborns.[49] It is defined by apnea lasting longer than 20 seconds, frequently accompanied by bradycardia. Apnea of prematurity is directly related to periodic breathing, which occurs in 25 to 50 percent of premature newborns. Periodic breathing, which presents as periods of apnea lasting 5 to 15 seconds followed by normal respiration at 50 to 60 times per minute, is considered a developmental delay in brain stem regulation of respiration in premature infants. Typically, it resolves by 36 to 37 weeks of gestation. Some investigators regard apnea as an extension of periodic breathing occurring when factors are present that prolong the apneic phase. Such factors include hypothermia, intracranial lesions, drugs, hypoxemia, acidosis, infection, gastroesophageal reflux, and metabolic disorders such as hypoglycemia and hypocalcemia. Another useful classification of apnea divides types into central, obstructive, and mixed disorders.[50] By this classification obstruction of the upper airway at the pharyngeal level gives rise to hypoxemia in the mixed and obstructive disorders. Treatment consists of sensory stimulation, changes in environment, oxygen supplementation, methylxanthine (theophylline or caffeine) administration, CPAP, or, if necessary, assisted ventilation. Prognosis is generally good.

Bronchopulmonary Dysplasia

The incidence of bronchopulmonary dysplasia (BPD) varies from 3 to 6 percent in all ventilated newborns to 30 to 40 percent in VLBW newborns.[51] It is clinically defined by oxygen dependency at 28 days following assisted ventilation, compatible radiographic findings, and appropriate clinical signs.[52] As determined by histologic examination, development of the disease progresses as necrosis with regeneration and proliferation of bronchiolar and alveolar epithelia, subsequent bronchiolar squamous metaplasia and interstitial fibrosis, and eventual obliterative bronchiolitis. The etiology is multifactorial and includes oxidant damage from prolonged oxygen therapy, barotrauma from positive pressure ventilation, secondary infections, occurrence of pulmonary interstitial emphysema, and intrapulmonary shunting via patency of the ductus arteriosus. Clinically, infants require prolonged respiratory support for hypoxemia and hypercarbia, thus contributing to the pathogenetic process. Treatment consists of weaning from respiratory assistance, diuretics, bronchodilators, optimal nutritional support, and methylxanthines. More recently, steroid therapy has offered promising improvements. In infants with severe BPD, mortality is 25 to 35 percent[53] and significant neurodevelopmental delays approach 60 to 80 percent.[54]

Diseases of the Gastrointestinal and Hepatobiliary Systems

Necrotizing Enterocolitis

Necrotizing enterocolitis (NEC) occurs with an incidence of about 2 percent in infants admitted to intensive care nurseries.[55] The most common factors associated with NEC are prematurity, history of asphyxia or shock, oral feedings, and overgrowth of gut flora. Other factors include umbilical catheters, clostridial enterotoxins, exchange transfusions, and polycythemia. Although etiologies appear multifactorial, a simplistic view of pathogenesis begins with ischemia of the intestine resulting in necrosis of epithelial mucosa, ensuing ileus, and overgrowth of bacterial flora in the presence of formula serving as substrate. Clinical presentations include feeding intolerance, abdominal distension, vomiting, gastric residua, hematochezia, or any of the signs of sepsis neonatorum. Intestinal perforation may present with septic shock, acidosis, or thrombocytopenia. Diagnosis is confirmed by radiographic examination. Treatment includes withholding oral feedings, gastric suction, systemic antibiotics, support of intravascular space with blood products, frequent radiographic examinations to detect perforation, and nutritional support by parenteral alimentation. In the event of perforation, elevated serum potassium, persistent acidosis, or thrombocytopenia, surgical intervention is indicated. Survival approximates 80 percent; however, a subpopulation of survivors suffer short gut syndrome resulting from insufficient bowel to provide adequate absorption of nutrients. Many of these infants require long-term parenteral alimentation.

Gastrointestinal Hemorrhage

The majority of gastrointestinal hemorrhages are undetermined. Possibilities include swallowed maternal blood, anorectal fissures, stress ulceration, NEC, and hemorrhagic disease of the newborn. The Apt test is useful for distinguishing maternal blood from newborn blood. Occasionally, intestinal volvulus, duplications, or hiatal hernias present with hematemesis. Supportive treatment is usually sufficient for most cases of gastrointestinal hemorrhage. Occasionally, surgery or specific treatment of clotting disorders is required. Overall, prognosis is good except for NEC.

Abdominal Wall Defects

Two types of abdominal wall defects occur in the newborn: omphalocele and gastroschisis. Omphaloceles result from failure of abdominal wall closure after return of the midgut into the abdominal cavity during the 10th to 12th weeks of gestation. Omphalocele presents as a midline defect with incorporation of the umbilical cord into the omphalocele sac. Nearly 70 percent of omphaloceles are associated with other major congenital anomalies.[56] The etiology of gastroschisis is less clear, but it presents as a defect in lateral closure of the abdominal wall. Intestine herniates through the defect in the absence of an enclosing sac. Unlike omphaloceles, gastroschisis is rarely associated with other congenital anomalies, but 60 percent of cases are associated with prematurity.[57] Management includes decompression of the gastrointestinal tract by gastric drainage that is followed by primary or staged surgical closure of the abdominal wall defect.

Obstruction of the Gastrointestinal Tract

Obstructive lesions of the neonatal gastrointestinal tract are divided by symptomatology into preampullary and postampullary small intestinal types and colonic types. Typically, infants with preampullary lesions present with salivation, nonbilious vomiting, and absence of abdominal distension. Etiologies include tracheoesophageal fistula, gastric web, lactobezoar, and hypertrophic pyloric stenosis. Postampul-

lary forms of gastrointestinal obstruction present with bilious vomiting and varying degrees of abdominal distension occasionally associated with delayed passage of meconium. Etiologies in this group include duodenal atresia, annular pancreas, small intestinal webs, malrotation, jejunoileal atresia, and meconium ileus. Occasional bilious vomiting, abdominal distension, and delayed passage of meconium characterize the last group of disorders. Examples of colonic obstruction include meconium plug syndrome, Hirschsprung's disease, functional immaturity of the gut and imperforate anus.

Despite the many causes of neonatal gastrointestinal obstruction, only a few are specifically associated with prematurity. Lactobezoars are more common in premature infants receiving 24 cal/ounce formulas. Contributing causes for the LBW infant's susceptibility to lactobezoars include decreased gastric emptying time and acidity, increased caloric density and calcium content, and increased transgastric absorption of formula fats—present as medium-chain triglycerides. Treatment rarely requires surgery. As many as 50 percent of infants with jejunoileal atresia are LBW newborns. In addition to other symptoms of postampullary small intestinal obstructive anomalies, polyhydramnios and jaundice may be associated. The anomalies occur as isolated or multiple atresia, and the etiology probably relates to intrauterine vascular accidents of mesenteric circulation. Surgical correction is required in all affected newborns. A common cause of delayed meconium passage in VLBW newborns is functional immaturity of the gut. Although rarely producing symptoms in the absence of attempted enteral feeding, it is often the reason behind slow attainment of a complete diet by the gastrointestinal route in VLBW newborns.

Gastroesophageal Reflux

Variable degrees of gastroesophageal (GE) reflux occur in many newborns. It is particularly frequent and more commonly severe in LBW newborns. The causes of neonatal GE reflux relate to developmental immaturity of the lower esophageal sphincter associated with lower pressures, prolonged sphincter relaxation, and shorter, predominantly intrathoracic sphincters, as well as reduced coordination of esophageal motility. Most cases of GE reflux are self-limited and resolve by the age of 6 months after adjusting for gestational age. Diagnosis may be confirmed by an esophageal pH probe, barium swallow examination, or gastric scintiscan. In severe cases complications include failure to thrive, aspiration pneumonia, recurrent vomiting, or esophageal bleeding. These complications are the usual indications for surgical intervention by the Nissen fundoplication. More commonly, however, GE reflux management consists of thickened feedings; frequent, small feedings; upright positioning; continuous orogastric or oroduodenal feedings; and, rarely, metoclopramide to facilitate gastric emptying. Except in the presence of severe neurologic injury, prognosis for recovery is very good.

Hyperbilirubinemia

Hyperbilirubinemia presents in the neonatal period as one of two types. Neonatal jaundice, or indirect (unconjugated) hyperbilirubinemia, occurs within the first 2 weeks of life and is the most common of the two types. Neonatal (infantile) cholestasis is the second type, and it presents as a direct (conjugated) hyperbilirubinemia after the first 2 weeks of life.

The most common cause of neonatal jaundice is physiologic jaundice. In premature newborns it peaks later and is more prolonged than in term newborns. It results from several factors, including an increased hepatic bilirubin load, decreased hepatic uptake and excretion of bilirubin, and reduced hepatic conjugation of bilirubin. It is a self-limited condition but occasionally requires phototherapy treatment, particularly in LBW infants. Another cause of neonatal jaundice is associated with the ingestion of breast milk. Although rarely causing hyperbilirubinemia that is significant enough to require phototherapy, elimination of breast milk from the diet for 24 to 48 hours resolves the condition. While etiology of breast milk jaundice is unknown, it is probably multifactorial.

In addition to physiologic jaundice and breast milk jaundice, there are many other causes that more typically require treatment by phototherapy or exchange transfusion. Indirect hyperbilirubinemia is treated to avoid excessively high serum concentrations of unconjugated bilirubin, which are associated with kernicterus and hearing loss. These additional causes are divided by pathogenesis into those producing increased loads of bilirubin, those associated with impaired hepatic ability to clear bilirubin, and those presenting with increased bilirubin loads as well as impaired hepatic function. Of those causes producing increased production of bilirubin, the most com-

mon are isoimmune hemolytic anemias, hematomas or internal hemorrhages, swallowed maternal blood, polycythemia, or increased enterohepatic circulation. Of those causes reducing hepatic clearance, the most common are prematurity, drugs, hepatic ischemia, and inborn errors of metabolism. Of the combined group of causes producing increased bilirubin production and reduced hepatic clearance, infections are the most common.

The differential diagnosis of neonatal cholestasis is extensive but, in general, etiologies are classified as intrahepatic or extrahepatic. The most common intrahepatic etiologies are idiopathic neonatal hepatitis, cholestasis associated with total parenteral alimentation administration, viral hepatitis, familial liver diseases, and inborn errors of metabolism. The most common extrahepatic causes are biliary atresia and choledochal cyst. The long-term prognoses of diseases causing neonatal cholestasis are generally worse than those causing neonatal jaundice—occasionally requiring immediate surgical intervention or eventual liver transplantation.

Diseases of the Genitourinary System

Urogenital Anomalies

The most common renal anomalies are horseshoe kidney, unilateral renal agenesis, and pelvic kidney. Bilateral renal agenesis, although relatively uncommon, has a striking presentation because of its frequent association with oligohydramnios and the fetal compression syndrome, consisting of Potter's facies, limb contractions, hypoplastic lungs, and IUGR. Other urogenital anomalies include poly- or multicystic kidneys, double collecting systems, Wilms' tumor, and hypo- or epispadias of the penis. None of the above anomalies have an identified association with prematurity.

Renal Insufficiency and Failure

Causes of acute renal failure in the newborn are classified as prerenal, renal, and postrenal. Prerenal failure in LBW newborns is common because of their predisposition to asphyxia, hypotension, congestive heart failure, hemorrhage, and infection. Renal causes include nephrotoxic drugs (i.e., aminoglycosides and indomethacin), renal vein thrombosis, and pyelonephritis. Less frequently, postrenal failure secondary to a neurogenic bladder or posterior urethral valves may occur. Treatment is supportive, with particular attention to restricted fluid and electrolyte administration in the early stages of failure. Peritoneal dialysis is an available therapy that is rarely necessary. The prognosis for recovery from prerenal failure is usually good, whereas that for renal or postrenal failure depends largely upon the etiology.

Renal Tubular Acidosis

Renal tubular acidosis (RTA) results from inadequate reabsorption of bicarbonate by proximal tubules or deficient secretion of hydrogen ions by distal tubules. It occurs as proximal, distal, and mixed forms. Therapy consists of bicarbonate supplementation in the diet. Prognosis is best for the proximal form.

Diseases of the Hematopoietic System

Anemia

The three types of neonatal anemias are hemorrhage, hemolytic anemias, and rarely, hypo- or aplastic anemia. Hemorrhage results from intrauterine twin-twin transfusion; chronic transplacental fetal-maternal transfusion in utero; acute fetal-maternal transfusion at the time of delivery; obstetric hemorrhage secondary to umbilical cord rupture, placenta previa, or abruptio placentae; sequestered hemorrhage as in cephalohematoma, intracranial hemorrhage, and pulmonary hemorrhage; or, frequently in sick VLBW newborns, iatrogenic anemia resulting from phlebotomy. Signs of clinical shock are most apparent in cases of acute hemorrhage. Treatment of shock requires rapid re-expansion of the intravascular space with volume expanders that include packed red blood cells. Treatment of more chronic forms of hemorrhage is eventual replacement of serum hemoglobin with packed red blood cell transfusions. Hemolytic anemias, in addition to isoimmune hemolytic anemia presented earlier, include hereditary spherocytosis, glucose-6-phospate dehydrogenase (G6PD), or pyruvate kinase deficiencies and occasional thalassemia syndromes. Hypo- and aplastic anemias are relatively uncommon in LBW newborns with the exception of physiologic anemia of prematurity, which becomes apparent by 6 weeks of life in the LBW infant. This anemia is explained by depression of erythropoietin activity following delivery from the relatively hypoxic intrauterine environment into the extrauterine oxygen-rich environment. Anemia of

this type spontaneously resolves by 3 to 4 months of age.

Polycythemia

The principal causes of polycythemia are twin-twin transfusion, placental insufficiency often associated with IUGR, maternal-fetal transfusion, and delayed cord clamping. Symptoms of polycythemia include respiratory distress, plethora, cyanosis, seizures, congestive heart failure, renal vein thrombosis, priapism, and hypoglycemia. In asymptomatic infants treatment remains controversial. However, in the presence of symptoms, partial exchange transfusion with fresh frozen plasma lowers the hematocrit. Prognosis is generally good.

Abnormal Hemostasis

The most common causes of hemostasis disorders in newborns are thrombocytopenia, disseminated intravascular coagulation (DIC), hemophilia, and hemorrhagic disease of the newborn (vitamin K deficiency). The differential diagnosis of thrombocytopenia is relatively extensive, but the most common etiologies are bacterial or viral infections, DIC, immune thrombocytopenias (including maternal idiopathic thrombocytopenia and isoimmune thrombocytopenia), and sequestration by hemangiomas or congested spleens. Platelet transfusions are administered to symptomatic patients. DIC most frequently occurs with cardiovascular collapse as from septic shock, cardiac arrest, or severe asphyxia. Treatment is directed at reversing cardiovascular collapse and replacement of platelets and clotting factors with fresh frozen plasma or cryoprecipitate. Hemorrhagic disease of the newborn is relatively rare in current practice because of prophylactic administration of vitamin K to all newborns.

Diseases of the Endocrine System and Inborn Errors of Metabolism

State Screens

Each of the 50 states employ neonatal screening programs for the early detection of relatively common and treatable endocrine disorders and inborn errors of metabolism. Although states vary in diseases for which they screen, the most common ones are phenylketonuria, hypothyroidism, galactosemia, G6PD deficiency, maple syrup urine disease, homocystinuria, congenital adrenal hyperplasia, and sickle cell disease.

Inborn Errors of Metabolism

Inborn errors of metabolism are relatively rare, occurring in about 1:15,000 to 1:20,000 newborns.[58] Phenylketonuria is the most common of the metabolic errors. Detailed discussion of these uncommon disorders is outside the scope of this chapter. However, disorders fall in the areas of carbohydrate, amino acid, lipid, organic acid, urea cycle, vitamin, mineral, glycogen, and lysosomal metabolism.

Hypoglycemia

Most cases of neonatal hypoglycemia do not result from inborn errors of metabolism. Idiopathic hypoglycemia, resulting from several factors including decreased oral or parenteral glucose intake, immature gluconeogenic and glycogenolytic pathways, and reduced glycogen deposition, occurs in as many as 5 to 14 percent of "appropriate-for-gestational-age" LBW newborns. In SGA newborns it may occur in as many as 60 percent.[59] Other contributing factors to the development of hypoglycemia in LBW newborns include asphyxia, hypoxemia, hypothermia, infection, and congestive heart failure. With supportive treatment this form of hypoglycemia usually resolves with a good prognosis.

Another major cause of hypoglycemia is hyperinsulinism. The most common etiology for neonatal hyperinsulinism is maternal diabetes. Perpetual fetal exposure to maternal hyperglycemia promotes islet cell hyperplasia and hyperinsulinism. Upon delivery, insulin levels remain high but exposure to high maternal glucose concentrations is truncated, thus resulting in hypoglycemia. Other less common diseases associated with hyperinsulinism include Beckwith-Wiedemann syndrome, Rh incompatibility, and nesidioblastosis. Treatment for all etiologies of hypoglycemia is early dietary supplementation with glucose.

Disorders of Calcium Metabolism

Neonatal hypocalcemia occurs in "early" and "late" forms. Early hypocalcemia is a disease of LBW newborns occurring in as many as 30 to 60 percent during the first days of life.[60] The etiology embraces multiple factors, including reduced calcium intake, transient hypoparathyroidism, hypercalcitoninemia,

and possibly abnormal vitamin D metabolism. Asphyxia and maternal diabetes also promote development of early neonatal hypocalcemia. Affected infants are usually asymptomatic, but symptoms include muscle hyperactivity and seizures. Treatment consists of early parenteral or enteral calcium supplementation. In contrast to early hypocalcemia, late hypocalcemia is primarily a disease of full-term newborns. It occurs after the first week of life and is the result of milk ingestion with high phosphate content, disordered intestinal calcium absorption, hypoparathyroidism, or hypomagnesemia.

Rickets of prematurity and osteopenia are diseases of VLBW infants occurring in as many as 20 percent of such infants.[61] The etiologies are multifactorial and include such factors as inadequate intakes of vitamin D, calcium, and phosphate, chronic diuretic therapy, and chronic acid-base disorders. Premature delivery of these infants prevents the substantial transplacental transfer of calcium and phosphate that otherwise occurs during the third trimester of pregnancy. The reduced availability of calcium and phosphate accounts for the direct association of osteopenia with rickets of prematurity. Rickets presents with typical bony changes observed upon radiologic examination and fracture occurrence at extremities and ribs. The incidence of rickets has decreased in recent years by virtue of parenteral and enteral dietary supplementation with increased quantities of vitamin D, calcium, and phosphate. Rickets usually presents at 2 to 4 months of age, and treatment is directed at increased dietary intake of vitamin D, calcium, and phosphate and stabilization of fractures. With treatment the prognosis is generally good.

Congenital Hypothyroidism

Congenital hypothyroidism occurs in about 1:4,000 births. Although the incidence is not particularly increased in LBW newborns, circulating concentrations of thyroxine and tri-iodothyronine are generally decreased because of decreased circulating concentrations of thyroxine binding globulin. The most common causes of congenital hypothyroidism are agenesis or hypoplasia of the thyroid gland, endemic goiter-associated hypothyroidism, drug-induced goiter, and inborn errors of thyroxine synthesis. Early treatment with thyroid hormone is vital for the attainment of normal mental development.

Adrenal Disorders

Detailed consideration of the various adrenal disorders is outside the scope of this chapter, particularly because they are relatively uncommon and not directly associated with prematurity. The two most common forms observed in the LBW neonate are adrenal hemorrhage and congenital adrenal hyperplasia. The etiologies of adrenal hemorrhage in LBW newborns are severe asphyxia, hypoxia, septic shock, and DIC. Clinical signs may be absent, nonspecific, or severe in association with hypovolemic shock, abdominal distension, seizures, or coma. Diagnosis is apparent by ultrasound examination, and blood transfusion for shock with steroid and mineralocorticoid replacement therapy constitutes treatment.

Ninety percent of congenital adrenal hyperplasias result from 21-dehydroxylase deficiency presenting as a simple virilizing form or salt-losing form. Virilization of the female newborn causes appearance of ambiguous genitalia, whereas virilization of the male may not be apparent. In the salt-losing form, virilization is present at birth and precedes the adrenal crisis that usually occurs at 1 to 4 weeks of age as failure to thrive, dehydration, hyponatremia, hyperkalemia, hypoglycemia, or acidosis. Without treatment shock, seizures or coma ensue. Treatment is directed at correction of metabolic disturbances and dehydration and replacement of corticosteroids and mineralocorticoids. Prognosis is good with early identification and treatment.

Diseases of the Musculoskeletal System

Malformations

Neonatal malformations are classified by failure of formation, failure of differentiation, duplication of limbs, and congenital constriction bands.[62] Formation failures occur as transverse congenital amputations of the distal extremities and hypoplasia or aplasia of the proximal and distal extremities. Treatment consists of prosthesis placement. Differentiation failures present as synostosis, syndactyly, skin webs, arthrogryposis, and other congenital joint contractures. Treatment is surgical separation of the fused parts. The most common example of duplications is polydactyly, in which case surgical removal of the extra digit is possible but not always advisable. Congenital constriction bands may present as digital rings

of constriction sometimes causing intrauterine distal ischemia and gangrene.

Skeletal Dysplasias

Skeletal dysplasias result from connective tissue disorders producing abnormal cartilage or bone formation. The majority of disorders are acquired through an autosomal recessive pattern of inheritance. The best known examples are achondrogenesis, achondroplasia (autosomal dominant), osteogenesis imperfecta, and asphyxiating thoracic dystrophy. Clinical presentations are too varied to provide a universal description. Of the above diseases, osteogenesis imperfecta is the only one associated with prematurity.

Congenital Hip Dislocation

The incidence of congenital hip dislocation is approximately 1:1,000 newborns.[63] It is seven times more common in females than males, and the left hip is dislocated three times more frequently than the right. Proposed etiologies for this multifactorial disease include congenital acetabular dysplasia, familial laxity of the muscular acetabular capsule, breech positioning of the fetus in utero, and a possible estrogen influence, particularly in females. Following birth and upon weight bearing, laxity of the acetabular capsule permits progressive erosion of the acetabulum and eventual posterior displacement of the femoral head from the acetabulum to the ilium. A false acetabulum may develop upon the ilium in association with reduction in femoral head size. Diagnosis is based upon physical, radiographic, and, more recently, ultrasound examinations. Early treatment consists of maintaining the hips in abduction and flexion with double diapers, splints, harnesses, or spica casts. Prognosis is excellent with early treatment, but permanent crippling is the outcome with late recognition.

Clubfoot

The incidence of talipes equinovarus deformities, the most common form of clubfoot, is 1:1,000 births. It is described by inversion and plantar flexion of the foot. Treatment usually consists of plaster casting. Surgery is rarely required and outcome is usually good. Other deformities of the foot are treated similarly unless the foot can be passively moved to the correct position, whereupon simple exercises suffice.

REFERENCES

1. Baucher H, Brown E, Peskin J: Premature graduates of the newborn intensive care unit: a guide to followup. Pediatr Clin North Am 35:1207, 1988
2. Battaglia F, Lubchenco L: A practical classification of newborn infants by weight and gestational age. J Pediatr 71:159, 1967
3. Lubchenco L, Searls D, Brazie J: Neonatal mortality rate: relationship to birth weight and gestational age. J Pediatr 81:814, 1972
4. Raju TNK: An epidemiologic study of very low and very very low birth weight infants. Clin Perinatol 13233, 1986
5. Cowett RM: Introduction. p 1. In Cowett RM, Hay WW (eds): The Micropremie: The Next frontier. Ross Laoratories, Columbus, OH, 1990
6. Hack M, Fanaroff. AA: How small is too small? Considerations in evaluating the outcome of the tiny infant. Clin Perinatol 15:773, 1988
7. Moore KL: Before We Are Born, Basic Embryology and Birth Defects. WB Saunders Co, Philadelphia, 1974
8. Battaglia FC, Meschia G: An introduction to Fetal Physiology. Academic Press, New York, 1986
9. Volpe JJ: Neurology of the Newborn. p 3. WB Saunders Co, Philadelphia, 1981
10. Teitel DF: Circulatory adjustments to postnatal life. Semin Perinatol 12:96, 1988
11. Fisher DJ, Towbin J: Maturation of the heart. Clin Perinatol 15:421, 1988
12. Wright JR, Clements JA: Metabolism and turnover of lung surfactant. Am Rev Respir Dis 135:426, 1987
13. Hollingsworth M, Gilfillan AM: The pharmacology of lung surfactant secretion. Pharmacol Rev 31:69, 1984
14. King RJ: Pulmonary surfactant. J Appl Physiol 53:1, 1982
15. Jansen AH, Chernick V: Onset of breathing and control of respiration. Semin Perinatol 12:104, 1988
16. Grand RJ, Watkins JB, Torti FM: Development of the human gastrointestinal tract. Gastroenterology 70:790, 1976
17. Lebenthal E, Lee PC, Heitlinger LA: Impact of development of the gastrointestinal tract on infant feeding. J Pediatr 102:1, 1983
18. Robillard JE, Nakamura KT, Matherne GP, Jose PA: Renal hemodynamics and functional adjustments to postnatal life. Semin Perinatol 12:143, 1988
19. Miller ME, Stiehm ER: Immunology and resistance to infection. p 27. In Remington JS, Klein JO (eds): Infectious Diseases of the Fetus and Newborn Infant. 2nd Ed. WB Saunders Co, Philadelphia, 1983
20. Khodr TM: Hypothalamic-like releasing hormones of the placenta. Clin Perinatol 10:553, 1983
21. Sparks J: Human intrauterine growth and nutrient accretion. Semin Perinatol 8:74, 1984
22. Battaglia F, Hay W: Energy and substrate requirements for fetal and placental growth and metabolism. p 501. In Beard R, Nathanielz P (eds): Fetal Physiology and Medicine, 2nd Ed. Marcel Dekker Inc, New York, 1984
23. Sinclair JC: Temperature Regulation and Energy Metabolism in the Newborn. Grune & Stratton, New York, 1978
24. Ladda RL: Prenatal genetic diagnosis. p 16. In Nelson NM (ed): Current Therapy in Neonatal-Perinatal Medicine — 2. BC Decker, Inc, Philadelphia, 1990
25. Grisoni ER, Gauderer MW et al: Antenatal ultrasonography: the experience in a high risk perinatal center. J Pediatr Surg 21:358, 1986
26. Finnegan JK: Amniotic fluid and midtrimester amniocentesis: A review. Br J Obstet Gynaecol 133:915, 1984
27. Rodeck C: Fetoscopy and chorion biopsy. p 84. In Nelson NM (ed): Current Therapy in Neonatal-Perinatal Medicine 1985–1986. BC Decker Inc, Philadelphia, 1985
28. Druzin ML: Antepartum fetal heart rate monitoring: state of the art. Clin Perinatol 16:627, 1989
29. Vintzileos AM, Campbell WA, Rodis JF: Fetal biophysical profile scoring: current status. Clin Perinatol 16:661, 1989
30. Schifrin BS: Fetal monitoring during labor. p 3. In Nelson NM (ed): Current Therapy in Neonatal-Perinatal Medicine — 2. BC Decker, Inc, Philadelphia, 1990
31. Torrance GW, Zipursky A: Cost-effectiveness of antepartum prevention of Rh immunization. Clin Perinatol 11:267, 1984
32. Blanchette VS, Zipursky A: Assessment of anemia in newborn infants. Clin Perinatol 11:489, 1984
33. Harmon CR: Fetal monitoring in the alloimmunized pregnancy. Clin Perinatol 16:691, 1989
34. Rock JA, Zacur HA: The clinical management of repeated early pregnancy wastage. Fertil Steril 39:123, 1893
35. Kochenow NK: Management of fetal demise. Clin Obstet Gynecol 30:322, 1987

36. Sullivan JM: Hypertension and Pregnancy. Year Book Medical Publishers, Chicago, 1986

37. Kochenour NK: Obstetric management of multiple pregnancy and postmaturity. p 149. In Fanaroff AA Martin RJ (eds): Neonatal-Perinatal Medicine: diseases of the Fetus and Infant, 4th Ed. CV Mosby Co, St Louis, 1987

38. Kurczynski TW: Congenital malformations. p 253. In Fanaroff AA, Martin RJ (eds): Neonatal-Perinatal Medicine: Diseases of the Fetus and Infant, 4th Ed. CV Mosby Co, St Louis, 1987

39. Gotoff SP, Behrman RE: Neonatal septicemia. J Pediatr 76:142, 1970

40. Gnehm H, Klein JO: Management of neonatal sepsis and meningitis. Pediatr Annu 12:195, 1983

41. Shohat M, Reisner SH: Retinopathy of prematurity: incidence and risk factors. Pediatrics 72:159, 1983

42. Volpe JJ: Intraventricular hemorrhage and brain injury in the premature infant: neuropathology and pathogenesis. Clin Perinatol 16:361, 1989

43. Volpe JJ: Intraventricular hemorrhage and brain injury in the premature infant: diagnosis, prognosis and prevention. Clin Perinatol 16:387, 1989

44. McCracken GH Jr, Freij BJ: Bacterial and viral infections of the newborn. p 927. In Avery GB (ed): Neonatology: Pathophysiology and Management of the Newborn, 3rd Ed. JB Lippincott Co, Philadelphia, 1987

45. Nelson KB, Ellenberg JH: Obstetric complications as risk factors for cerebral palsy or seizure disorder. JAMA 251:1843, 1984

46. Rowe RD, Freedom RM, Mehrizi A, Bloom KR: The Neonate with Congenital Heart Disease, 2nd Ed. p 271. WB Saunders Co, Philadelphia, 1981

47. Fyler DC: Report of the New England Regional Infant Cardiac Program. Pediatrics 65 (suppl):375, 1980

48. Stahlman MT: Acute respiratory disorders in the newborn. p 424. In Avery GB (ed): Neonatology: Pathophysiology and Management of the Newborn, 3rd Ed. JB Lippincott Co, Philadelphia, 1987

49. Daily WJR, Klaus M, Meyer HBP: Apnea in premature infants: monitoring, incidence, heart rate changes and an effect of environmental temperature. Pediatrics 43:510, 1969

50. Mathew OP, Roberts JL, Thach BT: Pharyngeal airway obstruction in preterm infants during mixed and obstructive apnea. J Pediatr 100:964, 1982

51. Mayes L, Perkett E, Stahlman MT: Severe BPD: A retrospective review. Acta Pediatr Scand 72:225, 1983

52. Bancalari E, Abdenour GE, Feller R, Gannon J: BPD: clinical presentation. J Pediatr 95:819, 1979

53. Markstad T, Fitzhardinge PM: Growth and development in children recovering from BPD. J Pediatr 98:597, 1981

54. Vohr BR, Bell CF, OH WM: Infants with BPD: growth pattern and developmental outcome. Am J Dis Child 136:443, 1982

55. Kleigman RM, Fanaroff AA: Necrotizing enterocolitis. N Engl J Med 310:1093, 1984

56. Yazbeck S, Ndoye M, Khan AH: Omphalocele: a 25 year experience. J Pediatr Surg 21:761, 1986

57. Martin LW, Torres AM: Omphalocele and gastroschisis. Surg Clin North Am 65:1035, 1985

58. Iafolla AK, McConkie-Rosell A: Prenatal diagnosis of metabolic disease. Clin Perinatol 17:761, 1990

59. Pildes RS, Pyati SP: Hypoglycemia and hyperglycemia in tiny infants. Clin Perinatol 13:351, 1986

60. Tsang RC, Oh W: Neonatal hypocalcemia in low birth weight infants. Pediatrics 45:773, 1970

61. Callenbach JC, Sheehan MB, Abramson SJ, Hall RT: Etiologic factors in rickets of very low birth weight infants. J Pediatr 98:800, 1981

62. Kay WH: A proposed international terminology for the classification of congenital limb deficiencies: the recommendations of the International Society for Prosthetics and Orthotics. Orthot Prosthet 28:33, 1974

63. Berman L, Klenerman L: Ultrasound screening for hip abnormalities: preliminary findings in 1001 neonates. Br Med J 293:719, 1986

Risks Associated with Diagnostic Examinations in the Neonate

2

Louis K. Wagner
Rodrigo Dominguez

Pharmaceuticals have side effects that a physician must understand to provide appropriate care for a patient. Such effects are studied and tested in both animals and humans before the medicine is approved by the United States Food and Drug Administration. Acute side effects become readily recognized in animal studies or in clinical trials but some potential long-term effects may not be uncovered until the drug has been in general use for some time. For this reason physicians must make decisions about the use of drugs for their patients based on a limited knowledge of their potential long-term side effects. This is a situation similar to that of the use of diagnostic radiation, except that in some cases extensive but incomplete human data on the potential long-term effects already exist.

Acute effects of radiation, as with pharmaceuticals, can be severe when the radiation is delivered in excessive amounts, well beyond the prescribed use. Ultrasound, for example, when used at very high intensities, can heat and destroy tissues, an effect that is exploited in some cancer therapies. This effect clearly does not occur at diagnostic levels.

When reviewing the potential harmful effects of diagnostic applications it is necessary to develop a perspective on the relationship between the harmful

potential and the amount of radiation applied. This applies equally well to radiography, nuclear medicine, magnetic resonance (MR), and ultrasound. The physician makes the judgment as to whether the use of diagnostic radiation is apt to be more important to patient care than the potential risks, known and unknown, much in the same way that a physician decides on the use of certain drugs.

Because of the sensitive health status of premature neonates, diagnostic examinations are most frequently performed at the bedside and should require as little preparation as possible, be brief, have few or no side effects, and be of negligible risk to other employees. Many ultrasound studies and mobile x-ray studies meet all of these criteria and, when they are of sufficient diagnostic value, are the modality of choice. Some conditions, however, can benefit only from other types of studies.

Nuclear scintigraphic imaging is also possible, in selected cases, in a mobile setting but may require some special preparation and radiation protection precautions. For example, diapers may require special handling for radionuclides excreted in the urine or through the digestive tract. Even though this radiation protection concern would also exist for studies done in the nuclear medicine department, the com-

25

promise for the mobile study is that the image quality may not be as high as that achieved by nuclear imaging cameras in their own department.

If computed tomography (CT) is required, the patient must be transported and anesthesia is required to prevent motion during imaging. If MR imaging is required, transport and anesthesia will be necessary but, in addition, special shielding devices are needed for monitors and support apparatus that may be affected by magnetic fields. There are also special concerns that must be addressed to prevent the potential for severe burns induced by electrical leads heated during MR imaging while the patient is under anesthesia and unable to respond to pain.

The physical size and biologic status of premature neonates are important factors in assessing risks during diagnostic examinations. Their size in many cases governs how much radiation must be applied to complete the study. Their biologic status may influence the mechanisms by which side effects from the studies may occur. They are susceptible to physical injury as a result of physical manipulation during procedures. In the following sections the potential risks associated with each type of study are reviewed, but they should not be construed as exhaustive.

ASSESSING RISKS FROM X-RAYS

The conventional radiograph is frequently utilized in diagnostic medical care of premature neonates because it is highly informative, is readily acquired, usually requires no special preparation, is minimally susceptible to motion artifacts, and is relatively inexpensive. The risks associated with the simple x-ray examination also appear to be quite small.[1] Fluoroscopically assisted studies and CT require more patient preparation and more radiation with concomitantly increased risks.

Early Effects of X-Ray Procedures

Early Radiation Effects

Acute deleterious effects of x-rays do not occur unless a certain threshold amount of radiation is delivered. The threshold amounts are far in excess of the radiation delivered during a diagnostic study. A biologically detectable early change that has occurred in patients following a high-dose examination, such as cardiac catheterization, is a slight increase in the number of chromosomal aberrations of peripheral lymphocytes.[2] Even for such an involved procedure, delivery of a dose sufficient to observe the effect would be uncommon in neonates because of their small size. Acute effects that may occur from diagnostic examinations are more likely to result from other factors associated with invasive procedures or from reactions to contrast agents or anesthesia.

Effects of Contrast Agents

Barium sulfate and iodinated salts are the two main types of radiographic contrast agents used. The chemical composition of these substances provides the x-ray absorption properties by which they are visualized under x-ray exposure. Neither of these compounds emits radiation but they may produce anaphylactoid reactions. In the case of barium, which is an inert substance, the reaction can be produced by the additives present in its suspension, but these reactions are usually mild and extremely rare.[3] Barium is only used orally or rectally to outline the gastrointestinal tract.

The intravascular injection of ionic iodinated contrast media for excretory urography, angiography, and other diagnostic purposes (CT and cardiac catheterization) can produce undesired side effects or reactions in a small number of patients. The cause of these reactions remains obscure; most of them are of the anaphylactoid type which are not life threatening, except for possible acute laryngeal edema. Other potential reactions are cardiac or vasovagal crisis and seizures. Occasionally, deaths have been reported.[4,5]

In neonates with immature renal function, another potential risk is pulmonary edema.[6] The hypertonicity of iodinated water-soluble intravascular contrast agents will produce transient osmotic imbalance with a significant effect on serum osmolarity. Because of the immature renal function of the premature infant, the intravascular injection of these iodinated salts should be avoided when possible; instead other less invasive diagnostic procedures, such as ultrasound, should be selected or the procedure should be delayed until the infant is a few weeks old. The patient should be well hydrated to reduce the likelihood of renal complications of pulmonary edema. New nonionic agents (which are low-osmolality iodinated media) significantly decrease the occurrence of adverse effects and are preferred.[7]

Barium is not to be used in cases of suspected gastrointestinal perforation or when aspiration by oral ingestion is a possibility.[8] The low-osmolality nonionic water-soluble contrast agents (isoiru-omnipaque) can be used to avoid the disadvantages of the water-soluble ionic iodinated agents: hypertonicity and shift of fluid from the blood to body tissues. Other iodinated water-soluble compounds used intra-orally in adults (Gastrografin and/or Hypaque) do not have the advantage of lower osmolality and their use is consequently not recommended in premature infants.

Delayed Effects of X-Rays

Delayed effects can occur years after exposure to ionizing x-rays. Radiation-induced neoplasm may be a potential long-term effect of exposure to radiation, as may cataracts and genetic effects that involve only the descendants of the individual. To gain a perspective on the level of risk it is necessary to understand, to some extent, the mechanisms involved and how the risks relate to the absorbed doses of x-rays, to which the patient is exposed.

Mechanisms for Delayed Effects

The mechanism by which x-rays can induce neoplasm starts with the ionization of molecules within tissue. This ionization induces a chemical disruption and, depending on how the cell manages this chemical disruption, there may or may not be adverse results. The chemical disruption could be completely repaired, could result in a benign change within the cell, could result in a change in the genetic information of the cell, or could result in other changes. Of these, it is thought that some specific heritable change in the genome of the cell is the principal means by which a neoplasm is initiated. The likelihood of this particular event occurring increases as the concentration of ionization produced in the tissues increases. It also depends on the time course of the delivery of this radiation, and on the biologic status of the irradiated tissue. This type of mechanism is also believed to be responsible for changes in the reproductive cells that could affect descendants.

Because the likelihood of inducing a neoplasm or a genetically important effect in the reproductive cells increases as the number of ionization events in the cells increases, the likelihood of any of these events occurring increases as the concentration of ionization produced in the tissues increases. The concentration of ionization as a result of exposure to ionizing radiation is proportional to the absorbed dose of x-rays, which is commonly expressed in units of milli-grays (mGy). However, it is not sufficient to simply know the radiation absorbed dose to the tissue because the time course of delivery of the radiation as well as the biologic status of the patient and other factors influence the potential effects of the radiation.

The time course of the exposure to the radiation is important because if sufficient time is provided between exposures, the concentration of ions at any one time is small and the tissues will have time to repair any small amount of injury. After complete repair, cells will be more capable of withstanding and repairing additional increments of exposure. In contrast, if the radiation is delivered acutely in a high exposure, then there is insufficient time during the exposure for repair to take place. The biologic changes induced by instantaneous and high concentrations of ionization are greater than those induced by the same cumulative concentration produced slowly over long intervals.

The biologic status of the patient is important because tissues show different susceptibilities to radiation depending upon their replicative capacity and their biochemical status, which may encourage or inhibit changes. The status is related to the sex and age of the patient as well as other factors.

For induced neoplasm and genetic effects on progeny, it is conceivable that only a single cell need be affected to start the process. Even though it is highly unlikely for the precise changes to occur as a result of exposure of a single cell to ionizing radiation, the possibility cannot be ruled out and even the very lowest of doses of x-rays are believed to pose some risk. For cataract to be induced many cells must be involved, and a threshold dose of x-rays does exist for this effect. There are, however, no data as to the threshold for neonates. For adults, the threshold is so great (about 2 Gy) as to render induced cataract of no concern for diagnostic studies.

Neoplasms induced by ionizing radiation require a long time (at least 2 years) to develop, and they may not develop until middle age or later if the individual is exposed as an infant. In general, younger individuals appear to be more susceptible to radiation-induced neoplasms than adults. Radiation-induced leukemia, thyroid neoplasm, and cancers of the digestive tract appear to be more prevalent in those exposed at younger ages. Radiation-induced cancer of the breast appears to occur only in women and may be more prominent in those exposed around the age of puberty, but the susceptibility of those exposed at younger ages is greater than those exposed as adults. Adults appear to be more susceptible than children to radiation-induced lung cancer, and this tends to be the exception in regard to susceptibility with age.

Radiation-induced cancers appear to follow the same time course of development as cancers that appear as a result of other causes. For example, even though girls exposed at very young ages are at risk for radiation-induced breast cancer, the cancer risk does not begin until they reach the age when breast cancers appear in the general population, at around age 30 or older. A similar pattern appears to hold for lung cancer. There also appear to be similarities in the susceptibility of each sex to radiation-induced cancer and the general cancer rates of the two sexes. For example, women have about twice to three times the risk of men for both radiation-induced thyroid cancers and thyroid cancers caused by other means.

Neoplasm

Data of greatest relevance to the patients of interest in this text are those from in utero exposure to low doses of radiation, in particular those from diagnostic roentgenographic pelvimetry. Multiple studies have shown an increase in childhood cancer, principally leukemia, of about 50 percent above the expected incidence when doses delivered in utero are approximately 10 mGy. Although a causal relationship between the radiation and leukemia is not confirmed, the benefit-versus-risk decision usually assumes the causal possibility. The expected incidence of childhood leukemia in one study in Great Britain was approximately 0.03 percent.[9] A 50 percent increase in this risk for a 10-mGy absorbed dose would represent an absolute increase of approximately 0.015 percent. Other estimates have suggested an increase in risk of 0.02 to 0.025 percent, or about two extra induced leukemias for every 10,000 children exposed prenatally to 10 mGy.

The absorbed doses delivered during screen-film pelvimetry are considerably larger than those delivered postnatally in a child because of the need to penetrate the enlarged abdomen of the mother with the radiation. In addition, pelvimetry examinations in many studies were performed with technology far different from contemporary devices that require much less radiation. The equivalent whole-body absorbed dose delivered to premature neonates from abdominal radiographs is on the order of 0.1 mGy or less for state-of-the-art radiography. Therefore, the risks involved with a single-film examination of the abdomen in the premature neonate should be at least 100 times less than those associated with a 10-mGy dose from pelvimetry. For childhood leukemia the radiation-induced risk is on the order of 0.0002 percent, which can certainly be considered trivial when compared to benefits to be derived from a needed abdominal x-ray. In some cases, patients can receive numerous single-film examinations during long-term intensive care. The risk of radiation-induced childhood leukemia following abdominal radiography of the premature neonate based on the best of estimates would not likely exceed 0.02 percent unless a hundred or more studies are performed.

Cancers among individuals exposed in utero at Hiroshima and Nagasaki appear to be increasing now that the individuals are middle aged. It is not known what the induced-cancer risks are once the individual matures past childhood. This remains one of those unknowns around which the physician must work when making a benefit-versus-risk judgment. The lifetime risk of induced cancer for a single abdominal film in a neonate, as estimated from those exposed in utero to atomic bomb radiation (principally gamma radiation) at Hiroshima and Nagasaki, may be 0.005 percent. For 100 films, using state-of-the-art low-dose technology, the risk might be 0.5 percent. The uncertainty in these estimates is great and the risk could be up to three times higher or as low as zero.

In some cases more aggressive roentgenographic studies of the neonate are required, such as cardiac catheterization or (CT). In these cases the patient is transported to a special imaging suite and absorbed doses may be on the order of 10 to 100 mGy. The risks to the neonate increase proportionately with the same uncertainties applying. Because of the risks of the invasive procedures and the risks associated with anesthesia or other drugs as well as the radiation exposure, such examinations are performed only after careful consideration of options.

Gastrointestinal disorders sometimes require fluoroscopic examination. It is commonly known that doses from such examinations in adults are much higher than those from single plain film studies. However, because of their small size, doses to neonates from fluoroscopy are greatly reduced when state-of-the-art low-dose technology is employed. Radiation risks from such studies would be less than those of CT or cardiac catheterization in neonates but more than those of plain film studies.

Developmental Risk

In utero exposures to atomic bomb radiation at Hiroshima and Nagasaki have also demonstrated that the developing child is vulnerable to radiation-induced developmental deficits such as mental retardation and reduced intellectual performance. The doses known to cause such deficits exceed 200 mGy. The developmental stages of gestation when the fetus is vulnerable start in the eighth week after conception and continue on through the 25th week after conception. After the 15th week postconception very high doses of radiation, well beyond the diagnostic range, are required to induce such effects. Since the premature neonate is at worst in the very late stages of the vulnerable period, the risk of such induced effects in the premature neonate from diagnostic examinations is negligible or nonexistent.

Risks to Future Descendants

The effects on descendants of premature neonates whose reproductive organs are exposed to diagnostic x-rays cannot be stated within any certainty but appear to be quite limited for several reasons. The primary reason is the small absorbed dose to the gonads for single plain film radiography of the pelvis. Studies that do not include the pelvis or wherein proper shielding of the gonads, either by collimation of the radiographic field or the use of gonadal shields, result in absorbed doses that may be considered trivial. Another reason the risk is small is that there has been no definitive demonstration of effects on descendants who were conceived following exposure of their parents at Hiroshima and Nagasaki, even for parents exposed to very high dose levels. It is important to consider that exposure to the gonads of neonates cannot be legitimately compared to exposure of mature individuals or even children. From all of the available data, however, it appears that if a risk to the descendants does exist, the risk is extremely small in comparison to the incidence of children born with severe birth defects as a result of other causes. The incidence of mental retardation in the population is approximately 0.8 percent, the incidence of severe birth defects in the general population is approxi-

mately 3 to 5 percent, and when all birth defects of moderate severity are taken into account the incidence in the general population has been estimated to be 10 percent. The increase in risks due to diagnostic examinations is much smaller than the general risks in the absence of radiation.

The previous discussion should not be construed to mean that shielding of the gonads is not an important practice in diagnostic radiology. Even though the risks are small on an individual basis, a large portion of the population receives diagnostic studies each year. The gonads should be shielded from the direct radiation during the examination whenever possible in order to reduce potential effects in the genetic pool of the population. This should be accomplished either through collimation or through the use of gonad shields. The only times that the gonads should be directly irradiated during diagnostic examinations are when shielding could interfere with diagnostic information or when the reproductive capability of the patient is absent.

Risks to Personnel

Radiography of the neonate is frequently performed at the bedside using mobile radiographic equipment. Risks to personnel in the area when such studies are properly done are too small to be a serious concern. At 2 m from the patient the risk to personnel from an abdominal radiograph of the neonate is much less than the equivalent risk from 1 day of natural background radiation.

ASSESSING RISKS FROM NUCLEAR SCINTIGRAPHY

Nuclear scintigraphy is infrequently used in premature neonates. Some applications include the use of xenon-133 gas to study ventilation and technetium-99m–labeled radiopharmaceuticals to study bone abnormalities, kidney function, and lung perfusion.

Absorbed Doses from Radiopharmaceuticals

Nuclear medicine employs the use of radioactive materials (radionuclides) as tracers attached to pharmaceuticals in order to study the function of tissues and organs. The radiation emitted is ionizing radiation and the biologic effects associated with these radiations are similar to those for x-rays. However, the types of radiations and manners in which the radiations are delivered are quite different from how x-rays are used during conventional radiography. The types of radiation include x-rays, gamma rays, beta rays, and electrons ejected from atomic orbitals. Usually, only the gamma rays are useful for diagnosis. The other radiations are an unavoidable by-product that unfortunately contribute only to the patient's radiation dose. Those radionuclides that emit few by-product radiations are preferred for imaging.

The radiopharmaceutical is introduced into the patient by injection, inhalation, or ingestion. The radioactive material emits radiation while inside the patient. The distribution of the radionuclides inside the patient depends on the biologic pathways of the radiopharmaceutical. Those organs in which the radiopharmaceutical concentrates are the organs that receive the highest doses. The amount of radioactivity used in neonates is much less than that used in adults. However, because of the biologic differences the absorbed dose per unit administered activity to neonates may be considerably different from, and usually greater than, that to adults.

For each injection, a limited number of radioactive particles are injected into the patient. Once a radioactive nuclide emits its radiation, no more radiation can be emitted from that nuclide. The nuclide is said to have "decayed." Therefore, the supply of radiopharmaceutical within the patient is continually reduced because of the natural radioactive decay. The rate at which the quantity of radionuclides decays depends on the physical constitution of the radioactive nucleus. For technetium-99m–labeled materials, the amount of radioactive material is, for all practical purposes, fully decayed within 48 hours.

Another mechanism by which radiopharmaceuticals are eliminated from the body is through natural biologic elimination. This depends on the biochemical nature of the radiopharmaceutical and on the health status of the individual being studied. Some radiopharmaceuticals are slowly eliminated from the body and therefore most of the radioactive material decays within the patient. Other pharmaceuticals are rapidly eliminated, often through the urinary tract.

The absorbed dosage to the patients from the incorporation of radiopharmaceuticals depends on the physical decay of the radionuclide, the biologic elimination of the radiopharmaceutical, and the types of radiations emitted by the radionuclide. These factors are taken into account when estimating the absorbed radiation dose and its related risk to the patient.

Xenon-133

Xenon gas used to assess lung ventilation is introduced either through breathing or by intravenous injection of the gas dissolved in saline. The radiation dose to the child is very small because the radioactive xenon gas is rapidly expelled from the lungs and exhausted into a breathing apparatus. Such studies are usually carried out within the imaging section of the nuclear medicine department and require transport of the child there. Risks to personnel in the area from such exposures are quite small because of the small amount of radioactive gas used in such studies and the fact that much of this is trapped in the breathing apparatus.

Technetium-99m – Labeled Compounds

Technetium-99m–labeled compounds are sometimes used to study organ function in the premature neonate.

Technetium-99m – Labeled Macroaggregated Albumin

Technetium-99m–labeled macroaggregated albumin (MAA) is used to study perfusion of the lung. The macroaggregate particles are trapped in the lung precapillary arterioles following intravenous injection. The particles subsequently break down and are translocated to the liver, where the albumin is metabolized as other proteins. The elimination of the radionuclide part of the molecule from the patient is mainly through physical decay, which takes about 2 days.

Technetium-99m – Labeled Methylene Diphosphonate

Technetium-99m–labeled methylene diphosphonate (MDP) is used to study the developing bones of the neonate. A large portion of the radiopharmaceutical concentrates in bone as a phosphate on the hydroxyapatite crystal or the organic matrix and is eliminated principally through natural radioactive

TABLE 2-1.   Absorbed Doses (in mGy) to Organs of a Healthy 4-kg Neonate from Selected Radiopharmaceuticals

Radiopharmaceutical	Administered Activity (μCi)	Whole Body	Bladder[a]	Kidney	Lung	Testes	Ovaries
99mTc-MDP	2,000	2.6	—	—	—	5.78	11.2
99mTc-MAA	500	0.9	—	—	16	0.3	0.6
99mDTPA	850	1.5	43	3.4	—	1.5	2.8

[a] Assumes 6-hour residence time.

decay. The rest of the radioactivity is eliminated through the urinary tract.

Technetium-99m – Labeled Diethylenetriaminepenta-acetic Acid

Technetium-99m – labeled diethylenetriaminepenta-acetic acid (DTPA) is a chelating agent used to study kidney function. It is rapidly eliminated through the urinary tract (glomerular filtration) of the patient. A large proportion of the initial radioactivity appears in the urine of the patient.

Absorbed Doses from Technetium-99m Studies

Absorbed doses to organs of a healthy 4-kg neonate from the above technetium-99m – labeled compounds are given in Table 2-1. The whole-body doses suggest a radiation related risk lower than what the child will experience from naturally occurring background radiation in 1 year. Selected organs receive higher doses that effectively elevate the risks to a range approximately equivalent to or even higher than that from annual background radiation. Doses to smaller neonates will increase approximately inversely with weight. That is, the dose to an infant weighing half as much as the 4-kg infant will be about twice as high.

The technetium studies can be done at the patient's bedside using mobile gamma camera scintigraphy. The risk to personnel in the area from the use of such radionuclides in neonates is trivially small since their exposures will be on the order of what individuals receive from natural background radiation in a few days. A small concern for personnel would be the handling of diapers of the babies who have been injected with such radionuclides. The Radiation Safety Officer should monitor the diapers and bedding of the child for the first few hours following the use of these materials and then as needed in order to avoid any potential for radiation exposure to personnel.

Other Labeled Compounds

Other radiopharmaceuticals such as indium-111 – labeled blood cells or gallium-67 are infrequently used in neonates to diagnose infections or neoplasms. When used in accordance with proper medical procedures the risks associated with these radionuclides are similar to those associated with the previously discussed radionuclides. The use of iodine-131 for diagnostic studies in neonates is discouraged because of the high radiation doses associated with small activities of this radionuclide. These high doses are due to a high-energy beta particle emitted as a by-product of the decay process and also due to the long-term physical decay of the radionuclide. Any studies that might require the use of iodine should consider the use of high isotopic purity 123I (i.e., radiocontaminants of 124I and 125I must be essentially zero). This latter isotope decays by electron capture and the concomitant radiation absorbed dose per unit administered activity is much smaller than that of 131I. However, it must be reiterated that the 123I must be of very high purity because very small contamination levels of other radioactive isotopes of iodine can result in high doses to the patient.[10]

MAGNETIC RESONANCE IMAGING

Magnetic resonance (MR) imaging employs the use of very intense static magnetic fields, rapidly changing gradient magnetic fields, and radiofrequency (RF) radiation. Each of these fields has a potential for risk, but precautions can be taken to markedly reduce the likelihood of an untoward event. For example, metallic objects that are attracted by a magnet must be prevented from entering the MR area lest the very strong field propel them into the air as dangerous projectiles. Another potential risk from MR scans relates to heating. The RF radiation can directly heat tissue and the rapidly switched gradient fields can also heat objects. Body heating by the RF radiation should not be a problem for a properly designed and properly controlled MR scanner. However, heating of metal leads that are attached to the patient either for monitoring or gating purposes can represent a considerable risk unless proper attention is given to minimize such effects, as will be discussed later.

Although MR imaging can be quite useful in the study of the central nervous system of a premature neonate, it is a very difficult study to perform for several reasons. The child must be transported to the scanning room, the child will have to be anesthetized in order to prevent motion during the scan, and the monitors to which the child may be attached must be specially designed and shielded in order to prevent interference by the magnetic and RF fields.

The child's ears should be plugged or otherwise shielded from sound during the examination because it is not known whether permanent hearing loss could be induced by the banging noises common to such examinations. These banging noises are caused by changing currents in the resistive gradient field magnets of the scanner and are a normal occurrence.

Of perhaps greatest concern are the leads that must be attached to the child for monitoring or gating purposes. These leads should be thermally and electrically insulated from the child because they may become heated during the examination. They also should be specially designed (coaxially shielded) to prevent the potential for heating during the examination. There should be no loops in any of the leads. All material not associated with or not required for the examination should be removed from the bore of the magnet. Such careful attention is necessary to prevent the potential of thermal burns resulting from leads heated during the examination. It is important to note that because the patient will be under anesthesia, the patient will not respond to pain caused by burning, thus rendering no indication that the examination should be terminated. Burns have been induced in patients on an infrequent basis, and some have been sufficiently severe to require surgical intervention.[11]

The use of a contrast agent in a premature neonate for MR scanning is not likely. Gadopentate dimeglumine (Gadolinium) is currently used to enhance contrast in MR imaging. A few minor anaphylactoid reactions have been reported for this agent,[12] but because of the limited experience with this agent it is not recommended for use in small children, term infants, or premature infants.

There are no known latent risks associated with this imaging modality as it is currently used. The mechanism known to induce cancer from ionizing radiation has not been demonstrated for MR. This is very encouraging; however, this should not lead one into a false sense of security about the safety of this examination. Electromagnetic fields have been implicated as a possible factor in an increased incidence of leukemia in children. There may be effects that have escaped our attention and our experience has thus far been brief. For example, the problem with burns took many by surprise. Still, the long-term latent risks are considered to be quite small and this diagnostic modality, as with all diagnostic modalities, must be employed with discretion and careful consideration given to the benefits and potential risks of such a study.

MR is still developing, with higher field strengths and more rapid imaging sequences being produced. There have been reports of headaches, transient effects of visual light flashes, and other sensations by individuals as a result of research with such devices. Research into potential adverse effects from exposures to such devices as well as from exposures to clinical units is continuing.

ULTRASOUND

Ultrasound is one of the primary diagnostic tools in premature neonates because it can be performed as a mobile examination at the patient's bedside, and it is very useful in studying the brain, blood flow, cardiac system, and abdomen. The primary limitation to an adequate study with ultrasound is the presence of gas. Therefore ultrasound is not used to study the airways of the lung and a study may be compromised by gas in the abdomen.

Ultrasonic imaging uses a pulsed beam of high-frequency sound (1 to 15 MHz) in order to sonographically outline tissues and organs of the body. Doppler ultrasound studies blood flow by analyzing frequency changes induced in the soundwave reflected by moving blood, much like radar is used to assess automobile speed. Ultrasound is a compression wave that rapidly stretches and compresses tissues as the soundwave propagates through them. This action heats tissue and can potentially disrupt molecules within cells. The likelihood of heating depends not only on the intensity of the soundwave, but also its duration and frequency. As the intensity, duration, and frequency of the ultrasound increase, heating increases. Under contemporary diagnostic use, heating should not be a problem.

The American Institute of Ultrasound in Medicine (AIUM) has synthesized reports from mammalian studies into a statement[13] on in vivo mammalian biologic effects as follows:

> In the low megahertz frequency range there have been (as of this date) no independently confirmed significant biological effects in mammalian tissues exposed in vivo to unfocused ultrasound with intensities[a] below 100 mW/cm², or to focused ultrasound[b] with intensities below 1 W/cm². Furthermore, for exposure times[c] greater than one second and less than 500 seconds (for unfocused ultrasound) or 50 seconds (for focused ultrasound) such effects have not been demonstrated even at higher intensities, when the product of the intensity and exposure time is less than 50 joules/cm².

---

[a] Free-field spatial peak temporal average (SPTA) for continuous wave exposures and for pulsed-mode exposures with pulses repeated at a frequency greater than 100 hertz.

[b] Quarter-power (−6-dB) beam width smaller than 4 wave lengths or 4-mm, whichever is less at the exposure frequency.

[c] Total time includes off-time as well as on-time for repeated pulse exposures.

Ultrasound can induce deep heating in tissues and is used in physical therapy for such purposes. However, the design of such ultrasound units for physical therapy is far different from that for diagnostic imaging, and the intensity levels are approximately 1,000 times higher with a continuous-wave rather than a pulsed-wave technique.

There is no known mechanism by which ultrasound might induce biologic effects when used at intensities and application regimens common to diagnostic levels. Although some studies have suggested biologic effects from diagnostic ultrasound, none of these reports has been reproduced independently by other investigators and it appears that reported suggestions of biologic effects may be associated more with experimental design of the studies than with truly biologically significant effects.

At this time diagnostic ultrasound when applied in accordance with accepted standard use is considered to be as close to safe as any modality can get. New instruments that exceed the regimens described in the AIUM statement may be developed for future use. Potential risks associated with future devices will have to be reviewed as they become available.

REFERENCES

1. Fletcher EWL, Baum JD, Draper G: The risk of diagnostic radiation of the newborn. Br J Radiol 59:165, 1986
2. Adams FH, Norman A, Bass D, Oku G: Chromosome damage in infants and children after cardiac catheterization and angiocardiography. Pediatrics 62:312, 1978
3. Feczko PJ: Increased frequency of reaction to contrast materials during gastrointestinal studies. Radiology 174:367, 1990
4. Cohan RH, Dunnick R, Bashore TM: Treatment of reactions to radiographic contrast material. AJR 151:263, 1988
5. Witten DM, Hirsch FD, Hartman GW: Acute reactions to urographic contrast medium. AJR 119:832, 1973
6. Wood BP, Smith WL: Pulmonary edema in infants following injection of contrast media for urography. Radiology 139:377, 1981
7. Wolf GL: Safer, more expensive iodinated contrast agents: how do we decide? Radiology 159:557, 1986
8. Foley MJ, Ghahremani GG, Rogers LF: Reappraisal of contrast media used to detect upper gastrointestinal perforations. Radiology 144:231, 1982
9. Stewart AM, Kneale GW: Radiation dose effects in relation to obstetric x-rays and childhood cancers. Lancet 1:1185, 1970
10. Romney B, Nickoloff EL, Esser PD: Excretion of radioiodine in breast milk (Editorial). J Nucl Med 30:124, 1989
11. Kanal E, Shellock FG, Talagala L: Safety considerations in MR imaging. Radiology 176:593, 1990
12. Tishler S, Hoffman JC Jr.: Anaphylactoid reactions to IV gadopentetate dimeglumine. AJNR 11:1167, 1990
13. Bioeffects considerations for the safety of diagnostic ultrasound. J Ultrasound Med 7 (Suppl):S4, 1988

Nuclear Medicine and the High-Risk Newborn

Lamk M. Lamki

Nuclear medicine has a limited role in the management of the premature infant; however, it can play a vital role in specific cases. The role of nuclear medicine can be divided into two general categories: (1) studies related to nuclear functional imaging and (2) in vitro blood and urine tests (e.g., radioimmunoassay of thyroid hormones and blood tests for enzyme deficiency disorders). The contents of this chapter are restricted only to the first category, nuclear medicine imaging in the premature and high-risk newborn.

Nuclear medicine imaging in these infants is often called upon as functional supplementation to the information obtained from anatomic imaging. Structural anomalies and other abnormalities detected by anatomic imaging, such as computed tomography (CT), magnetic resonance (MR) imaging, or ultrasonography, sometimes need the supplemental functional imaging offered by nuclear studies to establish the nature of the abnormal tissue without resorting to invasive procedures such as biopsy or surgical intervention. A typical example is the establishment of the nature of a mediastinal or pharyngeal mass as functioning thyroid tissue or an abdominal mass as functioning kidney tissue. There are, however, a few situations in which nuclear medicine is the preferred primary modality of imaging in the newborn, such as in the visualization of a clinically suspected Meckel's diverticulum.

The third general group of indications for nuclear medicine studies is when anatomic imaging shows no abnormality or minimal disturbance and nuclear studies show the abnormalities much more obviously. For example, CT or MR imaging of the premature brain (or traumatized brain) may be interpreted as normal but brain perfusion nuclear studies with technetium-99m–labeled exametazime (HMPAO) and single photon emission CT (SPECT) may show significant abnormalities. Likewise, positron emission tomography (PET) brain perfusion images with ^{13}N ammonia or neuroreceptor PET imaging may define the extent of brain perfusion abnormalities and the distribution and maturity of specific neurotransmitter receptors of the premature brain. This information cannot be obtained by anatomic tomographic studies such as CT, MR imaging, or ultrasound.

RADIOISOTOPES AND RADIATION DOSIMETRY

Several radioisotopes have been described in the literature as being suitable for nuclear investigation of the premature infant. However, the literature on this subject is relatively sparse, because of the general anxiety regarding use of radioisotopes in the newborn unless specifically indicated.

Technetium-99m

The most commonly used radioisotope in nuclear medicine both for adult and for pediatric indications is technetium-99m (^{99m}Tc). This may be used to label several pharmaceuticals depending on the nature of radiotracer desired. Technetium-99m may also be used as plain ^{99m}Tc pertechnetate (TcO_4^-), as in the investigation of thyroid tissue and in salivary gland imaging or gastric mucosa detections; all these tissues can concentrate the TcO_4^- metabolically and therefore can be visualized with the gamma cameras used in nuclear medicine departments. TcO_4^- is also useful for simple perfusion studies of several organs or tumors. There are several occasions when a small dose of radioisotope is sufficient for the diagnosis of abnormal drainage or passages (e.g., fistulas), with minimal radiation exposure to the infant. In such cases we use TcO_4^-. ^{99m}Tc more commonly is used to label specific tracers, such as ^{99m}Tc-labeled sulfur colloid for the investigation of ectopic spleen tissue, ^{99m}Tc-labeled HMPAO for brain perfusion imaging, or ^{99m}Tc-labeled diethylenetriaminepenta-acetic acid (DTPA) for renal perfusion and function imaging. These radiotracers are among the most commonly used for nuclear studies of the newborn.

^{99m}Tc is an excellent radionuclide for labeling biologic tracers used in nuclear medicine imaging because it is a pure gamma ray emitter of 140 kEv, the energy that is ideal for detection by the gamma cameras used today. Also because it has no beta emission, ^{99m}Tc results in very low radiation dose to the patient. It also has a short physical half-life of 6 hours, again giving it only a small radiation dose load to the patient.

Other Radioisotopes

Radioisotopes other than ^{99m}Tc are rarely used in the newborn. Others that are used include gallium-67, indium-111, iodine-123, and iodine-131. Gallium-67 (^{67}Ga) can be used as a simple citrate salt or to radiolabel other biologic tracers. Gallium citrate may be used to localize infection and on rare occasions to define the nature of an abnormal mass that is not accessible for biopsy (e.g., in efforts to rule out a neoplastic process). ^{67}Ga given intravenously as gallium citrate salt can be localized in many malignant tumors, but is is also localized in areas of infection or inflammation. Gamma camera images are typically obtained at 24 to 72 hours after injection, unlike ^{99m}Tc-labeled tracers, with which imaging is undertaken on the same day as injection.

Indium-111 (^{111}In) is another radioisotope that can be used in children, in the form of ^{111}In oxine–labeled mixed leukocytes or ^{111}In-labeled lymphocytes and occasionally labeled granulocytes. These labeled white cells can be either autologous (from the patient) or donor cells from a relative in case of premature infants. ^{111}In-labeled white blood cells localize in areas of infection and not in tumors, unlike ^{67}Ga citrate, and hence are better radiotracers for diagnosing osteomyelitis or intra-abdominal abscesses. However, like any other test, false positives may occur. Other ^{111}In-labeled compounds include ^{111}In-

labeled DTPA, used in cerebrospinal fluid flow studies. Rarely is ^{111}In used as a radioisotope by itself, although this may be the case in adults at times.

Radioiodine (^{123}I and ^{131}I) is also among the radioisotopes sometimes used in the premature baby to examine the thyroid gland; they are employed as sodium iodide solution or in a capsule because the thyroid gland can trap and organify iodide ion. Whenever possible ^{123}I is preferred to ^{131}I because of lower radiation dose to the baby. Radioiodide isotopes may also be used to label other biologic tracers. The later are very rarely used in the newborn but they include iodoamphetamines for brain imaging and other research agents (e.g., iodinated monoclonal antibodies). Other iodinated compounds such as radioactive iodinated serum albumin (RISA) and iodohippuran have now been generally abandoned in favor of new radiotracers that give better images and lower radiation dose to the patient.

Radiation Dosage

Both ^{111}In and ^{67}Ga can result in a relatively high radiation dose to the infant compared to ^{99m}Tc because of relatively long half-lives (nearly 3 days for each). ^{131}I has an even longer physical half-life (8 days) and it also emits beta particles as well as gamma photons, thus leading to a much higher radiation dose. (This aspect of nuclear imaging has been fully covered in Chapter 2. The reader is referred to that chapter for further details.) Suffice it to say that the minimum dose that will give the desired information should be used in the infant. This would be in keeping with the ALARA (as low as reasonably acceptable) Principle.[1,2] Thus, we try to use ^{99m}Tc as much as possible.

The dose of radiopharmaceuticals to be used in infants may be calculated by a complex formula[3] or simply by taking the adult dose and dividing that by 70 (presume that an ideal adult weight is 70 kg) and then multiplying the result by the child's weight in kilograms. However, in most cases the actual dose used in the newborn is larger than that calculated because of the very small weight of the premature newborn and the minimum dose requirement of these tests. A minimum dose is required to be able to obtain images, especially where a dynamic perfusion flow and other dynamic studies are required. For example, 0.5 mCi of gallium citrate is generally regarded as the minimum dose even though this may be higher than the calculated dose for a newborn infant.

BRAIN SPECT AND CEREBROSPINAL FLUID FLOW STUDIES

Planar nuclear brain scans have extremely limited roles in the newborn. However, lately brain SPECT has opened up new avenues of examining brain perfusion and function. The only role, perhaps, of planar brain scans with ^{99m}Tc-labeled DTPA is to diagnose viral encephalitis in older children. Brain SPECT imaging with perfusion agents such as ^{99m}Tc-labeled HMPAO have been used to define the degree of maturity of the brain.[4,5] HMPAO is a lipophilic agent that, when given intravenously, is taken up by the gray matter of the brain because it readily crosses the blood-brain barrier and enters the cells because of its lipophilicity. The distribution to the gray matter of the brain is proportionate to the regional perfusion and metabolism. If there is any perfusion abnormality or cortical thinning or cerebral atrophy in any localized area, this will be reflected in the SPECT tomographic slices. Cerebral cortical maturity and other functional disorders may be detected by this new functional imaging modality that would otherwise be missed in anatomic imaging such as CT or MR. Brain SPECT with ^{99m}Tc-labeled HMPAO will also detect perfusion/metabolic abnormalities of the cerebral/cerebellar cortex or subcortical gray matter (e.g., basal ganglia and thalamus) that may have resulted from birth trauma[6,7] or cerebrovascular accidents (Figs. 3-1 and 3-2).

Other neurologic nuclear medicine studies that may be helpful in the management of the premature newborn are those tests that relate to cerebrospinal fluid (CSF) flow. Nuclear medicine tests are most helpful in assessing the function of CSF drainage shunts (e.g., ventriculoperitoneal and rarely ventriculoatrial shunts) used to drain obstructive hydrocephalic conditions. The dose of the radiopharmaceutical (e.g., ^{99m}Tc-labeled sulfur colloid or ^{99m}Tc-labeled DTPA) used in these cases is minimal, just enough to establish patency of the shunt—typically less than 500 μci of ^{99m}Tc-labeled sulfur colloid injected directly into the reservoir of the shunt while the distal limb is manually obstructed by finger pressure. Re-

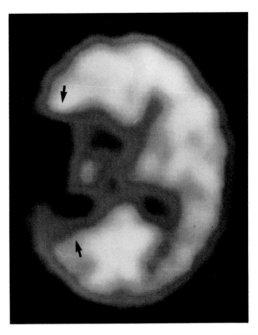

Fig. 3-1. ^{99m}Tc-labeled HMPAO brain SPECT. A transverse slice showing a large perfusion defect (arrows) in the gray matter, a result of either birth trauma or a cerebrovascular accident from other causes.

flux of radioactivity into the ventricles is followed by spontaneous flow of the radioactive CSF from the ventricles to the peritoneal cavity if the ventriculoperitoneal shunt is patent. If no spontaneous flow is observed then pumping the shunt (a small pump is part of the shunt) may be necessary to start the flow and establish that impaired CSF drainage from the ventricular system is not the cause of the symptoms of the infant.

In the rare cases in which a ventriculoatrial shunt is used, the ^{99m}Tc-labeled sulfur colloid is injected into the reservoir and, if the shunt is patent, the radioactivity will be detected in the liver in a few minutes after circulating via the right atrium. ^{99m}Tc-labeled sulfur colloid is taken up by the reticuloendothelial (Kupfer) cells in the liver. The liver radioactivity increases with time as the ventricular activity decreases.

Radiopharmaceuticals have also been used to establish the diagnosis of brain death in the newborn. A small molecule that is lipophilic and can normally cross the blood-brain barrier and is retained intrace-

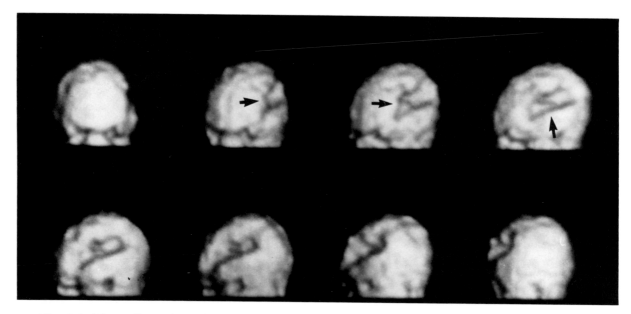

Fig. 3-2. Three-dimensional (3D) reconstruction of brain SPECT. A series of eight images created from transverse SPECT slices at a variety of angles using surface rendition 3D software showing a large perfusion defect (arrows) in the left cerebral frontoparietal lobe from a cerebral infarct in an infant.

rebrally, such as ^{99m}Tc-labeled HMPAO, is well suited to this purpose. It is likely to be more accurate than the planar imaging undertaken with ^{99m}Tc-labeled DTPA or TcO_4^- for brain flow in the diagnosis of brain death in the adults, but is also more expensive. Brain death is identified by total absence of intracranial radioactivity (e.g., in the blood vessels if ^{99m}Tc-labeled DTPA or TcO_4^- is used or in the gray matter if ^{99m}Tc-labeled HMPAO is used).

GASTROINTESTINAL AND HEPATOBILIARY STUDIES

Gastrointestinal bleeding[18] and abnormalities of the hepatobiliary tree[9-12] form the major indications for nuclear medicine studies in the neonatal gastrointestinal (GI) tract. There are several other indications for nuclear medicine examination of the GI tract.[13-16]

Abnormalities of the Hepatobiliary Tree

Examination of the hepatobiliary tree using nuclear medicine tests has been accepted as very helpful in the management of the newborn with persistent jaundice for differentiation between biliary atresia

and neonatal hepatitis (Fig. 3-3). The agent used for this study is iminodiacetic acid (IDA) labeled with [99m]Tc.

There are several analogues of ^{99m}Tc-labeled IDA that are currently being used, including DISIDA and BRIDA. These agents are injected intravenously and are taken up by the functioning hepatocytes. They are then excreted through the biliary canaliculi to the intrahepatic bile ducts and eventually drain into the common bile duct and on to the intestines. In the presence of biliary atresia and good hepatocyte function, there is prompt initial visualization of the liver (hepatic phase) because of preserved hepatocyte function, but no activity leaves the liver. There is no visualization of the common bile duct or the intestines even after acquiring delayed images as late as 24 hours after the injection. Typically, the activity normally reaches the intestine in less than 1 hour and there is good visualization of the intra- and extrahepatic bile ducts and gallbladder before that. In cases of neonatal hepatitis, there is typically a delayed hepatic phase due to poor hepatocyte function. However, with delayed imaging, the radiotracer is seen to eventually reach the intestines, albeit in small amounts. Liver visualization remains poor throughout the study. Occasionally, it is difficult to differen-

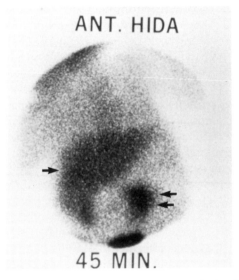
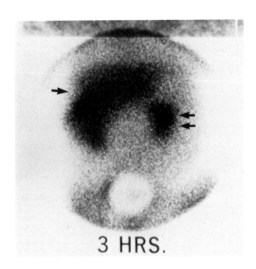

Fig. 3-3. Neonatal biliary atresia. IDA cholescintiscan images of an infant with neonatal jaundice from biliary atresia. There is good liver uptake (hepatocyte function) but the radioactivity remains in the liver (single arrows) with no appearance of radioactivity in the intestines even in delayed images (3 hours), suggesting complete obstruction to flow of bile from the biliary atresia. Extra activity in the circulation is excreted via kidneys (double arrows).

tiate intrahepatic cholestasis from obstruction due to biliary atresia when the hepatocyte function is still reasonably well preserved. A repeat study after 10 to 14 days of phenobarbital therapy at 5 mg/kg/day usually settles the uncertainty because the intestines will usually be visualized after phenobarbital enzyme stimulation.

^{99m}Tc-labeled IDA hepatobiliary studies may also be used for other congenital abnormalities (e.g., choledochal cyst[17] formation to determine whether there is a complete obstruction to bile flow). Also, abnormal drainage and leakage of bile due to congenital malformations or other reasons, such as postoperative complications with bile leaks and biloma formation, can be established by using this radiotracer. Any radioactivity accumulation outside the gallbladder, ducts, or intestines is abnormal. The dose of ^{99m}Tc-labeled IDA is determined according to pediatric dose charts, but there is a minimum dose of 0.5 mCi intravenously and 1 mCi if the bilirubin is elevated.

Gastrointestinal Bleeding

Gastrointestinal bleeding in the newborn is a rare clinical condition but it may present a major problem with respect to localizing the site of the bleed. Radio-

nuclide studies may help in localizing a bleeding ectopic gastric musosa of Meckel's diverticulum (Fig. 3-4). This is established by intravenous injection of TcO_4^-, which is normally excreted by the gastric musosa. Focal increased radioactivity seen in the right lower quadrant at about 5 to 20 minutes after the injection would suggest the presence of Meckel's diverticulum. It appears simultaneously with the normal visualization of the stomach in the left upper quadrant. This test will also detect duplication of the small bowel.

Rarely is there reason to try to localize bleeding sites from other causes, but this may be achieved by intravenous injection of ^{99m}Tc-labeled sulfur colloid, a very sensitive test for lower GI bleed. Normally within a few minutes of IV injection, the sulfur colloid will be extracted from circulation by the reticuloendothelial system (RES) cells of the liver, spleen, and bone marrow. Any activity outside the RES system in the abdominal area indicates a focal GI bleed because the radiolabeled sulfur colloid must have left the circulation. The site of a GI bleed can also be diagnosed by labeling the red blood cells of the patient with TcO_4^- and stannous ion so that the patient can be observed for many hours for intermittent GI bleed. Normally technetium-labeled red blood cells must re-

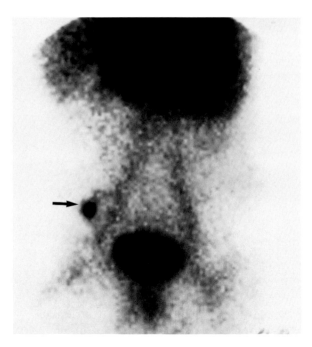

Fig. 3-4. Meckel's diverticulum. A very early appearance (a few minutes after the injection of the radiopharmaceutical) of radioactivity in the right lower quandrant from a bleeding Meckel's diverticulum (arrow) that had ectopic gastric mucosa.

main within the confines of the cardiovascular tree (Fig. 3-5).

CARDIOVASCULAR NUCLEAR STUDIES

There are several circumstances in which nuclear medicine studies can be helpful in diagnosing congenital abnormalities in the premature infant. These may be related to myocardial function or to abnormal venous return and other vascular structural abnormalities. Several of these may be and commonly are diagnosed by other existing methods, specifically echocardiography and angiography. Nuclear medicine, however, may be helpful in difficult cases (e.g., detection of an abnormal communication between flow channels when this cannot be achieved by anatomic imaging of echocardiography). Also, the quantification of left-to-right or right-to-left shunts may be

undertaken readily by nuclear medicine studies without the use of cardiac catheterization or contrast agents and their potential hazards.

Any radioactive agent that results in minimal radiation dose to the infant, such as ^{99m}Tc-labeled DTPA or TcO_4^-, may be injected intravenously (preferably near a central vein) and used for first-pass studies to sequentially follow the passage of the bolus from the peripheral veins to the right heart, the lungs, and eventually the left heart and aorta. This may be achieved in a noninvasive manner.[18-20] From the first-pass studies, ejection fractions of the right and the left ventricles may be quantified and wall motion during each ventricular contraction may be assessed in a dynamic and temporally isolated mode.

This nuclear medicine modality is not to be considered to compete with echocardiography but rather to be complimentary to it.[21,22] However, when accurate measurement of left ventricular ejection fraction is critical (and this is rare in the newborn), then the radionuclide method is regarded as more accurate by many cardiologist as compared to the echocardiographic method.

Gated first-pass studies usually result in a lower radiation dose to the infant than gated equilibrium studies, which also can be utilized for evaluation of ventricular wall motion and ejection fraction studies. The gated equilibrium studies are achieved by labeling the patient's red blood cells with TcO_4^- and a small amount of stannus ion (obtained from pyrophosphate vials).

Cardiac shunt studies can be quantified by nuclear methods using first-pass studies of computer-determined regions of interest and gamma-variate analysis of the bolus passage over the lung areas for left-to-right shunts and using ^{99m}Tc-labeled macroaggregated albumin (MAA) (size approximately 40 μ) for right-to-left shunts. ^{99m}Tc-labeled MAA injected intravenously should normally all be trapped in the lung precapillary arterioles, but these particles will go to the brain, kidneys, and other systemic circulation organs and be trapped there, bypassing the lung capillaries, if there is a right-to-left shunt. Counting the radioactivity in the total body minus the lung activity and taking appropriate ratios of the two will quantify the shunt. With a good radiopharmaceutical preparation, radioactivity counts of the rest of the body that are greater than 3 percent of the lung counts are regarded as abnormal.

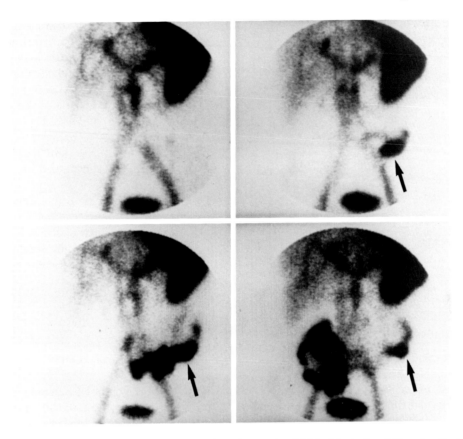

Fig. 3-5. Active GI bleeding. The study was undertaken using ^{99m}Tc-labeled red blood cells. It shows that the blood leaves the circulation at the site of the GI bleed (arrow). The top left image was acquired soon after injection of radiolabeled red blood cells and the last image at the bottom right (60 minutes) shows massive GI bleeding in the left lower quadrant.

RENAL FUNCTION STUDIES

Radionuclide studies of the genitourinary system of the premature infant can play a vital role in identifying renal masses and in the differential diagnosis of obstruction to urine drainage.[23-28]

Identification of Renal Masses

The nature of an abdominal mass in the newborn is often easy to establish but, if difficulty exists, intravenous injection of ^{99m}Tc-labeled mertiatide (MAG3) or ^{99m}Tc-labeled DTPA will often identify the functioning nature of the mass if it is renal. This is particularly helpful because contrast agents used in intravenous pyelography (IVP) studies are not concentrated in the premature or very young kidney. For practical purposes, the intravenous pyelogram is not a viable option in these babies when ultrasound fails to define the nature of an abdominal mass.

Sometimes an intrauterine ultrasound diagnosis of dilated ureters and calyces is made prenatally and, when such a baby is born, a renal functional study is needed to establish whether the dilation is from active obstruction or not (Fig. 3-6) and the relative function contribution of each kidney. Renal scanning using (IV) ^{99m}Tc-labeled DTPA or MAG3 is very helpful in these cases. Often it is necessary to give a diuretic (flurosemide) during the study to differentiate a passively dilated collecting system with megaureters produced by congenital anomaly from an actively obstructed drainage system (Fig. 3-6). This test is usually done by giving an IV injection of ^{99m}Tc-labeled DTPA and then IV Lasix at 20 minutes into the test. When

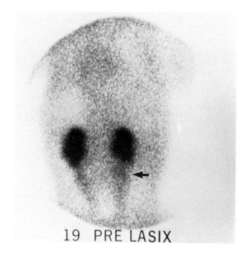
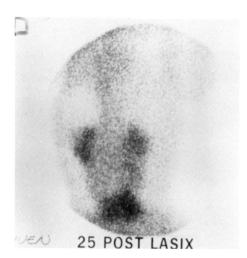

19 PRE LASIX   25 POST LASIX

Fig. 3-6. Megaureters but no active obstruction. 99mTc-labeled DTPA study in a neonate who had an intrauterine diagnosis of megaureters made by ultrasonography shows the megaureters well (arrow). However, following Lasix administration the kidneys and ureters drained almost completely (more than half of the activity clearing in less than 10 minutes is the criterion used usually). Here they cleared in 6 minutes (19- to 25-minute images).

the function of the kidneys is poor, 99mTc-labeled MAG3, a new tubular function agent that is a better radiotracer than the glomerular filtered 99mTc-labeled DTPA, is preferred. 99mTc-labeled MAG3 has replaced the old 131I-labeled iodohippuran, which had a higher radiation dosimetry from the 131I and should be now avoided in children. It has also replaced 99mTc-labeled DTPA in most institutions as the routine imaging agent. It can be used with diuretics such as Lasix or with Captopril (renovascular hypertension test) when necessary.

Obstruction to Urine Drainage

Radionuclide renal studies are also helpful in detecting abnormal urine drainage and fistulas and in cases of bladder exstrophy or other anterior abdominal wall defects. It is extremely rare that the knowledge of the existence of vesicoureteral reflux is of interest in the newborn, but should this be necessary, then the instillation of radioactivity into the bladder and observation by a gamma camera connected to a computer will determine the presence of and quantify of reflux back into the ureters. The radioactivity (99mTc-labeled DTPA) in the bladder may be instilled by the retrograde method using a catheter or, where gross reflux is suspected, it may be given intravenously (indirect voiding cystogram) as part of renal

scanning. At the end of 1 hour the bladder, now full from the renal excretion of the radiotracer into it, is used for evaluation of this type of reflux, but this is less accurate than the direct method. The direct radionuclide method compares favorably to contrast cystography, a higher radiation dose radiographic method that needs to be done only once for anatomic details and should never be used for follow-up studies during therapy.

For anatomic functional evaluation of the renal cortex, 99mTc-labeled gluconate may be used to examine masses or cystic disease of the kidney (e.g., multicystic dysplastic kidney). Also, 99mTc-labeled gluconate is used to evaluate scarring from pyelonephritis when it is difficult to do so by ultrasonography.

MUSCULOSKELETAL IMAGING

The radionuclide bone scan is a very common nuclear study in adults but is used much less in the premature neonate. The most common indications in the newborn would be focal osteomyelitis and birth trauma or child abuse.[29,30] Nuclear medicine has been shown [31-33] to be a sensitive indicator of acute osteomyelitis and it is much more reliable than just planar radiographic films. The three-phase bone scan (perfusion phase images obtained at the time of injection,

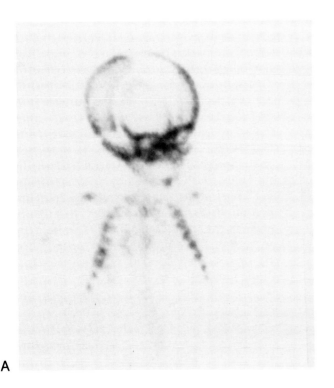

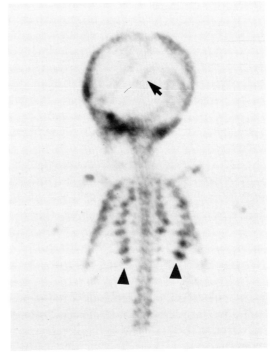

A

Fig. 3-7. (A) Bone scan acquired using ^{99m}Tc-labeled MDP. The skull shows abnormal uptake in the bone and widening of sutures, suggesting intracranial abnormality. **(B)** Corresponding CT scan showing hygroma accumulation (arrow). (From Howard et al,[30] with permission.)

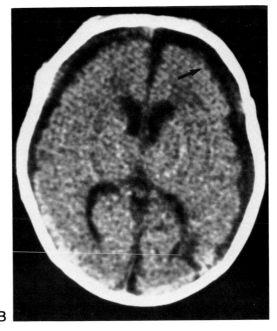

B

blood pool images obtained immediately at the end of the flow study, and two-hour delayed static images) is necessary in acute osteomyelitis and also in child abuse and birth trauma (Fig. 3-7). In examination of the joints, the three-phase bone scan will also help diagnose bone involvement in septic arthritis. Bone neoplasms may also be detected by bone scanning, although this is rarely necessary. Calcific soft tissue abnormalities (inflammatory and neoplastic) may also be detected. In fact, the three-phase bone scan is very helpful in differentiating cellulitis from osteomyelitis.

Sequential dynamic perfusion images and early

blood pool images may also be used to diagnose focal vascular abnormalities as seen in avascular necrosis of bones, even though this is normally not a high-risk problem in newborn babies. Arteriovenous malformations may also be detected by the three-phase bone scan. ^{99m}Tc-labeled methylene diphosphonate (MDP) is the standard radiopharmaceutical for bone imaging. It is taken up actively by the metabolically active stimulated osteoblasts involved in repair of infection, tumor, or trauma. ^{99m}Tc-labeled MDP is filtered through the glomerulae, and therefore during the IV injection, images of the abdomen will indicate renal perfusion status and in the ensuing 3 minutes the glomerular filtration rate.

LUNG VENTILATION AND PERFUSION

In adults pulmonary embolus is the number one indication for lung perfusion and ventilation studies. However, in the newborn perfusion lung scan is used more for cystic disease of the lung and in establishing areas of the lung that are perfused not by the pulmonary arteries but rather by the bronchial arteries or systemic circulation, as in lung sequestration. The later appears as a "cold" area in lung perfusion scans. The ^{99m}Tc-labeled MAA is given intravenously with a minimum dose of 0.5 mCi; this will be trapped in lung precapillary arterioles in the distribution of pulmonary artery. Less than a 1-mg dose of MAA is given to block only 1:1,000 terminal arterioles to avoid any complication.[34-36] Similarly, although very rarely needed, establishment of ventilation abnormalities of certain areas of the lung can be achieved by using xenon-133 gas or by using xenon solution intravenously and observing and recording the ventilation as the xenon leaves the circulation and enters the alveoli.

Both global and regional abnormalities may be detected during wash-in (first breath) and washout phases. Computer enhancement is called upon when quantification of regional perfusion and ventilation is required. This may be particularly important preoperatively in cases of pneumonectomy or lobectomy in patients with already compromised global ventilatory function.

THYROID SCAN

If there is a doubt as to the presence or absence of thyroid tissue in the newborn, TcO_4^- or ^{123}I may be used to establish the function of the thyroid tissue.[37,38] These radioisotopes may also be used to establish whether or not a mass identified in the mediastinum, the neck, or the back of the tongue is indeed functioning thyroid tissue. The thyroid gland or part of it may be trapped in the thyroglossal tract or in the back of the tongue (Fig. 3-8), and this may be identified by using one of these radioisotopes, preferably ^{123}I because of the high background activity found in TcO_4^- scans.

Both isotopes are normally metabolized in the thyroid tissue, but iodine is organified and therefore stays longer in the thyroid to allow delayed imaging when the background has cleared, and also higher uptake in the thyroid gland. TcO_4^- is only trapped and not organified in the thyroid. As indicated earlier, these radionuclides are primarily used to establish the functioning nature of a clinically discovered mass. Occasionally they are also used to search for functioning thyroid tissue in ectopic areas (e.g., struma ovarii) and even functioning thyroid cancer tissue following thyroidectomy in cases of differentiated papillary-follicular cancers.

MISCELLANEOUS NUCLEAR IMAGING

The nuclear medicine studies described in this chapter are relatively commonly called upon, so the tests described are structured as standard studies. There are, however, special needs for which a specific test is tailored to study a specific abnormality, such as a fistula or diaphragmatic hernia,[39] or to study the perfusion status of certain organs and abnormal masses, or to study the dynamic behavior of certain organs under pharmacologic stimulation or suppression. The choice of the radioisotope is dependent on the nature of the custom-designed study, the nature of the clinical question, and the physiology of the organ to be studied. For example, recording a dynamic study over an organ during an injection of 1 to 5 mCi of TcO_4^- or some other ^{99m}Tc-labeled radiotracer will give the physician an idea of the perfusion or function status of that organ.

It is relatively easy to create a custom-designed nuclear study with the knowledge of the function of the organ in question and some knowledge of radiopharmacy. ^{111}In-labeled leukocytes[40] and ^{67}Ga scans for infection and tumors have already been discussed earlier in this chapter. Other special studies include a metaiodobenzylguanidine (MIBG) scan of the adrenal medulla (e.g., for pheochromocytomas and neu-

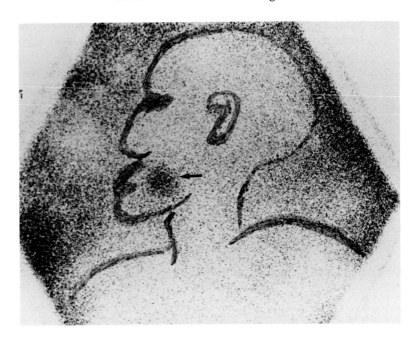

Fig. 3-8. Ectopic thyroid. A TcO_4^- study shows a focus of abnormal uptake (arrow) in the back of the tongue (lingular thyroid) and no activity in the thyroid bed. The body outline was drawn in for purposes of identification.

roblastomas) and radiolabeled monoclonal antibody studies.[41-43]

NUCLEAR COMPUTERIZED TOMOGRAPHY

Single photon emission computed tomography (SPECT) is closely related to transmission x-ray computed tomography (CT). However, in SPECT, the source of radioactivity (gamma rays) is emissions from the internally administered radiopharmaceutical. The "gantry" is formed by one or more rotating gamma camera heads (up to four heads currently). The back-projection algorithm used in reconstruction of the images is also slightly different. SPECT is acquired by volume acquisition and therefore reconstruction and presentation of all three planes (transverse, coronal, and sagittal) is almost instantaneous. SPECT helps in three-dimensional localization of a lesion and it is also more sensitive because of the isolation of the lesion against the background activity. SPECT can be applied to enhance almost any nuclear static study—for example, ^{99m}Tc-labeled HMPAO brain SPECT, bone SPECT using ^{99m}Tc-labeled MDP, and ^{67}Ga scan to localize infection foci or tumors.

Positron emission tomography (PET) is the dual-photon version of emission tomography. PET uses radioisotopes that decay by emitting positron particles. These antimatter positively charged particles collide with negatively charged electrons very quickly, and annihilation of the masses of both particles result in release of two gamma rays of 511 kEv each at 180° to each other. These are then detected by the PET camera gantry for back-projections and reconstruction. The interesting aspect of this test is that several positron emitters are isotopes of elements of physiologic interests (e.g., oxygen-15, carbon-11, and nitrogen-13). These can thus be incorporated in biochemical tracers such as $[^{11}C]$glucose, $[^{13}N]$ammonia, and $[^{15}O]$water for metabolic/perfusion studies or even in ligands such as $[^{11}C]$methylspiperone for imaging of serotonin neuroreceptors.

Functional images of SPECT or PET may be compared to CT or MR images or even superimposed slice upon slice for accurate correlative imaging of anatomy and function of the brain and other body organs.

Acknowledgments. The author wishes to thank his colleagues, Drs. Bruce Barron and Huyen Tran, for reviewing this chapter and for their constructive criticisms; and Dr. Barron for supplying Figure 3-7. Also, he wishes to thank Adlene Rehfeld for her assistance in the preparation of this chapter.

REFERENCES

1. Protection of the patient in nuclear medicine. Ann ICRP 52:8,1987
2. Radiation protection. Ann ICRP 26:3, 1977
3. Shore RM, Hendee WR: Radiopharmaceutical dosage selection for pediatric nuclear medicine. J Nucl Med 27:2287, 1986

4. Fockele DS, Bauman RJ, Shih WJ, Ryo Uy: Tc-99m HMPAO SPECT of the brain in the neonate. Clin Nucl Med 15:175, 1990

5. Denays R, Van Pachterbeke T, Tondeur M et al: Brain single photon emission computed tomography in neonates. J Nucl Med 30:1337, 1989

6. Rubinstein M, Denays R, Ham HR et al: Functional imaging of brain maturation in humans using iodine 123. J Nucl Med 30:1982, 1989

7. Galaske RG, Schober O, Heyer R: 99mTc HM PAO and 123I amphetamine cerebral scintigraphy: a new, non invasive method in determination of brain death in children. Eur J Nucl Med 14:446, 1988

8. Sibler G: Lower gastrointestinal bleeding. Pediatr Rev 12:85, 1990

9. Urgancioglu I, Kapicioglu T, Vardareli E, Sayman HB: Observation of hepatobiliary systems in joined twins by Tc-99m EHIDA. Clin Nucl Med 15:273, 1990

10. Oddo SM, Ziessman HA: Cholescintigraphy for assessing the separation potential of thoracomphalopagus twins. Clin Nucl Med 15:243, 1990

11. Freeman LM, Lan JA: Radiopharmaceutical evaluation of the hepatoiliary pathway. Int J Rad Appl Instrum [B] 17:129, 1990

12. Hunt FC: Potential radiopharmaceuticals for the diagnosis of biliary atresia and neonatal hepatitis: EHPD and HBED chelates of 67Ga and 111In. Int J Rad Appl Instrum [B] 15:659, 1988

13. Miller JH: Technetium 99m labeled red blood cells in the evaluation of hemangiomas of the liver in infants and children. J Nucl Med 28:1412, 1987

14. Kumuar D, Miller JH, Sinatra FR: Septo-optic dysplasia: recognition of causes of false-positive hepatobiliary scintigraphy in neonatal jaundice. J Nucl Med 28:966, 1987

15. Castronovo FP: Gastroesophageal scintiscanning in a pediatric population: dosimetry. J Nucl Med 27:1212, 1986

16. Lamki L, Sullivan S: A study of gastrointestinal opiate receptors: the role of the mu receptor on gastric emptying: concise communication. J Nucl Med 24:689, 1983

17. Aburano T, Taniguchi M, Hisada K: Bile ascites from a ruptured choledochal cyst detected by hepatobiliary imaging. Clin Nucl Med 13:366, 1988

18. Flynn B, Wernovsky G, Summerville DA et al: Comparison of technetium-99m MIBI and thallium 201 chloride myocardial scintigraphy in infants. J Nucl Med 30:1176, 1989

19. Roguinn N, Lam M, Frenkel A, Front D: Radionuclide angiography of azygos continuation of inferior vena cava in left atrial isomerism (polysplenia syndrome). Clin Nucl Med 12:708, 1987

20. Lopez Majanno V, Sansi P, Colter R: Nuclear medicine in the diagnosis of cardiac contusion. Eur J Nucl Med 11:290, 1985

21. Orzel JA, Monaco MP: Inadvertent ligation of the left pulmonary artery instead of patent ductus arteriosus. Noninvasive diagnosis by pulmonary perfusion imaging. Clin Nucl Med 11:629, 1986

22. Houzard C, Andre M, Guilhen S et al: Perfusion lung scan in patients operated for transposition of the great arteries. Clin Nucl Med 14:268, 1989

23. Sfakianakis GN, Sfakianaki E, Paredes A et al: Single dose captopril scintigraphy in the neonate with renovascular hypertension: prediction of renal failure, a side effect of captopril therapy. 54:246, 1988

24. Heyman S, Duckett JW: The extraction factor: an estimate of single kidney function in children during routine radionuclide renography with 99m technetium diethylenetriaminepentaacetic acid. J Urol 140:780, 1988

25. Sfakianakis GN, Sfakianaki ED: Nuclear medicine in pediatric urology and nephrology. J Nucl Med 29:1287, 1988

26. Lamki L, Haynie T: Role of adrenal imaging in surgical management. J Surg Oncol 43:139, 1990

27. Meglin AJ, Balotin RJ, Jelinek JS et al: Cloacal exstrophy: radiologic findings in 13 patients. AJR 155:1267, 1990

28. Keating MA, Escala J, Snyder HM et al: Changing concepts in management of primary obstructive megaureter. J Urol 142:636, 1989

29. Traina GC: Congenital dislocation of the hip. A protocol for early diagnosis. Ital J Orthop Traumatol 15:393, 1989

30. Howard JL, Barron BJ, Smith GG: Bone scintigraphy in the evaluation of extraskeletal injuries from child abuse. Radiographics 10:67, 1990

31. Ruppert D, Barron BJ, Madewell JE: Osteomyelitis, acute and chronic. Radiol Clin North Am 25:1171, 1987

32. Bressler EL, Conway JJ, Weiss SC: Neonatal osteomyelitis examined by bone scintigraphy. Radiology 152:685, 1984

33. Lamki L: Bone scintigraphy: current trends and future prospects. J Nucl Med 26:312, 1985

34. Dowdie SC, Humann DG, Mann MD: Pulmonary ventilation and perfusion abnormalities and ventilation perfustion imbalance in children with pulmonary atresia or extreme tetralogy of Fallot. J Nucl Med 31:1276, 1990

35. Jeanndot R, Lambert B, Brendel AJ et al: Lung ventilation and perfusion scintigraphy in the follow up of repaired congenital diaphragmatic hernia. Eur J Nucl Med 15:591, 1989

36. Lamki L, Cohen P, Driedger AA: Malignant pleural effusion and Tc-99m MDP accumulation. Clin Nucl Med 7:331, 1982

37. Brooks PT, Aarchaard ND, Carty HM: Thyroid screening in congenital hypothyroidism: a review of 41 cases. Nucl Med Commun 9:613, 1988

38. Singh A: Impaired trapping of Tc-99m pertechne-

tate in the salivary glands of patients with congenital hypothyroidism. Clin Nucl Med 15:257, 1990

39. Williamson SL, Williamson MR, Golladay ES et al: Use of technetium 99m albumin colloid to assess competency of hemidiaphragms in children. Clin Nucl Med 12:373, 1987

40. Lamki LM, Kasi LP, Haynie TP: Localization of indium-111 leukocytes in noninfected neoplasms. J Nucl Med 29:1921, 1988

41. Stewart RE, Grossman DM, Shulkin BL, Shapiro B: Iodine 131 metaiodobenzylguanidine uptake in infantile myofibromatosis. Clin Nucl Med 14:344, 1989

42. Gordon I, Peters AM, Gutman A et al: Skeletal assessment in neuroblastoma—the pitfalls of iodine 123 MIBG scans. J Nucl Med 31:129, 1990

43. Lamki L, Murray J, Rosenblum M et al: Effect of unlabelled monoclonal antibody (moAb) on biodistribution of [111]Indium labelled (MoAb). Nucl Med Commun 9:553, 1988

Diagnostic Imaging in Perinatal Brain Pathology

4

Rodrigo Dominguez
Mauricio Castillo

Studies on the physiology and pathology of the neonatal brain have advanced quite dramatically in the last 15 years secondary to the following three important factors:

1. A proportionate and absolute increase in the population of high-risk neonates (mainly prematures) in our developed Western societies, resulting in a rise of perinatal morbidity and mortality rates. This is mainly the result of negligent prenatal care in an increasingly larger population of pregnant adolescents, and of more selective pregnancies in working women close to menopausal age.
2. The development of sophisticated neonatal intensive care units in tertiary hospitals to care for these prematures.
3. The arrival of computers and of microchip technology, which have spun off new imaging modalities such as real-time ultrasound and advanced computed tomography (CT) and magnetic resonance (MR) imaging, revolutionizing the field of diagnostic radiology and consequently allowing a better look into the perinatal brain.

The increasing costs of these new imaging methods and other technological breakthroughs in intensive care medicine, and the severe cerebral and pulmonary sequelae seen in some surviving premature infants, have raised serious ethical and social questions that have yet to be resolved.

High-risk newborns are usually premature or have a low weight for gestational age. They may have suffered significant perinatal asphyxia, or may carry life-threatening congenital anomalies. They suffer more frequently from cerebral stroke, hyaline membrane disease (leading to hypoxia), intraventricular hemorrhages, and cerebral birth injury. Certain maternal diseases place the fetus at risk; for example, viral diseases such as rubella, AIDS, and herpes may produce congenital malformations and prematurity.[1] Diabetes and hypertension, with decreased placental perfusion, can alter the growth of fetal organs,[2] and can have a definitive teratogenic influence on the developing fetus.

The brain of a premature baby (Fig. 4-1) is characterized by a high water content, a relative lack of myelin (deposited centrally only in the posterior limbs of the internal capsule/dorsal brain stem and cerebellar peduncles), a poorly developed cortex with few convolutions, and a very prominent and temporary subependymal germinal matrix with rich and loosely attached vessels that lacks the autoregulatory mechanism of the adult cerebral blood flow. Also, the subependymal circulation is preferentially ventriculopetal or basal ganglia directed, which distinguishes it from the centrifugal or cortically oriented adult type of cerebral flow.[3] Thus, the premature brain is, in particular, very prone to anoxic-ischemic insults, enhanced by other immature liabilities such as surfactant deficiency, pulmonary insufficiency, and patency of the ductus arteriosus.

49

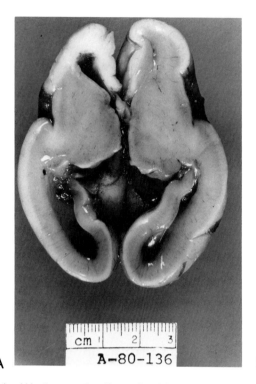
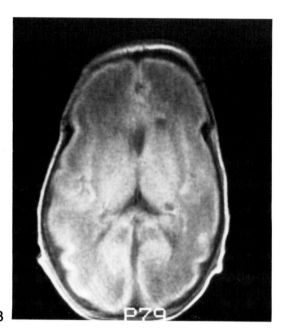

Fig. 4-1. (A) Anatomic slice of a 28 weeks' gestation premature infant's brain. **(B)** Comparative T_1-weighted MR image of another premature brain of similar age. Notice the ribbonlike thin cortex and the lack of developed gyri and myelin; the subcortical, not yet myelinated, white matter is hypointense in this MR image.

In the field of diagnostic radiology, we have gone beyond invasive and consequently inadequate examinations for these tiny babies (such as angiograms and pneumoencephalograms), past the conventional radiology of skull roentgenograms (although they still have value in certain clinical conditions), and into the realm of portable real-time ultrasound, fast-scanning CT, and the spectacular MR imaging, allowing us a definitive, clearer insight and evaluation of the intracranial structures. Each method does, however, have its advantages, inconveniences, and cost containment factors.

CT was the first technology used in peering inside the skull, but portable real-time ultrasound, with its lack of ionizing radiation and using the anterior fontanelle as an acoustic window, allows more frequent evaluations of the neonatal brain to better monitor the evolution of intraventricular bleeds. The later application of Doppler-duplex ultrasound technology offered further insights on the status of cerebral blood flow.

Puzzling questions incompletely resolved by CT and ultrasound regarding the unstable premature

brain are now better understood by utilizing the enhanced soft tissue contrast resolution capabilities of MR imaging. This method can depict the degree of cerebral maturation and of the pregressive differentiation between subcortical white and gray matters through the display of the extension and degree of myelination; the earlier and more precise assessment of infarctions and other ischemic or anoxic derangements at the white and gray matters; and the better detection of aberrant development of the brain.

The diagnosis of perinatal brain pathology is better approached by correlating the stage in the cerebral morphogenesis or development with the time of the insult. Most neurologic disabilities in childhood result from congenital malformations or brain damage in the perinatal period and are usually nonprogressive.[1] Any brain insult during embryogenesis, regardless of the inductive agent, results in a congenital malformation. If we consider that the premature infant is still in the process of active growth to achieve complete development of its anatomy, any derangement of its immature brain caused by its increased lability to a harsh environment can be classified within the spectrum of the so-called congenital cerebral anomalies or malformations.

CLASSIFICATION OF CONGENITAL CEREBRAL, CEREBELLAR, AND SPINAL MALFORMATIONS

A classification of congenital cerebral anomalies based on etiology is not as valuable because the various presumed causes may lead to similar pattern of malformations. The abnormalities reflect the time at which the noxious agent interfered with neural development, rather than the nature of the noxious agent. To the extent possible, we note the time at which each malformation had its onset. The classification presented in Table 4-1 is based on the morphologic abnormalities shown by MR and CT at the time at which the derangement of neural development occurred.

In over 60 percent of congenital central nervous system (CNS) structural anomalies, the underlying etiology is unclear, but inherited factors account for 20 percent, chromosomal anomalies for 10 percent, and environmental factors for 10 percent.[7] Many teratogenic agents have been experimentally proved as causal factors when given during early pregnancy, including retinoic acid (which induces abnormalities of migration of the neural crest cells),[8,9] x-ray radiation,[10] thalidomide,[11] and carbon monoxide.

While the distinct disruptive events may be obscure, the great significance of these lesions is not, since one third of all major anomalies involve the CNS. Our classification is as complete as possible, but not all the entities listed are described in detail in this chapter since this would be beyond the scope of this book.

NEUROCRISTOPATHIES

The development of the human nervous system commences with the development of the notochordal process, which extends from the primitive knot to the cranial end of the embryo. The notochordal process induces the neural plate, a thickened area of embryonic ectoderm. The neural plate invaginates, forming the neural groove, which is lined on each side by a neural fold. The neural crest is a transient embryologic entity derived from early neural fold that appears at 15 to 18 days of embryologic life. Because the neural crest contributes to the development of multiple cell types, abnormalities of its development affect such varied structures as the peripheral nervous system, eyes, skin, hair, thymus, parathyroid glands, and gastrointestinal tract.[8] Anomalous development of these structures provides possibilities for a variety of clinical expressions.

The term *neurocristopathy* is today used for identification of neural disorders arising from aberrations in neural crest cell migration, growth, and differentiation. The definition has been expanded to include disorders associated with other affected tissues of the head, neck, and abdomen.[9,10]

DISORDERS OF DORSAL INDUCTION

The neural plate forms the neural tube, which eventually gives rise to the spinal cord and brain. These events are referred to as dorsal induction. In these processes distinction is made between primary and secondary neurulation. Primary neurulation refers to the formation of the neural tube from approximately the L1-L2 level, which corresponds to the caudal end of the notochord, upward to the cranial end of the embryo. These events occur during the third and fourth weeks of gestation. Secondary neurulation refers to the formation of the caudal neural tube below the caudal end of the notochord by canalization and retrogressive differentiation. The distinction between derangements of primary and secondary neurulation is unclear.[11]

Primary Neurulation

Anencephaly

The bulk of the cerebral mantle is absent in anencephaly, whereas the basal ganglia are usually well formed but the brain stem is atrophic. The affected infants die at birth or within a few days.[1]

Cephaloceles

A cephalocele is a defect in the midline of the cranium and the dura matter with extracranial herniation of intracranial structures. The term *meningocele* is reserved for conditions in which the herniated sac contains only the leptomeninges filled with cerebrospinal fluid (CSF). The term *encephalocele* designates herniation of brain tissue frequently associated with agenesis of the corpus callosum and brain heteroto-

TABLE 4-1. **Classification of Congenital Cerebral, Cerebellar, and Spinal Malformations**

Malformation	Gestation Time
Neurocristopathies	15–20 days
Disorders of dorsal induction	
Neural tube defects	4 weeks
Anencephaly	
Myelomeningocele	
Chiari malformation	
Occult dysraphic states	
Diastematomyelia/diplomyelia	4 weeks–postpartum
Dermal sinus	
Lipoma	
Tethered cord	
Caudal regression	
Disorders of ventral induction. Midline cerebral defects	6 weeks
Holoprosencephaly	
Septo-optic dysplasia	
Agenesis of the septum pellucidum	
Cerebellar hypoplasia	
Dandy-Walker syndrome	
Craniosynostosis	
Disorders of neuronal proliferation, differentiation, and histogenesis	
Neurofibromatosis	7 weeks and beyond
Tuberosclerosis	
Sturge-Weber syndrome	
Other neurocutaneous syndromes	
Congenital vascular malformations	
Congenital brain tumors	
Aqueductal stenosis	
Meningeal cysts	
Errors of neuronal migration	8 weeks
Schizencephaly	
Lissencephaly	
Pachygyria	
Polymicrogyria	
Neuronal heterotopias	
Dysgenesis of the corpus callosum	
Encephaloclastic disruptions	
Hydranencephaly	Second trimester
Porencephaly	
Cerebral atrophy	
Multicystic encephalopathy	
Hydrocephalus	
Secondary acquired injuries	
Porencephaly	Third trimester
Subependymal hemorrhage	
Periventricular leukomalacia	
Congenital brain infarction	
Defects of myelination	
Decreased myelination	Perinatal
Retarded myelination	
Degenerative diseases of the developing brain	
Demyelination (usually caused by a biochemical defect)	Perinatal
Severe anoxic-ischemic insult	
Neonatal meningitis and encephalomyelitis	

(Data from van der Knaap and Valk,[4] Volpe,[5] and Poe et al.[6])

pias (Fig. 4-2). Geographic differences in the distribution of encephaloceles suggest that there may be additional racial and environmental factors in its pathogenesis. Encephaloceles are most often occipital in location in Europe and America and frontal or sphenoidal in Asia.[12]

Meningomyelocele and Arnold-Chiari Malformations

Spina bifida with meningomyelocele, a midline defect of the skin, posterior vertebral arches, and neural tube, usually occurs in the lumbrosacral region. It is one of the most common developmental anomalies of the CNS.[1] It presents at birth as a skin defect with bony prominences laterally (unfused posterior arches of the vertebrae) and later a bulge of the covering membrane with CSF until a sac is formed. In nearly all cases an Arnold-Chiari type II malformation is also present, with an associated craniolacunae (bone dysplasia) (Fig. 4-3). The brain anomaly consists mainly of maldevelopment and downward displacement of parts of the cerebellum, fourth ventricle, and medulla oblongata into the cervical spinal canal.[13] Aqueductal stenosis with hydrocephalus and migrational disorders of the cerebral mantle and syringomyelia are also frequently present.

Malsegmentation of the Craniovertebral Junction

Chiari I malformation, basilar impression, Klippel-Feil anomaly, and other vertebral errors of segmentation at this level are usually present in association with a moderate herniation of the cerebellar tonsils (more than 3 mm) below the foramen magnum and a small or absent cisterna magna. Hydromyelia is present in 20 to 70 percent of cases.[14]

Secondary Neurulation: Spinal Dysrasphisms

Secondary neurulation refers to the formation of the caudal neural tube below the caudal end of the notochord by canalization and retrogressive differentiation.[15] The lower lumbar, sacral, and coccygeal segments are thus formed. This canalization starts at 4 weeks and continues until the seventh week of gestation. The retrogressive differentiation lasts from the seventh week until some time after birth. These occult dysraphic abnormalities (lipoma, diastematomyelia, epidermoid cyst, and tethering of the cord) can be checked by portable ultrasound of the spinal canal or, when possible, they can much more thoroughly be studied by multiplanar MR imaging.

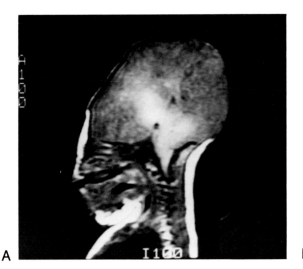
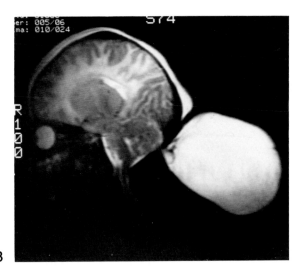

A   B

Fig. 4-2. (A) T_1-weighted midsagittal MR image of a premature infant with partial herniation of the brain through the posterior fontanel; notice abnormal distribution of gray matter, irregularly in the subcortical area (heterotopia), and the absence of corpus callosum. **(B)** T_2-weighted midsagittal MR image of a midline posterior occipital meningocele and intact normal intracranial structures.

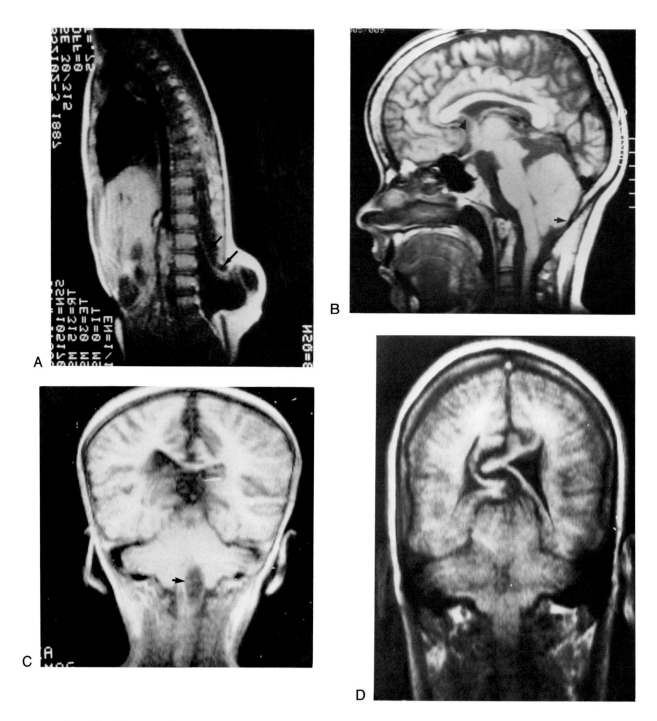

Fig. 4-3. **(A)** T_1-weighted midsagittal MR image of a lumbar meningomyelocele with tethering of the spinal cord (arrows) in a newborn. **(B)** Chiari type II malformation on T_1-weighted midsagittal MR image. Notice the tight posterior fossa with downward herniation of the cerebellum beyond the craniocervical junction (arrow), decreased anteroposterior diameter of the pons, posterior kinking of the medulla (open arrow), elongated fourth ventricle, beaking of tectum, and hypoplasia of the rostral part of the corpus callosum (arrowhead). **(C)** Chiari type II malformation on T_1-weighted coronal MR image demonstrating a tight posterior fossa with a towering central cerebellum partially herniated through the incisura and syrinogobulbia (arrow). **(D)** Coronal T_1-weighted image of Arnold-Chiari type II malformation with upward cerebellar herniation through the incisura and a fenestrated falx, allowing interdigitations of the cerebral hemispheres. (*Figure continues.*)

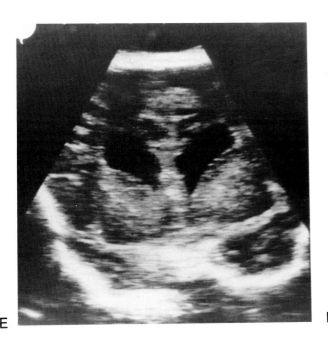

E

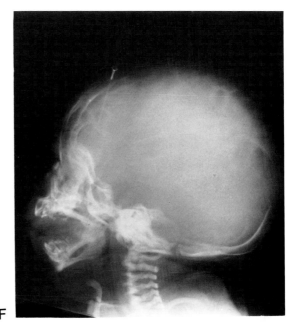

F

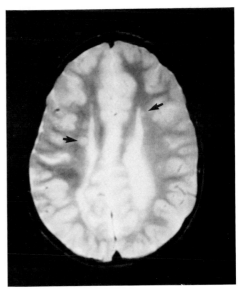

G

Fig. 4-3 (*Continued*). **(E)** Brain ultrasound in mid-coronal plane showing Arnold-Chiari type II malformation with typical downward pointing of the dilated bodies of the lateral ventricles. **(F)** Radiograph of Calvarial manifestations of Arnold-Chiari type II malformation: shallow posterior fossa, craniomegaly, and craniolacunae (dysplastic changes in the membranous bone). **(G)** T₂-weighted axial MR image of Arnold-Chiari type II patient with heterotopic islands of gray matter in periventricular locations (arrows).

DISORDERS OF VENTRAL INDUCTION

Ventral induction refers to the induction of events in the rostral end of the primitive brain that are intimately tied to the development of the face. These inductive events lead to the formation of the prosencephalon (forebrain), mesencephalon (midbrain), and rhombencephalon (hindbrain). The forebrain becomes the telencephalon, which will divide into two cerebral hemispheres. These events also lead to the development of the optic vesicles, the olfactory bulbs, the third ventricle, the hypothalamus, and the thalami. These major events occur between the fifth and 10th weeks of gestation. The cerebellum develops from the dorsal part of the metencephalon.

The disorders of ventral induction include the holoprosencephalies, septo-optic dysplasia, agenesis of the septum pellucidum, congenital malformations of the posterior fossa, and craniosynostosis. In contrast to the classification of Volpe,[5] we include the congenital malformations of the posterior fossa in this section, since the ventral inductive events comprise the formation not only of the prosencephalic structures, but also of the mesencephalic and rhombencephalic structures. The cerebellar vermis develops into a rostrocaudal direction, as is the case with the corpus callosum.

Holoprosencephaly

Holoprosencephaly is a disorder characterized by incomplete segmentation of the primitive forebrain (prosencephalon) into the cerebral hemispheres, with abnormal continuity of gray and white matters across the midline.[16] The development of the face is intimately related to development of the brain, so a spectrum of facial defects occurs, ranging from mild hypotelorism to large midline clefts and cyclopia.

When there is no diverticulation of the prosencephalon, the anomaly is further classified as "alobar." Alobar holoprosencephaly is characterized by the following: a central large single ventricle with associated posterior band of white matter, agenesis of the corpus callosum, absence of the falx or interhemispheric fissure, and undivided diencephalon resulting in fused thalami, no midline third ventricle, and posterior outpouching of the incompletely developed third ventricle, which forms a large dorsal cyst or sac above or below the incisura. The "semilobar" type of holoprosencephaly demonstrates partial separation of the primitive forebrain into temporo-occipital lobes, with partial differentiation of the monoventricle into occipital and temporal horns. The third type, or "lobar" holoprosencephaly, has a nearly normal anatomy. However, the gray and white matters remain fused across the midline at the base of the frontal lobes, with the frontal horns of the ventricles close together and no septum pellucidum[7] (Fig. 4-4).

Alobar holoprosencephaly must be distinguished from both massive hydrocephalus and hydranencephaly. In massive hydrocephalus, unlike alobar holoprosencephaly, the falx and interhemispheric fissure are present. In hydranencephaly, unlike alobar holoprosencephaly, the thalami are not fused.

Septo-optic Dysplasia

Septo-optic dysplasia is a rare anterior midline anomaly that is often considered to be a mild form of lobar holoprosencephaly. It results from an insult during the fifth to seventh week of gestation, during the for-

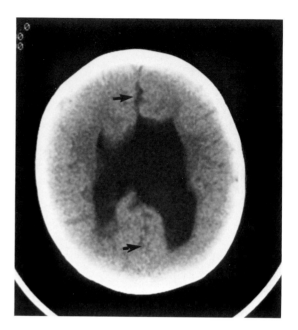

Fig. 4-4. Noncontrast CT scan in a child with lobar holoprosenephaly. There is a single, horseshoe-shaped ventricle. The corpus callosum is absent but the interhemispheric fissure is present (arrows), distinguishing this case from the more severe forms of holoprosencephaly.

mation of the anterior wall of the diencephalon (which gives origin to the septum pellucidum and the optic vesicles).[17] Clinical findings include optic nerve hypoplasia, hypotelorism, hypopituitarism (with diabetes insipidus in 50 percent of patients), seizures, nystagmus, and hypotonia. There is no consistent relationship between the clinical findings and the findings on MR imaging or CT, and septo-optic dysplasia may occur with no accompanying findings.

Isolated absence of the septum pellucidum has been said to be a normal variant, but in a review of 200 cases examined by MR imaging, Barkovich and Norman found none in which it occurred as an isolated entity.[18] Absence of the septum pellucidum should therefore alert us to the possibility of other structural midline cerebral defects such as dysgenesis of the corpus callosum and schizencephaly. Coronal and axial imaging sections show to best advantage the absence of the septum pellucidum, flattening of the roofs of the ventricular frontal horns, downward pointing of the floor of the lateral ventricles (as seen in the coronal plane), enlargement of the suprasellar cistern, and hypoplasia of the optic nerves and optic

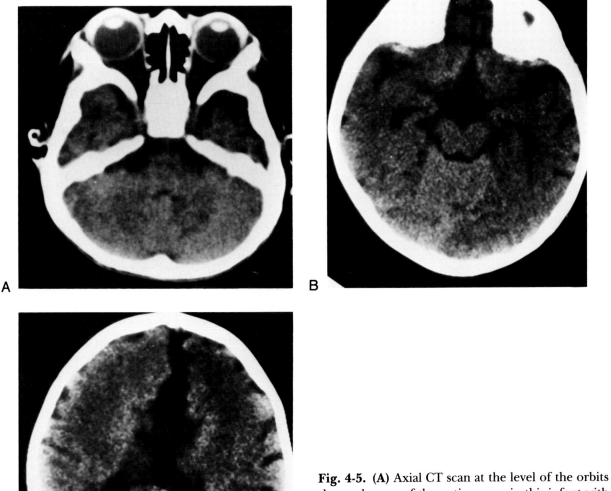

A

B

C

Fig. 4-5. (A) Axial CT scan at the level of the orbits shows absence of the optic nerves in this infant with septo-optic dysplasia. **(B)** Axial CT section through the suprasellar cistern in the same patient shows absence of a well-formed optic chiasm. **(C)** Axial CT image in the same patient at the level of the lateral ventricles. Note that the anterior aspect of the corpus callosum is absent and that the splenium is probably hypoplastic.

chiasm.[19] The corpus callosum can be absent or hypoplastic (Fig. 4-5).

Dandy-Walker Syndrome

The Dandy-Walker syndrome is a hindbrain malformation characterized by variable hypoplasia of the vermis and cystic dilation of the fourth ventricle. This cyst also displaces anteriorly and laterally the cerebellar hemispheres, which may be hypoplastic. The posterior fossa is enlarged, and there is elevation of the insertion of the tentorium and the torcula. Over 60 percent of cases of Dandy-Walker cyst or variant will have other associated congenital CNS anomalies, including agenesis of the corpus collosum, neuronal migration anomalies, and encephaloceles (Fig. 4-6). Differentiating between a Dandy-Walker variant and a mega cisterna magna may not be possible, and therefore the term *Dandy-Walker complex* has been suggested to encompass these anomalies.[20]

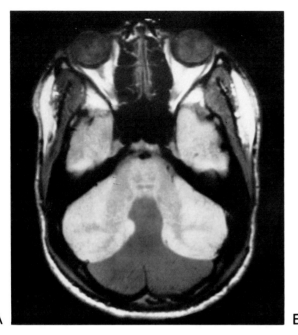 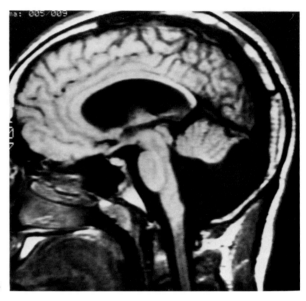

A   B

Fig. 4-6. Axial **(A)** and midsagittal **(B)** T_1-weighted MR images of a Dandy-Walker malformation. Notice the hypoplastic cerebellar lobes and absent vermis, anterolateral displacement of this organ, and communication between the fourth ventricle and the large posterior fossa cyst.

Craniosynostosis

Craniosynostosis appears to result from an early embryonic disturbance in the formation of the skull base and as such can be included in the disorders of ventral induction.

DISORDERS OF NEURONAL PROLIFERATION, DIFFERENTIATION, AND HISTOGENESIS

Histogenesis refers to the organization of cells into tissues. Once the essential external form of the brain has been established, complex processes of neuronal proliferation, differentiation, migration, and organization follow. Major events initially occur between 2 and 5 months of gestation, although after this time the processes continue into the postnatal period.

Although migrational processes occur simultaneously with proliferation and differentiation, in a number of conditions pathology is predominantly a derangement of migration; therefore, these malformations are classified as a separate subset.

Aqueductal Stenosis ("Congenital Hydrocephalus")

We are not sure whether aqueductal stenosis is a disorder of histogenesis, but we classify it here because of its probable time of onset. Aqueductal stenosis can be a congenital entity, transmitted as an X-linked recessive trait that produces obstructive hydrocephalus. It can also be secondary to other congenital anomalies or perinatal events (infection or subdural hematoma in the posterior fossa). Axial and sagittal MR imaging is the best diagnostic modality for visualization of the aqueduct and periaqueductal region and evaluating possible causes for stenosis (Fig. 4-7). Flow-sensitive MR imaging sequences through the aqueduct may help document its patency.

Vascular Malformations

Formation of arteriovenous malformations, congenital aneurysms, and angiomas date back to early developmental stages, but the precise time of onset is controversial and possibly differs for the various types of vascular abnormalities.

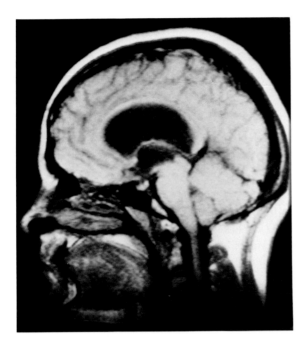

Fig. 4-7. T_1-weighted midsagittal MR image of "congenital" aqueductal stenosis, showing not only the extremely narrowed aqueduct but the dilatation of the ventricular system above.

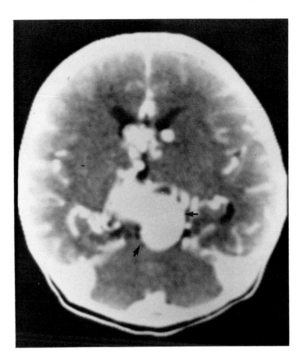

Fig. 4-8. Axial contrast-enhanced CT scan in an infant with a vein of Galen arteriovenous fistula. There is aneurysmatic dilatation of the vein of Galen (arrows) and multiple enlarged vessels in its vicinity.

Arteriovenous Fistula of the Vein of Galen

This high-flow fistula results in a large vein of Galen (hence the name "aneurysm"), which compresses the surrounding cerebral tissue and may cause periventricular leukomalacia, vascular thrombosis, and/or hemorrhagic infarctions. Hydrocephalus can also be present.[21-23] Clinically it usually presents by shunting excessive blood to the lungs, and causing high-output congestive heart failure and a systolic bruit heard over the entire head. Diagnostic studies will show a cystic structure in the region of the pineal gland. Doppler-duplex ultrasound and CT will assert its vascular origin[22] (Fig. 4-8). Treatment can be accomplished via transtorcular or arterial embolizations.

Congenital Brain Tumors

Various types of tumors have been found in the CNS at birth that are due to remains of embryonic neural cell proliferation (e.g., craniopharingoma, medulloblastoma, and chordomas) and to residual embryonic cells normally present in the cranial cavity but alien to nervous tissue (e.g., teratomas, germinomas, dermoids, epidermoids, and lipomas).

Meningeal Cysts

Meningeal cysts develop between the cerebral surface and the cranial base or vault; they can also be extracranial along the spinal canal. They arise in the septum posticum from misplaced nests of arachnoid cells or by herniation of the arachnoid through congenital dura diverticula. This more generic category of meningeal cysts also includes the so-called arachnoid cysts.[24] The membrane of the cyst has a single layer of arachnoid cells; intracranially they may communicate with the pericerebral cisterns.

Symptomatic cyst may be revealed in the neonatal period through cranial deformations or macrocephaly.

Ectodermal Dysplasias

Ectodermal dysplasias present as congenital lesions in many organs and regions of the body, but more specifically in the CNS, eyes, and skin, hence the name "phakomatosis." We shall briefly review the most important intracranial perinatal manifestions in three of the main phakomatoses.

Sturge-Weber Syndrome

Sturge-Weber syndrome is a congenital capillary hemangioma involving the facial and or cervical skin as well as the intracranial meninges and choroids. The capillary hemangioma of the skin is clinically manifested as a port-wine nevus that involves the trigeminal nerve distribution and generally the ipsilateral parieto-occipital lobes. The intracranial parts lead to anoxic cerebral injury with later development of calcifications in a curvilinear "railroad track" pattern[25] (Fig. 4-9).

Tuberous Sclerosis

Tuberous sclerosis is an autosomal-dominant phakomatosis. The intracerebral lesions are sclerotic patches or "tubers" (hamartomas) scattered through the brain. They consist of neurons, astrocytes, and giant cells without a normal organization. Glial nodes are also present in the periventricular region and have a tendency to calcify later in life.[26] Obstructive hydrocephalus may ensue. When these subependymal nodules are located near the foramen of Monro and develop a tendency to enlargement and enhance-

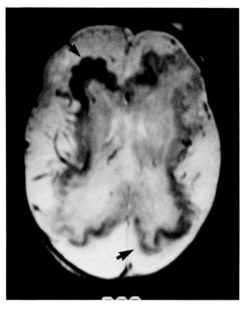

Fig. 4-9. T_2-weighted axial MR image in an infant with Sturge-Weber disease. Anoxic cerebral injury and severe brain atrophy are present, secondary to the meningeal and diffuse capillary hemangiomata. Note the hypodense calcified crust around the cerebral cortex (arrows).

ment, they are called giant cell astrocytomas. Adenoma sebaceum is the most common facial skin lesion, but other organs such as the kidneys can be involved with fibrous and fatty tumors.

The hamartomas have MR relaxation times similar to that of white matter if they are not calcified. Calcifications of these lesions are better identified by CT than by MR imaging. These lesions are frequently and characteristically of high signal intensity on T_2-weighted MR images and present central low signal intensity secondary to calcifications; on T_1-weighted imaging their signal intensities are equal to or less than that of white matter. Hamartomas can be situated anywhere from the periventricular regions to the subcortical areas; the latter are said to be the most characteristic lesions of tuberous sclerosis.

Neurofibromatosis

Neurofibromatosis is the most common of the phakomatoses and may occur either spontaneously or as a result of an autosomal-dominant inheritance with variable expressivity. In the CNS this disorder affects the mesodermal and ectodermal tissues. A classical mesodermal change includes hypoplasia of the sphenoid wings. Traditionally, neurofibromatosis has been divided into central and peripheral types, with many cases presenting findings in both groups. Currently two distinct types of neurofibrotosis are recognized according to chromosomal relationship: type I (identified at chromosome 17) and type II (identified at chromosome 22). Some authors describe a third type in order to classify those cases with characteristics of both types I and II.

Optic nerve glioma is one manifestation of type I neurofibromatosis (Fig. 4-10). It is the most common tumor in the CNS, being found in up to 30 percent of neurofibromatosis patients. Approximately 75 percent of these lesions are identified in the first decade of life and many are bilateral. The majority of those discovered on MR imaging or CT scanning are in asymptomatic patients. Multiple focal areas of abnormally increased signal intensity are found in the majority of neurofibromatosis type I patients on proton density and T_2-weighted MR images. The exact nature of these lesions is unclear. They may represent dysplastic hamartomas, and some cases may represent gliomatosis or dysmyelinations. Both schwannomas and meningiomas tend to occur in a younger age group in those patients with neurofibromatosis type II than in those without; intraventricular menin-

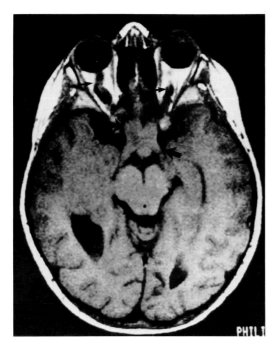

Fig. 4-10. T_1-weighted axial MR image in a young patient with neurofibromatosis type 1. There is marked enlargement of the optic chiasm (large arrows) that was presumed to represent an optic glioma. The optic nerves are enlarged (small arrow) and hypointense, probably secondary to accumulation of fluid underneath the sheaths.

gioma is more common in these patients than in the general population.

ERRORS OF NEURONAL MIGRATION

Migration of the nerve cells from the germinal matrix to the superficial cortex and deep nuclei of the brain occurs predominantly in the third, fourth, and fifth months of gestation. Likewise, in this period the cerebellar nuclei and cortex are formed.

Lissencephaly

The terms *agyria* and *lissencephaly* refer to a flat, smooth brain surface caused by the absence of cortical gyri. This is the most severe of the neuronal migrational disorders. *Pachygyria* refers to multiple areas of broad, flat, shallow gyri. A totally agyric brain is a rarity, and most cases display mixed areas of lissencephaly and pachygyria, the difference between the two entities being merely one of severity. The

sylvian fissures are shallow, creating a so-called figure-8 deformity. The temporal lobes tend to be less involved than other portions of the brain. The white matter is significantly thinned, leading to the absence of interdigitation at the gray-white matter junction and hypoplasia of the white matter tracts, including the corticospinal tracts[27] (Fig. 4-11).

Polymicrogyria

Polymicrogyria is characterized by excessive thickening and excessive convolutions of the cerebral cortex.

Heterotopias

Islands of gray matter known as heterotopias can be encountered along the neuronal migrational path to the cortex, usually localized in the subependymal or subcortical white matter (Fig. 4-12).

Schizencephaly

Schizencephaly is a form of migrational disorder characterized by a full-thickness transcerebral column of gray matter that extends in continuity from the subependymal layer of the ventricle to the cor-

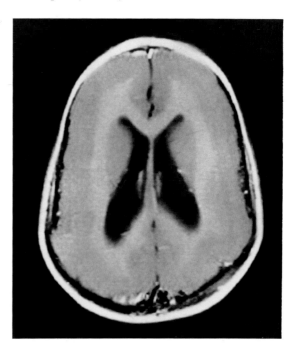

Fig. 4-11. T_1-weighted axial MR image in an infant with lissencephaly shows a very smooth cortical surface as well as abnormally thickened gray matter and a relatively thin mantle of white matter.

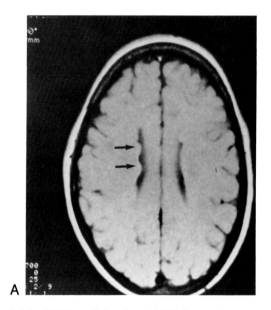 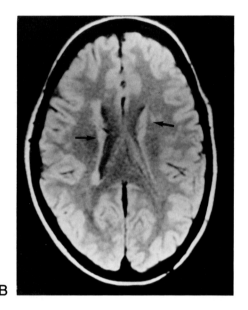

Fig. 4-12. (A) T_1-weighted axial MR image in a young patient with intractable seizures and heterotopia. Note that the outer borders of the lateral ventricles appear to be lobulated (arrows). **(B)** MR proton density image of the same patient and at the same level as Fig. A shows heterotopic gray matter lining the outer border of the lateral ventricles (arrows). The signal intensity from the ectopic gray matter is similar to that of the cerebral cortex.

tex.[28] This disorder is thought to arise during the second month of gestation when the developing wall of the brain should differentiate into several layers. A small, ependyma-lined ventricular diverticulum extends into the gray column, as the glial lining of the cortex surrounds the dimple or arrested cerebral wall segment. The pia and ependyma merge within the sleeve of gray matter, forming a transcerebral cleft, which may be closed (closed lips schizencephaly) (Fig. 4-13). If the involved area is larger and there is associated hydrocephalus, then the central part of the abnormal zone is pushed outward and thinned, creating a large defect in the cerebral mantle (open lips schizencephaly) (Fig. 4-14). This wedge-like transcortical defect should not be confused with porencephaly or an arachnoid cyst, because the transcerebral column of gray matter can be identified at its edges by MR imaging.[29] The lesion is usually bilateral and symmetric, placed in the central or sylvian fissures, and is seen in association with septo-optic dysplasia and gray matter heterotopias.

Dysgenesis of the Corpus Callosum

Complete callosal presence appears to be dependent upon the successful closure of the anterior neuropore and the induction of the precursors of the commissural plate (i.e., the massa commissuralis) from the rostral wall of the telecephalon (the primitive lamina terminalis). This disorder is included with migrational disturbances because, presumably, dysgenesis of the corpus callosum in a sense results not only from abnormal induction but from migration of cells and their axons away from the midline or paramidline regions.[4] Thus, this is a generic term for a spectrum of abnormalities ranging from partial or complete absence of the corpus callosum to lipomas of the interhemispheric fissure.[19] Patients with isolated callosal dysgenesis can be asymptomatic.

Since the axons from the hemispheres cannot cross the midline in the commissural plate, they course longitudinally instead, to establish paired longitudinal bundles (of Probst) along the medial borders of the lateral ventricles. The coronal imaging plane will show a steer horn configuration of the frontal ventricular horns (widely separated with concave medial borders) because they are indented by the abnormal bundles. The third ventricle is high in location. Sagittal midline MR images will demonstrate the abnormal location of the pericallosal arteries, a vein of Galen not curving around the splenium, and the internal cerebral veins separated by the high-riding third ventricle. This malformation is commonly associated with a wide spectrum of anomalies (Fig. 4-15).

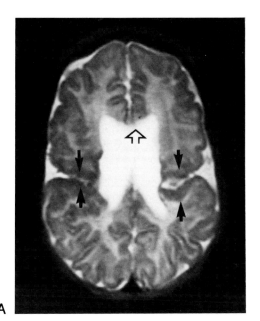 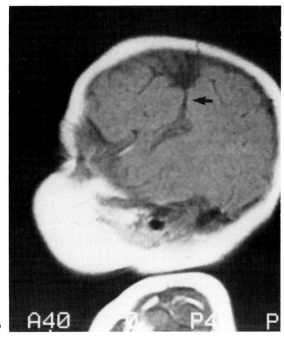

Fig. 4-13. (A) T_2-weighted axial MR image of a newborn with bilateral midparietal closed lips schizencephaly. Notice the transcerebral columns of heterotopic gray matter along the clefts (arrows) and also the associated absence of the septum pellucidum and a shallow anterior angle of the frontal horns of the lateral ventricles as an expression of hypoplasia of the corpus callosum (open arrow). **(B)** T_1-weighted parasagittal MR image of same infant demonstrating the coronal plane of the cleft connecting the subarachnoid space with the lateral ventricle (arrow).

ENCEPHALOCLASTIC DISRUPTIONS

Vascular insults in the forming brain will have different clinicopathologic outcomes according to the stage of development at which they happen. Some researchers have observed cerebral architectural changes when the vascular insult takes place in the very early stages of pregnancy, resulting in congenital malformations such as polymicrogyria and schizencephaly.[30] Strokes taking place during late fetal morphogenesis will disturb the brain at a borderline period between late malformative and early destructive physiopathogic mechanisms (early second trimester). The resulting brain lesions constitute a series of deformities called encephaloclastic disruptions or structural defects, representing the destruction of a previously normally formed brain.

The capacity of the astrocytes to react to the ischemic insult with proliferation and hypertrophy does not appear until the end of the pregnancy. On histo-

logic examination, reaction of immature nervous tissues to necrosis is fast and consists of liquefaction and dissolution of the necrotic tissue with no proliferation of fixed elements and no gliosis around the scar. The resulting lesion, or porus, is lined by a thin, smooth layer devoid of neurons.[31]

A cerebrovascular insult during the second trimester of pregnancy will form a CSF-filled cavity or porus in contact with the ventricules or the subdural space (porencephaly). During the third trimester (or in premature infants) such an insult may present with a mixed appearance of ischemic leukomalacia (porencephaly of the third trimester) or a hemorrhagic component (perinatal stroke).

Hydranencephaly

Hydranencephaly is a giant porus that results from an early gestational vascular insult. There is nearly complete destruction of the cerebral hemispheres, which are replaced by CSF-filled bubbles. The membrane forming the wall of the bubbles is smooth with-

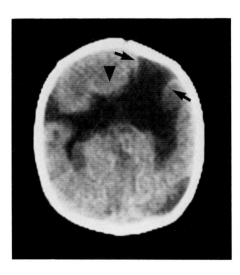

Fig. 4-14. Open lips schizencephaly in a 1-month-old infant as seen on axial CT scan of the brain without contrast. Notice the presence of corpus callosum (arrowhead) and the thin rim of heterotopic gray matter surrounding the margins of the bilateral cleft (arrows) as features that differentiate this lesion from lobar holoprosencephaly or hydrocephalus.

out convolutions. It may have some islands of glial tissue, but no ependymal layer corresponding to the ventricular walls. Preservation of the basal ganglia and the inferior part of the temporal and occipital lobes is frequent[32] (Fig. 4-16). There is absence of the main cerebral arteries but preservation of the basilar one and its cerebral branches. This can be documented by arteriography or a less invasive procedure such as MR angiography.

Porencephalies

Porencephalies formed in the second trimester of pregnancy extend across the cerebral hemisphere and communicate between the ventricles and the brain surface. They are located in the territory of the main cerebral arteries and often are associated with absence of the septum pellucidum[33] (Fig. 4-17A).

Atrophy and Encephalopathy

Intrauterine placental insufficiencies, anemias, and/or chorioamnionitis can also influence the development of the brain, resulting in cortical embolism and diffused infarctions with brain atrophy, cysts, cystic encephalomalacia, calcifications, and microcephaly (Fig. 4-18).

SECONDARY ACQUIRED INJURIES

Porencephalies

When porencephalies occur during the third trimester or in the perinatal period the cyst does not necessarily involve the entire thickness of the cerebral mantle and it is associated with some degree of homolateral or diffuse cerebral atrophy[34] (Fig. 4-17B).

Brain Lesions of Circulatory Origin in the Premature Infant

The development of the brain requires a higher metabolic rate of glucose consumption in its central areas where maturation and myelination first start; consequently fetal hypoxia affects primarily these central structures (cerebellum, basal ganglia, periventricular white matter), where subependymal (SEH) and intraventricular (IVH) hemorrhages and periventricular leukomalacia (PVL) can take place and are the most common vascular lesions in the brain of very low-birthweight infants. SEH occurs in the germinal matrixes, which are the areas known as the ventricular and subventricular zones in neurodevelopmental studies of the brain. These zones are present in subependymal locations at all levels of the developing CNS. They are the sites of proliferation of neuronal and glial precursors. These cells migrate from their subependymal location to the various layers of cortex by a complex and only partially understood process during the third to fifth months of gestation. In the last 12 to 16 weeks of gestation this area becomes less and less prominent, and it has nearly vanished by term.

The site of SEH is characteristically over the body of the caudate nucleus before 30 weeks' gestation, over the head of the caudate near the foramen of Monro after 30 to 32 weeks, and the choroid plexus at term. The vessels of the capillary bed in the germinal matrix change with gestation and are the sites of hemorrhage.[35] The incidence of germinal matirix hemorrhage averages approximately 67 percent from 28 to 32 weeks' gestation and drops to less than 5 percent at 40 weeks as the germinal matrix disappears in the normal maturation of the neonatal brain.[36]

Hemorrhagic brain lesions were originally diagnosed mainly by clinical criteria and postmortem examination. In the late 1970s, CT scans began to provide much more in vivo information.[34] However, CT scanning is inherently difficult in the newborn, especially in the labile premature infant, in whom there is

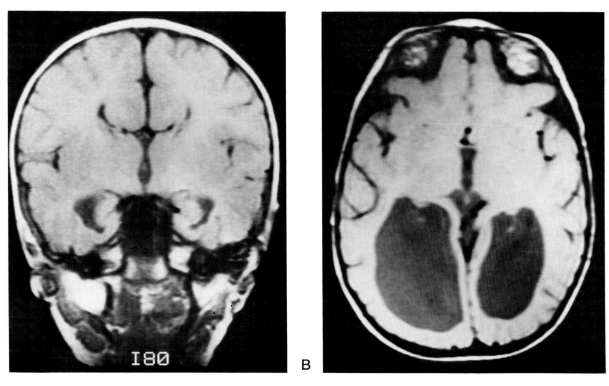

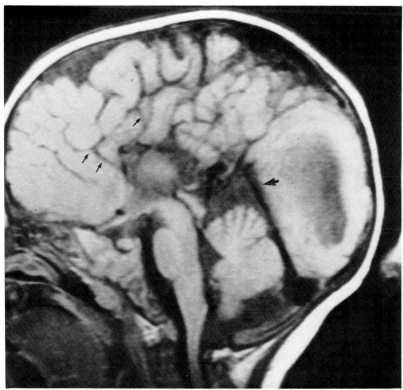

Fig. 4-15. T$_1$-weighted MR images of the brain in a child with agenesis of the corpus callosum. **(A)** Coronal image: notice the longitudinal bundles of Probst along the medial borders of the lateral ventricles, producing a steer horn configuration. Also, the third ventricle has a high location. **(B)** Axial image: notice dilatation of the occipital horns of the lateral ventricles (colpocephaly). **(C)** Midsagittal image: notice the abnormal location of the pericallosal arteries (small arrows) and a vein of Galen not curving around the splenium (arrow).

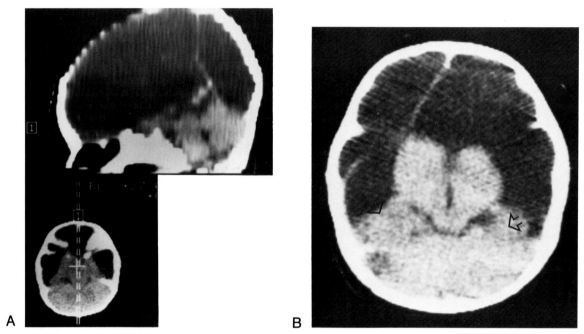

Fig. 4-16. Axial **(A & B)** and midsagittal **(A)** CT scans of a newborn with hydranencephaly and almost complete destruction of the cerebral hemispheres; the basal ganglia and structures of the posterior fossa are intact. The falx (arrow) is deviated but present along with residual parts of the occipital lobes (arrowheads).

an incompletely developed cerebral mantle. Early CT machines produced a significant amount of radiation and the infants had to be transported to a radiology unit. CT interpretation, with its diffuse hypodensity of the white matter, was and still is quite unreliable in depicting parenchymal abnormalities.[37] These problems meant that a limited number of scans were done and infants were rarely sequentially exposed.

Papile and colleagues performed the first population study of infants weighing less than 1500 g.[38] Their study indicated that the classic clinical signs of IVH were not always associated with hemorrhage into the brain and that "silent" events could be of major size. The development of portable real-time ultrasound scanners allowed a grading and description of the evolution of hemorrhagic lesions. This led to the discovery that hemorrhage occurs primarily in the first few days of extrauterine life. Therefore, it is logical to look at events during this relatively short time in an attempt to explain the lesions.

Our understanding of pathogenic mechanisms is not yet settled and it has undergone major changes during the last decade.[39] Hambleton and Wigglesworth first pointed out that the major site of hemorrhage in the preterm infant was within the capillary bed of the germinal matrix. They hypothesized that

arterial hypertension was a potential mechanism.[40] Shortly thereafter, theories of arterial hypotension with subsequent rebleeding and loss of autoregulation were proposed.[41] The term *autoregulation* is used to describe the maintenance of constant perfusion pressure to the brain in spite of varying arterial pressures. It is known, in both animals and humans, that this autoregulatory mechanism is disrupted and can be abolished by moderate to severe asphyxia. Accordingly, loss of autoregulation became a plausible explanation for hemorrhagic lesions because it encompassed both increased and decreased flow as pathogenic mechanisms. In a condition of pressure-passive flow the brain could be underperfused, causing infarction and a secondary hemorrhage into the area with reperfusion. It is also possible that the full strength of a normal systemic blood pressure delivered to an immature germinal matrix could produce a hemorrhage from overperfusion, a model similar to hypertensive stroke but occurring at normal or slightly elevated blood pressure in a situation of pressure-passive flow.[39]

Technology has not been as effective in measuring cerebral blood flow. Several workers have used Doppler cerebral blood flow velocity, a derived value, to estimate perfusion.[37] The ultrasound system com-

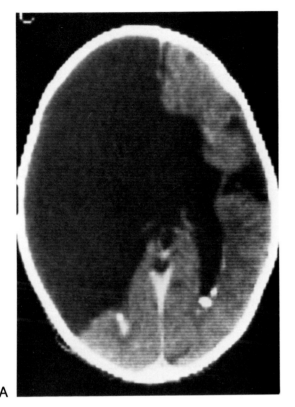
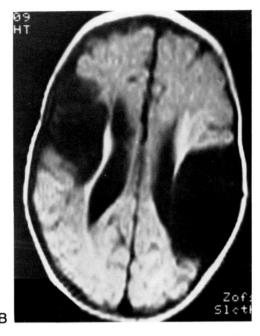

Fig. 4-17. Axial CT scan of **(A)** second trimester porencephaly. Notice the absence of midline cerebral structures such as the septum pellucidum and corpus callosum. **(B)** T_1-weighted axial MR image of third trimester bilateral porencephaly. Notice a similarity to open lips schizencephaly, but normal midline cerebral structures are present and there is absence of gray matter heterotopia along the porencephalic clefts.

bining real-time images and pulsed Doppler technique with syncronized phase allows the possibility of monitoring the vascular structure originating the ultrasound signal and at the same time obtaining the appropriate reading for the blood flow velocity (by readjusting the sonic Doppler angle and vascular blood flow).[42-44] These and other indirect methods of assessing cerebral blood flow depend on certain assumptions, most particulary that vessel size remains constant and there is no intracranial redistribution of flow. This is an important limitation because few actual arterial sites (the most widely used are the anterior cerebral arteries) can be sampled by most techniques and significant intracranial redistribution affects accuracy.[45]

The absence or presence of intracranial hemorrhage in the brain of the premature infant does not keep a constant relationship with the specific type of Doppler flow pattern (Fig. 4-19). Velocity profiles of Doppler readings in the internal carotid, basilar, and anterior and middle cerebral arteries have been useful in classifying brain edema in infants and at times can predict outcome.[46,47] Doppler can also be used to detect lenticulostriate vasculopathy and to document brain death.[48] Color Doppler enhances the identification of the usual blood flow in the circle of Willis.[49]

Not surprisingly, a single unifying cause of hemorrhage has not been found, although most would agree that hemorrhages are most likely to develop in sick babies and that sick babies have more adverse events during the critical neonatal period.[39]

Imaging of Circulatory Brain Lesions

On CT scans and MR images acute SEH presents as a high-density lesion; it may also present as isointense to mildly hypointense areas on the T_1-weighted MR images (Fig. 4-20). If the lesion is older than 3 days (subacute), there is bulging in the wall of the ventricle, usually adjacent to the frontal horn, and the lesion

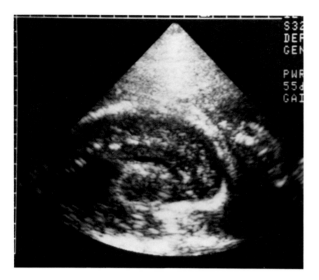

Fig. 4-18. Intrautero sagittal ultrasound scan of an eight month fetal brain demonstrating microcephaly and periventricular echogenicities (calcifications) (arrows) due to chorioamnionitis and diffuse infarction caused by cytomegalovirus infection.

becomes hyperintense on T_1-weighted images. On ultrasound, SEH is diagnosed by increased echogenicity in the region of the caudate-thalamic groove. Small subependymal hematomas may resolve or progress (grade I). As the hematoma enlarges, ventricular extension is most common (grades II and III); with progressive enlargement the hematoma can extend into the brain parenchyma (grade IV).

Acute IVH will be seen as high-density material within the ventricles on CT scans. CSF-blood levels may also be evident on any diagnostic modality in the dependent portions of the ventricles, usually the occipital horns. Acute IVH is best diagnosed by CT or ultrasound but often will be difficult to diagnose by CT after 2 to 3 weeks because the ventricular clot resolves and looses diagnostically valuable density. However, after IVH the ventricular surfaces become very echogenic on ultrasound in what seems to be a chemical ventriculitis in response to blood in the CSF. The ventricular wall will be quite echogenic on ultra-

sound but is usually isodense on CT.[50] The extension of the subacute hemorrhage is well outlined by MR imaging, as is the degree of accompanying edema and infarction (see Fig. 4-21A).

PVL is defined as an ischemic infarction of the white matter located around the lateral ventricles of the premature infant's brain, with coagulation necrosis and edema and, later, reactive astrocytosis and cystic cavities.[51] PVL is caused by the hypoperfusion of end arteries that supply the white matter in the watershed areas between the two different vascular systems of the maturing brain: the centripetal type (a prominent temporary vascular system around the ventricles in the subependimal matrix) and the centrifugal adult type of the developing cerebral cortex.[37]

PVL is the second most common cause of cerebral injury in premature infants and has an incidence of approximately 7 to 22 percent.[52,53] There is a high mortality rate for patients with the more severe grades of the often accompanying IVH. Subependymal and small intraventricular hemorrhages (grades I and II) do not have neurologic sequelae. Conversely, PVL is rarely fatal but usually results in severe neurologic damage, commonly including spastic diplegia, spastic quadriplegia, cortical blindness, deafness, and mental retardation. The clinical findings of this disease are not sufficiently distinctive in the neonatal period to allow a specific diagnosis to be made.[54] Hemorrhage ranging in size from microscopic to massive may occur into regions of PVL, as demonstrated in postmortem examinations by Armstrong and Norman.[54] Prominent hemorrhage into PVL is indicative of a major degree of brain infarction[55] (Fig. 4-21B).

Real-time ultrasound is currently the most accepted method for establishing the diagnosis of PVL. Several authors have documented four pathologic and sonographic stages in the evolution of PVL.[56-58] The first stage occurs within a few days after an ischemic insult to the neonatal brain and is characterized by coagulation necrosis of the periventricular white matter. Sonograms obtained during this period show an increase in periventricular echoes (Fig. 4-22A).

Fig. 4-19. Ischemic diffuse encephalomalacia. **(A)** Doppler-duplex ultrasound of the brain in a 3-week-old premature infant with cursor applied to middle cerebral artery. Notice absence of diastolic flow with a waveform of a high-resistance appearance. The peak systolic velocities are not uniform, indicating loss of cerebral blood flow autoregulation (a sign of poor prognosis). **(B)** Similar examination in a healthy newborn with cursor on the posterior cerebral artery. Compare the normal arterial flow of rapid systolic upstroke and sharp systolic peak with arterial flow of patient in Fig. A.

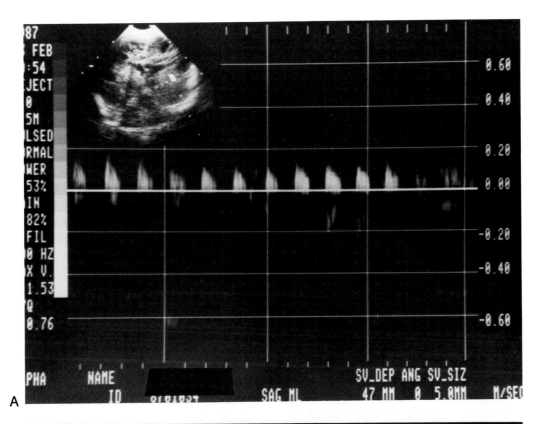

A

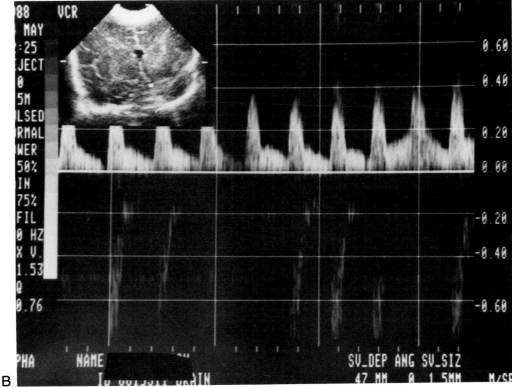

B

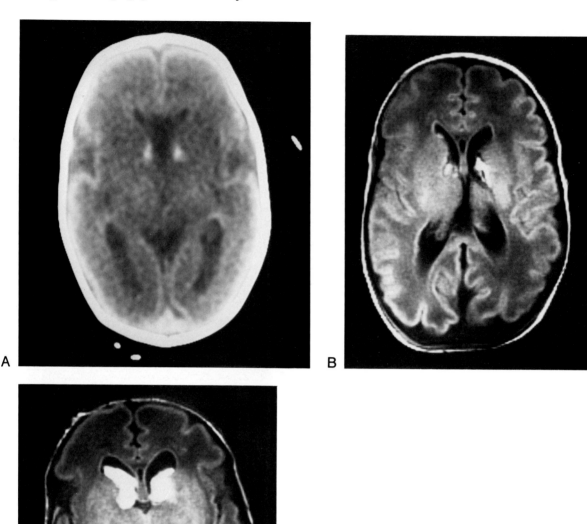

Fig. 4-20. (A) A 28-weeks' gestation premature infant with a subependymal hemorrhage studied by axial noncontrast CT. **(B)** Same patient studied by T$_1$-weighted axial MR image. Both modalities demonstrate well the abnormalities at the head of the caudate nuclei. **(C)** Same patient 10 days later with intraventricular bleeding and acute hydrocephalus on T$_1$-weighted axial MR image.

The second stage follows in 1 to 2 weeks and consists of a proliferation of astrocytes and macrophages. Sonograms obtained during this phase may appear relatively normal (Fig. 4-22B). Approximately 3 to 4 weeks after the ischemic event, fluid-filled cavities form in the periventricular white matter, and sono-grams obtained during this third stage of evolution reveal numerous periventricular cysts (Fig. 4-22C). Over the next several months the cysts gradually decrease in size, and many of them disappear. The white matter becomes much thinner and a dense gliotic scar develops. Sonograms obtained during this final phase

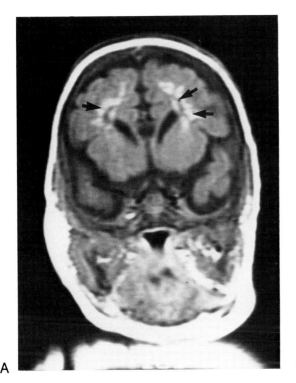
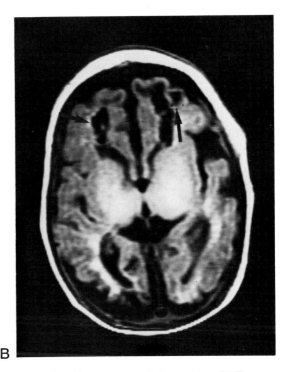

Fig. 4-21. **(A)** Coronal photon density MR image of a 1-month-old premature infant whose PVL was detected by ultrasound at 12 days of life. Notice the increased signal intensity in the subcortical white matter surrounding the periventricular cysts (arrows) as an expression of later hemorrhage into the areas of PVL. **(B)** Axial photon density MR image shows major degree of brain damage with cystic infarctions accompanied by brain atrophy (arrows).

reflect ventriculomegaly and prominent sulci in the areas affected by brain atrophy (Fig. 4-22D). Ultrasound has been and still is the preferred modality in excluding this type of parenchymal changes in the premature brain.

The ability to depict cerebral infarctions will depend on the stage of the development of the brain at the time when the insult occurs; therefore the hydration and myelination states of the cerebral white matter have bearing on the imaging modality used.[35] In preterm infants, the CT appearance of subcortical white matter is less evident than that of full-term infants because of the high brain water and minimal myelin contents. Consequently, edema, acute cerebral infarctions, and PVL may be suboptimally depicted at that stage of brain growth by CT, and better evaluated with MR imaging. Subacute infarctions of the white matter are shown by MR imaging because of the changes in relaxation times for the different metabolites of the extravasated blood.

DEFECTS OF MYELINATION

Decreased or retarded myelination can still be considered within the classification of congenital cerebral malformations when the inductive agent operates during the perinatal period (Table 4-1).

Delayed Patterns of Brain Maturation

Developmentally delayed children will present a neonatal or infantile brain myelination pattern; Malnutrition will have similar effects. Pelizaeus-Merzbacher disease is an idiopathic disease that will produce retarded myelination.

Normal and Abnormal Patterns of Brain Maturation

One of the most important contributions of MR imaging in perinatology has been the demonstration of the dynamic process of brain maturation. The pre-

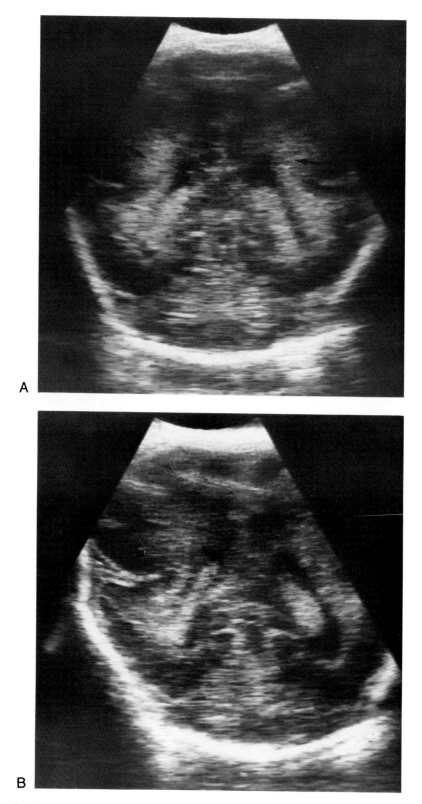

Fig. 4-22. Evolution of PVL as monitored by ultrasound in the same premature infant's brain using coronal scans at the level of the ventricular atria; follow-ups made chronologically at different stages of evolution. **(A)** Periventricular increased echogenicity (arrows). **(B)** Improvement of this abnormality. (*Figure continues.*)

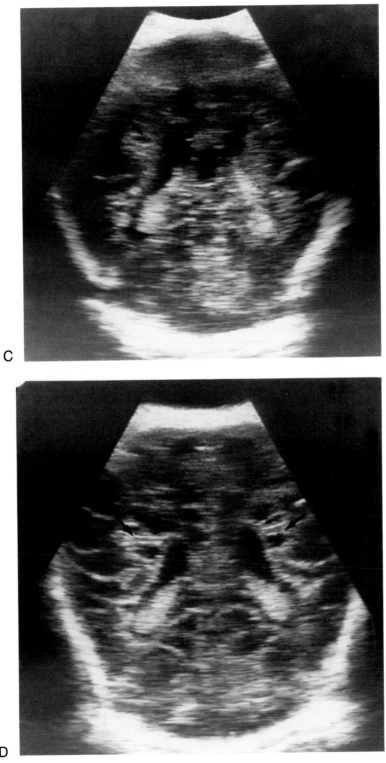

C

D

Fig. 4-22 (*Continued*). (**C**) Fluid-filled cavities appear (arrow). (**D**) Gliotic scars around the periventricular cysts (arrows).

mature brain (28 to 34 gestational weeks) has a very thin and hypodeveloped layer of gray matter and the nonmyelinized and hypointense subcortical white matter predominates on T_1-weighted MR images because of its excessive water content. Only the more central structures are bright, because of the presence of myelin (Fig. 4-23A). Upon reaching 42 weeks of gestation, the brain of the normal newborn will have, using the same T_1-weighted MR imaging sequence (Fig. 4-23B), an appearance similar to that of an adult brain as displayed on a T_2-weighted MR imaging sequence (i.e., gray matter is brighter than white matter) (Fig. 4-24). On T_1-weighted imaging the changeover to the adult pattern is observed at 6 months of age (Fig. 4-25); on T_2-weighted imaging the changeover does not happen until 10 months, reflecting in this manner the development of T_1 contrast prior to T_2 contrast.[59] Myelin, in contrast, spreads from its original forming places (cerebellum, dorsal brain stem, and posterior internal capsules) in the premature brain to the centrum semiovale and corona radiata in the full-term brain. Complete myelination along the subcortical white matter is fully accomplished by 18 months of age when the brain reaches the adult normal MR pattern. Milestones of normal progression in myelination can thus be identified and correlate with age[59] (Fig. 4-26). Gray matter–subcortical white matter differentiation correlates with age regardless of underlying brain insults; myelination will be delayed or altered in certain pathologic conditions. Using T_1- and T_2-weighted MR imaging sequences it is then possible to standardize normal brain patterns according to age.

Although Barkovich and Jackson[59] and other authors have described a detailed table of milestones for the maturation of the brain by MR imaging, we think that five basic patterns should be considered as landmarks that may help differentiate the normally growing brain from the brain with pathology.

Premature Pattern. This pattern is revealed on a T_1-weighted image (Fig. 4-23A) as a thin and poorly developed layer of gray matter, hyperintense relative to the prominent nonmyelinized and water-rich subcortical white matter. Only bright and myelinized central brain structures are visualized.

Neonatal Pattern. This pattern is revealed on a T_1-weighted image (Fig. 4-23B). Subcortical white matter is still less bright than gray matter, and central

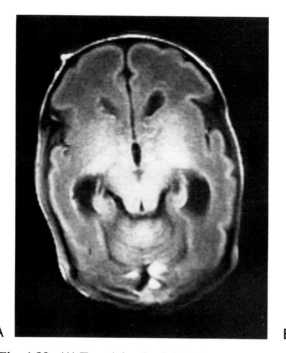
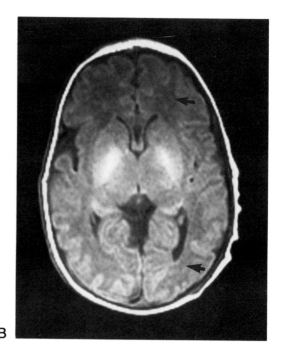

A   B

Fig. 4-23. (A) T_1-weighted axial MR image of a 28-weeks' gestation premature infant with few sulcii formations, myelin in the central nuclei and brain stem only, and prominent, hypointense subcortical white matter. **(B)** Similar image of a full-term newborn with normal development of the gray matter and its interdigitation with the not-yet myelinized subcortical white matter (arrows).

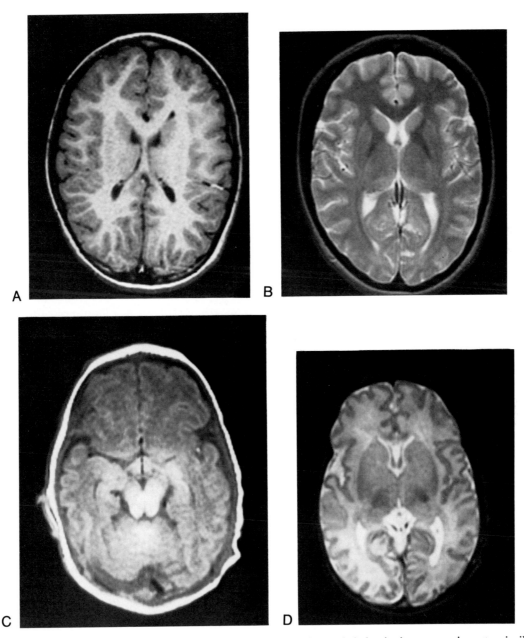

Fig. 4-24. T_1- (**A**) and T_2-weighted (**B**) axial MR scans of an adult brain in comparison to similar images (**C & D**) of a full-term newborn brain. Notice that the gray and subcortical white matter contrast is in an inverse relationship: gray matter is brighter than subcortical white matter in the T_1-weighted image of the infant (**C**) and the T_2-weighted image of the adult (**B**), whereas the reverse is true in the T_2-weighted image of the infant (**D**) and the T_1-weighted image of the adult (**A**).

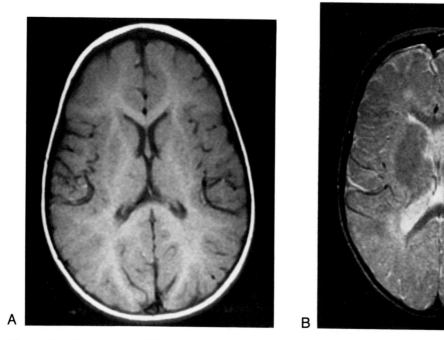

Fig. 4-25. T_1-weighted (**A**) and T_2-weighted (**B**) axial MR images of a 6-month-old infant. The differentiation between subcortical white and gray matter is already present in the T_1-weighted image, but this is not the case in the T_2-weighted image.

white matter is hyperintense. Development of convolutions and sulci on the gray matter is noted, with the appearance of interdigitations along boundaries with the subcortical white matter.

Early Infantile Pattern. First seen at the age of 6 months, on a T_1-weighted image the early infantile pattern reveals white matter with a nearly mature, adult appearance (Fig. 4-25A). On a T_2-weighted image there is isointense brightness of the subcortical white and gray matter and the central white matter is hypointense (Fig. 4-25B).

Late Infantile Pattern. This pattern is revealed on a T_2-weighted image in which gray matter progressively becomes brighter than white matter. It defines the progression of myelination (hypointensity in this sequence) along the limbs of the internal capsule, corpus callosum, and arborization of the subcortical white matter at the frontal horns (Fig. 4-26).

Adult Pattern. At about 18 months of age the adult pattern, in which gray matter is brighter than white matter, is visualized on the T_2-weighted image. The myelination of gray matter parallels the myelination of subcortical white matter in its complete peripheral extension and fine arborization (Fig. 4-27).

DEGENERATIVE DISEASES OF THE DEVELOPING BRAIN

Demyelination

Demyelination may have patchy and diffuse distribution; usually secondary to a severe anoxic-ischemic insult, infection, or certain metabolic diseases, such as subacute necrotizing encephalomyelitis (Leigh's disease) (Fig. 4-28). The MR image will demonstrate irregular areas of destruction in both white and gray matters either in a generalized pattern in cases of metabolic diseases or localized mainly at the watershed regions between the circulations of the brain major arteries (with cystic changes and localized or generalized brain atrophy, subdural hygromas, and asymmetric or symmetric ventricular dilatation) in cerebral infarctions secondary to septic emboli or anoxic-ischemic insults.

Leukodystrophies can be categorized according to loss of white matter. Diffuse loss of white matter in specific areas of the brain is characteristic of Alexander's disease (frontal lobes) (Fig. 4-29), adrenoleukodystrophy (occipital and parietal lobes) (Fig. 4-30),

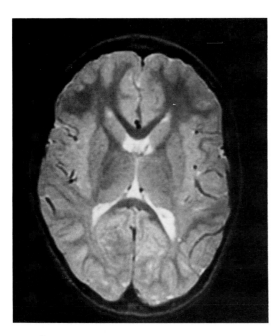

Fig. 4-26. Progression of cerebral myelination at 14 months of age using T_2-weighted MR image. Myelin is present in the central ganglia, outlining clearly the splenium and genu of the corpus callosum, further defining both anterior and posterior limbs of the internal capsule, and progressing into the subcortical white matter of the frontal lobes.

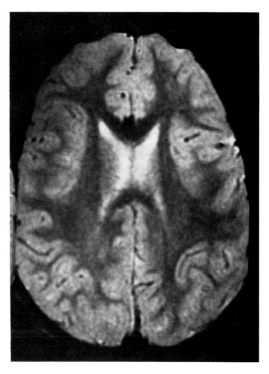

Fig. 4-27. Complete myelinization of the brain at 18 months of age (T_2-weighted MR image).

and Krabbe's disease (thalami). Patchy loss of white matter is noted in progressive multifocal leukoencephalopathy, early multiple sclerosis, and other metabolic diseases such as mucopolisaccharidosis with accompanying pachymeningitis and meningeal cysts.

Cerebrovascular Insults in the Full-Term Infant

The nonhemorrhagic forms of damage that occur in the brain of the term infant in association with birth asphyxia are usually described as "anoxic," "hypoxic," or "ischemic." [60] The use of these names in itself encourages us to think that we are faced with two alternative types of damage. However, the mechanisms leading to cessation of function and ultimate death of an individual cell in the CNS are similar, irrespective of whether the initial event is pure ischemia or pure hypoxia. In either case there will be failure of oxidative phosphorylation with increased anaerobic glycolysis, resulting in a local increase in lactic

acid concentration and decreasing pH until cellular activities are inhibited.[37] The patterns of injury are likely to be determined by the extent to which cerebral blood flow is maintained or enhanced by compensatory vasodilation due to hypoxia and hypercarbia, at what point the blood-brain barrier breaks down in the face of a falling pH, and for how long fetal cardiac function and blood pressure are preserved throughout asphyxial episodes.

In view of these variables it is not surprising that a considerable variety of patterns of damage in the cortex, white matter, basal ganglia, cerebellum, and brain stem have been described following fatal birth asphyxia in the term infant.[61] However, there is now evidence from both animal and human studies that certain patterns of injury occur regularly following particular sequences of events.

Patterns of Damage

There appear to be three distinctive patterns of major damage that merit separate consideration: (1) cerebral edema and cortical necrosis, (2) boundary zone infarctions, and (3) necrosis of thalamic and brain stem nuclei.[61]

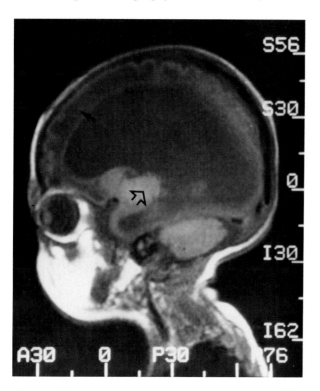

Fig. 4-28. Sagittal T_1-weighted MR image of the brain of a 15-month-old infant with severe subacute necrotizing encephalomyelitis, complicated with hydrocephalus. The subcortical white matter has a low signal intensity, discordant with the child's age (arrow); bright myelin is only seen in the cerebellum and basal ganglia (arrowhead).

Cerebral Edema and Cortical Necrosis. The most frequent finding in the brain of a term infant who dies following birth asphyxia is generalized swelling with flattening of convolutions (Fig. 4-31). The predominantly cortical flow of the more mature brain puts the cortex at increased risk of damage in these conditions. Eventual breakdown of the blood-brain barrier would result in cerebral edema with consequent impairment of cerebral blood flow. This sequence is similar to that recognized in the adult with hypertensive encephalopathy.

Watershed Zone Infarction. This infarction most frequently is of the adult type, involving the cortex and subcortical white matter at the boundaries of the regions supplied by the anterior and middle, and the middle and posterior cerebral arteries (Fig. 4-32A&B). Less commonly in a full-term infant, the infarction may be of the fetal type, involving the peri-ventricular boundary zones (Fig. 4-32C&D). One can see the development of either type of watershed zone lesions during birth asphyxia as a consequence of failing fetal circulation with falling blood pressure.

Necrosis of Thalamic and Brain Stem Nuclei. These lesions are seen consistently in infants who have died following a single acute asphyxial episode or a cardiac arrest.[62] The damage appears to be due to total failure of circulation to the CNS and involves selectively those central (brain stem, thalami) regions that have the greatest metabolic requirements and normally receive the greatest blood flow. Kernicterus may represent another example of damage of these most metabolically active nuclear regions. These become stained more readily by bilirubin in conditions of asphyxia and ischemia.[63]

Thus, it is possible to define three regions of vulnerability of the term infant brain[61]:

1. The region most susceptible to blood-brain barrier breakdown in prolonged hypoxia, hypercarbia, and acidosis is primarily the cerebral cortex.
2. The regions most susceptible to prolonged hypotension are the cortical and white matter boundary zones.
3. The regions most susceptible to impaired metabolism are the thalami and brain stem nuclei.

In most infants who die as a result of birth asphyxia, a mixed pattern of lesions is seen, although there is usually an accentuation of one or other of the above groupings. One of the important contributions of Volpe[61,64] to the clinical study of birth asphyxia is documentation that the clinical state varies in a recognizable manner with the length of time after insult. Initially, the baby presents with hypotonia, depressed spontaneous movements, or frank coma. Seizures are common, usually commencing 8 to 12 hours after birth. From 12 to 24 hours of age there is often a transitory improvement. Although the frequency and severity of seizures may increase, the baby becomes more responsive in the interictal periods. The time period from 24 to 72 hours marks a definite turning point. The infant may continue to show steady improvement, although at a very variable rate. Alternatively, there may be a secondary deterioration with increasing stupor, signs of increased intracranial pressure, brain stem compression, and finally respiratory arrest. Most deaths directly attributed to birth asphyxia occur during the second or third day.

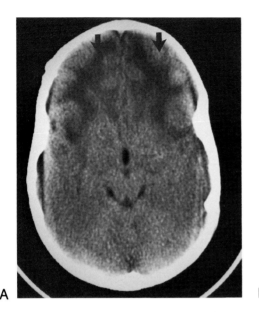 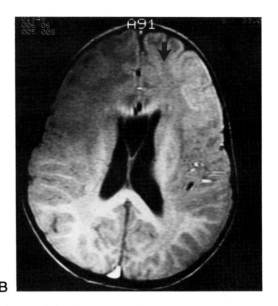

Fig. 4-29. Axial CT scan **(A)** and T_1-weighted MR image **(B)** of the brain of a child with Alexander's disease. Notice the obvious lack of myelin in the frontal regions on both modalities (arrows).

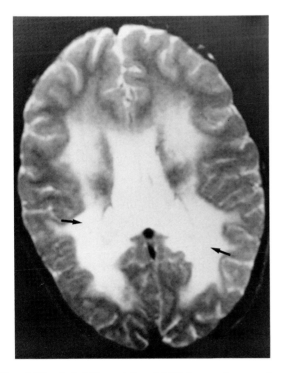

Fig. 4-30. Axial T_2-weighted MR image in a patient with proven adrenoleukodystrophy shows symmetrically increased signal intensity from the occipitoparietal regions extending anteriorly (arrows). These findings in a young child are characteristic of this disease.

Prevention is the best approach to birth asphyxia; thus consideration of the underlying pathophysiology allows a rational prevention plan to be developed. The single most important requirement relates to meticulous supportive care. Cerebral edema is to be expected in all severe cases as discussed above. Myocardial damage is a common result of severe asphyxia and may lead to congestive cardiac failure. If unrecognized, this can accentuate brain injury by further decreasing cerebral perfusion. In view of this, fluid overload must be avoided, particularly until adequate renal function is assured.

Seizures must be treated because convulsive activity has been shown to increase cerebral metabolic rate. Neonatalogists now favor phenobarbital as the drug of first choice because it has been shown to be effective and safe and has the additional benefit of directly decreasing cerebral metabolic requirements.

Imaging of Cerebrovascular Insults

The appearance of the neonatal brain on CT scans has been the subject of much controversy because it is thought that CT is not entirely reliable in depicting parenchymal abnormalities.[65,66] Hypodense white matter has been attributed to PVL and hypoglycemic or hypoxic-ischemic brain injury.[67-69] In some cases the hypodensity resolves without explanation. Other

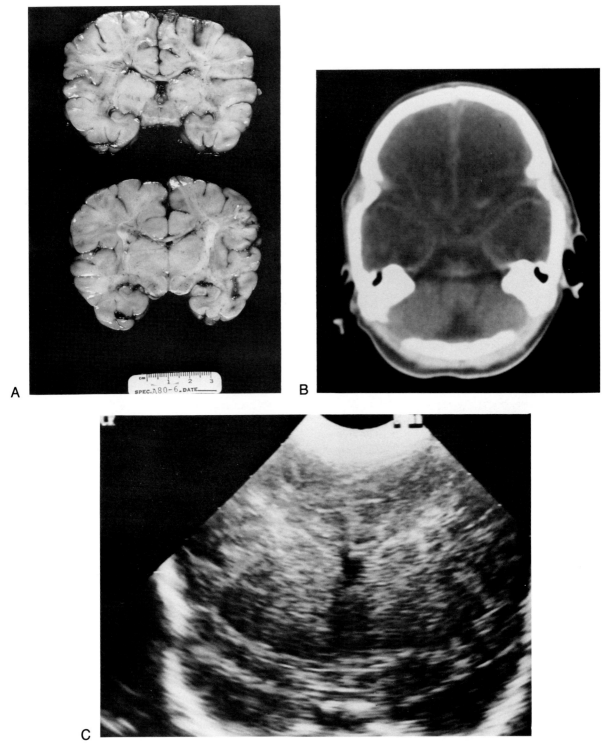

Fig. 4-31. Cerebral edema in asphyxia neonatorum. **(A)** Full-term neonatal brain specimen in coronal slices, showing flattening of cerebral convolutions and narrowing, by swollen and compression effect, of the lateral ventricles. **(B)** Contrast-enhanced axial CT scan of a newborn with a similar clinical condition. Note the diffuse decrease cerebral density, with lack of visualization of the sulci or lateral ventricles; only the cerebellum retains a fair parenchymal perfusion. **(C)** Coronal ultrasound scan of the brain of the infant in Fig. B demonstrating a diffuse increased echogenicity due to the presence of edema.

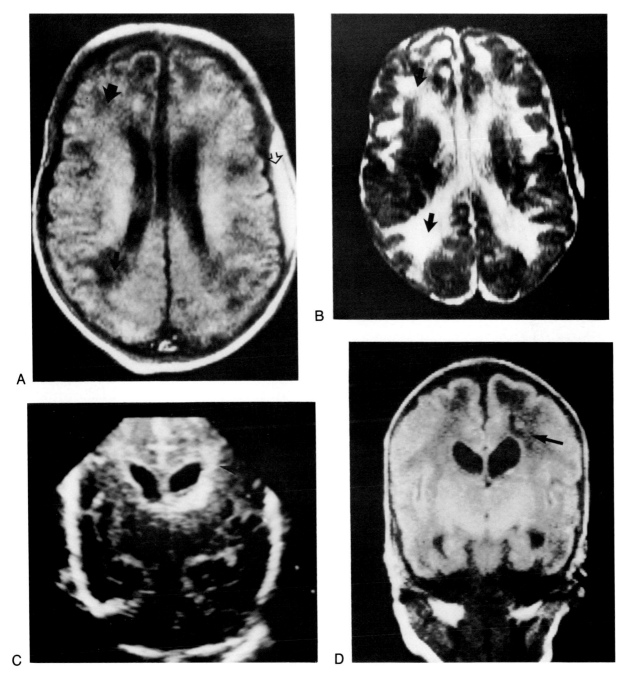

Fig. 4-32. T₁-weighted **(A)** and T₂-weighted **(B)** axial MR images of a neonatal brain with subacute and extensive anoxic-ischemic insult. The pattern of tissue damage (decreased signal intensity on T₁-weighted image and increased signal in T₂-weighted image) follows the adult type of cerebral infarctions at the watershed areas between the left superior and middle and posterior cerebral arteries (arrows). Notice that the T₂-weighted image has better delination of the stroke extent. An associated right-sided subdural hematoma is also present (open arrow). **(C & D)** Brain of a 29-weeks' gestation premature infant with periventricular infarction and subependymal bleeding seen by coronal ultrasound scan **(A)** and by coronal T₁-weighted MR image **(D).** Notice the areas of fresh ischemia in the subcortical white matter of the frontal horn demonstrated by decreased MR signal intensity (arrow); they are more extensive and consequently more accurately depicted than by the ultrasound scan, on which the abnormal areas are documented by increased periventricular echogenicity (arrow). Notice, however, that the subependymal bleeding is still better outlined by ultrasound scan.

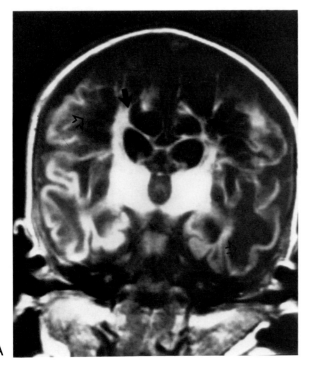
A

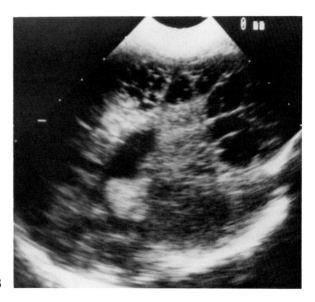
B

Fig. 4-33. (A) Coronal T_1-weighted MR image of a full-term infant suffering from severe multicystic encephalomalacia. Notice the delayed and altered myelination, diffuse low-signal infarctions (open arrows), periventricular and subcortical cysts (arrows), and sulcal effacement. (B) Right parasagittal cerebral ultrasound scan demonstrates similar but less distinct changes.

studies have noted that hypodense white matter is normal in premature infants.[66] However, marked hypodensity in a full-term infant has a high correlation with poor neurologic outcome. A frequently given explanation for the decreasing hypodensity of white matter in the neonatal period is the "myelination process." This explanation is by necessity vague because CT does not directly depict myelin.[37]

CT scanning, real-time ultrasound, and MR imaging demonstrate cerebral edema in the brain of the full-term infant by (respectively) decreased brain density, increased echogenicity, and decreased signal intensity on T_1-weighted images with accompanying compression of the ventricles (Fig. 4-31). The response of the infant to treatment may be monitored with Doppler-duplex sonography. In the chronic phase of the event, cerebral atrophy with ventricular dilation or atrophy with widened sulci may be found at follow-up ultrasound, with CT, or MR scans of infants with perinatal asphyxia.

In multicystic encephalomalacia, multiple cysts in the greater part of the two cerebral hemispheres

(mainly at the external white matter and the internal cortical layers) are seen. The territories of the anterior and medial cerebral arteries are most commonly involved and the central brain structures are spared (Fig. 4-33).

MR imaging is very capable of depicting infarcts in the brain of the full-term neonate.[37] The prenatal brain water content has decreased and edema becomes more distinct. The higher intensity of white matter on T_1-weighted images provides good contrast to highlight the low signal of infarcts. The shift of infarct location from the periventricular white matter to the cortical region also makes edema easier to appreciate. A mass effect is manifested as spread of the gyri and sulcal effacement. Normal white matter can be separated from edematous infarcted white matter on T_1-weighted images, but heavily T_2-weighted images depict more subtle lesions. (Fig. 4-32A&B). The typical infarction on MR images corresponds to low signal areas in the cortex with decreased, delayed, or abnormal subcortical myelination. In later follow-up studies, cortical thinning with persistent hypo-

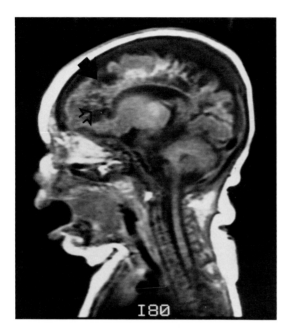

Fig. 4-34. Midsagittal T_1-weighted MR image of a 5-week-old full-term neonate suffering from initial, severe birth asphyxia. Notice brain atrophy and cerebral infarctions, represented by cortical thinning, and persistent hypodense and demyelinated subcortical white matter areas (arrow), along with strands of glial tissues (arrowhead).

dense and demyelinated subcortical white matter areas can be seen, along with glial strands traversing these hypodense areas, which are characteristically located in the frontal and parietal watershed regions (Fig. 4-34). Accompanying cystic changes can also be present. These infarcts are more difficult to see on CT, especially when only nonenhanced technique is used. In general, the older the infant and the lower the brain water content, the easier it becomes to see these lesions on MR imaging as well as on CT.

Infections

Neonatal meningitis is the term used for those cases of meningitis with onset during the first month of life; the incidence may vary according to geographic distribution but overall it reaches 0.4 percent of newborns.[70] It is more common in premature and other high-risk neonates, after complicated deliveries, or in infected mothers. *Escherichia coli, Proteus mirabilis, Klebsiella, Pseudomonas,* and streptococcus B are the most frequent pathogens. The inflammatory meningeal exudate during the first days after the

onset gives way to progressive fibroblast proliferation and strands of collagen by the second week, resulting in communicating hydrocephalus and obstruction of the basal cisterns (Fig. 4-35). Cerebral infarctions of the underlying brain with irregular distributions are seen in 30 percent of cases, and they may lead to abcess formation. CT with and without contrast enhancement and MR imaging are the diagnostic methods of choice.

Herpes simplex viral infection in the neonatal period may result in visceral, cutaneous, and encephalitic manifestations, which can occur together or in isolation. The disseminated viral infection results in lethargy, poor feeding, apnea, and seizures during the first days after birth. The mucocutaneous lesions may be absent and the diagnosis may be masked in these very important first few days when an adequate antiviral treatment should be started. CT has been useful in demonstrating areas of decreased density corresponding to cerebral edema, which may have prolonged contrast enhancement (Fig. 4-36). Porencephaly or localized brain atrophy may appear relatively fast in these affected areas.

BIRTH TRAUMA

Delivery by forceps or a spontaneous difficult passage through the vaginal canal may produce cranial molding (a temporary abnormality without clinical significance), skull fractures (important to investigate if depressed), cephalohematomas, and subdural hematomas. Epidural hematomas are uncommon in the newborn. If the localized swelling of the head is otherwise asymptomatic, conventional radiographs may be all that is necessary to confirm the clinical impression. In cephalohematomas the subperiosteal hemorrhage will limit the swelling to the suture edges of the underlying cranial bone; in caput succedaneum the swelling will cross the sutures. Subdural hematoma and/or intracerebral hemorrhage can be associated with skull injury, and depending upon the seriousness of the birth trauma they may lead to chronic subdural hygromas (Fig. 4-37) and cerebral atrophy with cerebral palsy. The differential diagnosis from an old anoxic-ischemic perinatal insult is almost impossible when the patient's neurologic problems are brought to clinical attention later during infancy and no clear abnormal perinatal history can be elucidated.

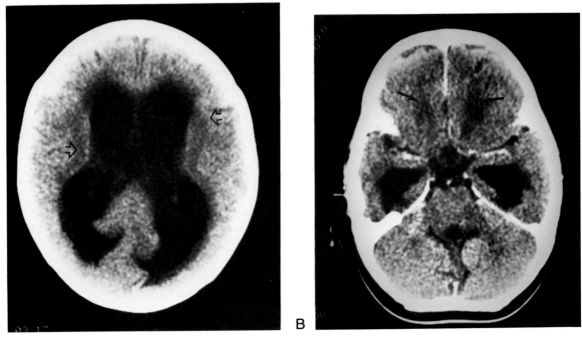

Fig. 4-35. Contrast-enhanced axial brain CT at two different levels **(A & B)** showing neonatal meningitis with communicating hydrocephalus. Notice abnormal parenchymal densities (arrows) and periventricular halo (open arrows) of edema secondary to acute ventricular obstruction.

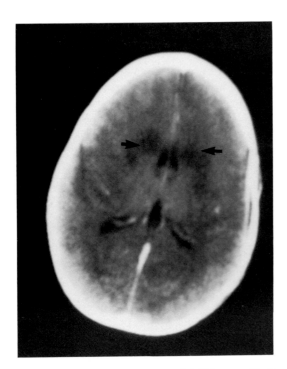

Fig. 4-36. Contrast-enhanced axial CT scan of infant with acute neonatal herpes encephalitis. Notice diffuse cerebral edema and infarction in the basal ganglia (arrows).

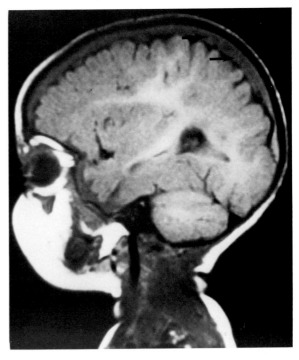

Fig. 4-37. T$_1$-weighted axial cerebral MR image of diffuse subdural hygroma and associated cerebral atrophy in a 10-month-old infant. Notice the low signal intensity of the pericerebral old fluid collection and the veins crossing through the subdural space (arrows).

REFERENCES

1. Behrman RE, Vaughn DC, Nelson WE: Nelson Textbook of Pediatrics. 13th Ed. WB Saunders Company, Philadelphia, 1987
2. Becerra JE et al: Diabetes mellitus during pregnancy and the risks for specific birth defects. Pediatrics 85:1, 1990
3. Wiggleworth JS, Pape KE: An integrated model for hemorrhage and ischaemic lesions in the newborn brain. Early Hum Dev 2:179, 1978
4. van der Knaap MS, Valk J: Classification of congenital abnormalities of the CNS. AJNR 9:315, 1988
5. Volpe JJ: Neurology of the Newborn: Major Problems in Clinical Pediatrics. Vol 22. 2nd Ed. WB Saunders, Philadelphia, 1987
6. Poe LB, Coleman LL, Mahmud F: Congenital central nervous system anomalies. Radiol Clin North Am 9(5), 1989
7. Faerber EN: Cranial Computed Tomography in Infants and Children. JB Lippincott, Philadelphia, 1986
8. Oelberg DG, Dominguez R, Hebert AA: Neurocristopathy syndrome: review of four cases. Pediatr Dermatol 7:87, 1990
9. Lammer EJ, Chen DT, et al: Retinoic acid embryopathy. N Engl J Med 313:837, 1985
10. Lieuw Kie Song SH, Been W, Van Limborgh J: Developmental deficiencies of the upper facial skeleton due to partial elimination of mesencephalic neural crest cells in the chick embryo. Acta Morphol Neerl Scand 21:253, 1983
11. Brent RLP: Radiation teratogenesis. Teratology 21:281, 1980
12. Naidich TP, Zimmerman RA: Common congenital malformations of the brain. In Brant-Zawodki M, Normal D (eds): Magnetic Resonance Imaging of the Central Nervous System. Raven Press, New York, 1987
13. Caviness VS: The Chiari malformations of the posterior fossa and their relationship hydrocephalus. Dev Med Child Neurol 18:103, 1976
14. Hardwood-Nash DC, Fitz CR: Neuroradiology in Infants and Children. CV Mosby Co, St. Louis, 1976
15. Naidich TP, Radkowski MA, Bernstein RA et al: Congenital malformation of the posterior fossa. In Taveras JM, Ferucci JT (eds): Radiology. JB Lippincott, Philadelphia, 1986
16. Fitz CR: Holoprosencephaly and related entities. Neuroradiology 25:225, 1983
17. Hale BB, Rice P: Septooptic dysplasia; clinical and embryological aspects. Dev Med Child Neurol 16:812, 1974
18. Barkovich AJ, Norman D: Absence of the septum pelucidum: a useful sign in the diagnosis of congenital brain malformations. AJNR 9:1107, 1988
19. Byrd S, Naidich T: Common congenital brain anomalies. Radiol Clin North Am 26:755, 1988
20. Barkovich AJ: Pediatric Neuroimaging: Contemporary Neuroimaging. Vol 1. Raven Press, New York, 1990
21. Norman MG, Becker LE: Cerebral damage in neonates resulting from arteriovenous malformation of the vein of Galen. J Neurol Neurosurg Psychiatry 37:252, 1974
22. Saliba E, Santini J et al: Retentissement cardiaque et cerebral de l'aneurysme de l'ampoule de galien. Neurochirurgie 33:296, 1987
23. Milhoret TH: Hydrocephalus and the Cerebrospinal Fluid. Williams & Wilkins, Baltimore, 1972
24. Nabors MW, Pait TG, Byrd E et al: Updated assessment and current classification of spinal meningeal cysts. J Neurosurg 68:366, 1988
25. Peterman AF, Hayles AB, Dockerty MB et al: Encephalotrigeminal angiomatosis (Sturge-Weber disease): clinical study of 35 cases. JAMA 167:2169, 1958
26. Hurwitz S, Braverman IM: White spots in tuberous sclerosis. J Pediatr 77:587, 1970
27. Zimmerman RA, Bilaniuk LT, Grossman RI: CT in migratory disorders of human brain development. Neuroradiology 25:257, 1983
28. Barth PG: Disorders of neural migration. Can J Neurol Sci 14:1, 1987
29. Yakovlev PI, Wadsworth RC: Schizencephalies. A study of the congenital clefts in the cerebral mantle. II Clefts with hydrocephalus and lips separated. J Neuropathol Exp Neurol 5:169, 1946
30. Barkovich J, Norman D: MR Imaging of schizencephaly. AJR 150:1391, 1988
31. Spats H: Über die Vorgänge nach experimentaler Rückenmarchdurchtrennung mit besouderer Berücksichtigung der Untershiede der Reaktionsweise des reifen und unreifen gewebes nebsdt Beziehungen zur menschlichen. Pathologie (Porencephalie und Syringomyelie) Nissl Alzheimer Histolog Histopath Arb 49-367, 1921
32. Lange-Coosak H: Die Hydranencephalie (Blasenhiorn) als Sonderform der Grosshirnlosigkeit. Arch Psychiatr Nervenker 117:595, 1944
33. Dekaban A: Large defects in cerebral hemispheres associated with cortical dysgenesis. J Neuropathol Exp Neurol 24:5121, 1965
34. Diebler C, Dulac O: Pediatric Neurology and Neuroradiology: Cerebral and Cranial Diseases. p.186, Springer-Verlag, New York, 1986
35. Allan W, Volpe J: Periventricular intraventricular hemorrhage. Pediatr Clin North Am 36:47, 1986
36. Krishnamoorthy RS, Fernandez RA, Moiusse KI et al: Evaluation of neonatal intracranial hemorrhage by CT. Pediatrics 59:165, 1977
37. McArdle D, Richardson CJ et al: Abnormalities of

the neonatal brain: MR imaging. Radiology 163:395, 1987

38. Papile L, Burstein G, Burstein R et al: Incidence and evaluation of subependymal hemorrhage: a study of infants with birth weights less than 1500gr. J Pediatr 92:529, 1978

39. Pape K: Etiology and pathogenesis of intraventricular hemorrhage in newborns. Pediatrics 84:382, 1989

40. Hambleton G, Wigglesworth JS: Origin of intraventricular hemorrhage in the preterm infant. Arch Dis Child 51:651, 1976

41. Lou CL, Lassen NA, Frills-Hansen B: Impaired autoregulation of cerebral blood flow in the distressed. J Pediatr 9:118, 1979

42. Costeloe K, Rolfe P: Techniques for studying cerebral perfusion in the newborn. In Pape KE, Wigglesworth JS (eds): Perinatal Brain Lesions. Blackwell Scientific Publications, London, 1989

43. Grant EG, White EM, Schellinger D et al: Cranial duplex sonography of the infant. Radiology 163:177, 1987

44. Periman JM: Neonatal cerebral blood flow velocity measurement. Clin Perinatol 12:179, 1985

45. Yordy M, Harrigan WC: Cerebral perfusion pressure in the high-risk premature infant. Pediatr Neurosci 12:226, 1985

46. Deeg KH: Colour flow imaging of the great intracranial arteries in infants. Neuroradiology 31:40, 1989

47. Deeg KH, Rupprecht T, Zeilinger G: Dopplersonographic classification of brain edema in infants. Pediatr Radiol 20:509, 1990

48. Ben-Ami T, Yousefzadeh D, Backus M et al: Lenticulostriate vasculopathy in infants with infections of the central nervous system: sonographic and Doppler findings. Pediatr Radiol 20:575, 1990

49. Mitchell DG, Merton DA, Mirsky PJ, Needleman L: Circle of Willis in newborns: color doppler imaging of 53 healthy full-term infants. Radiology 172:201, 1989

50. Rumack C, Johnson M: Neonatal brain scanning: choosing between modalities. Diagn Imag 00:28, 1983

51. Wilson D, Steiner R: Periventricular leukomalacia: evaluation with MR imaging. Radiology 160:507, 1986

52. Levene MI, Wigglesworth JS, Dubowitz V: Hemorrhagic periventricular leukomalacia in the neonate: a real-time ultrasound study. Pediatrics 71:794, 1983

53. Bowerman RA, Donn SM, DiPietro MA et al: Periventricular leukomalacia in the preterm newborn infant: sonographic and clinical features. Radiology 151:383, 1984

54. Armstrong D, Norman MG: Periventricular leukomalacia in neonates: complications and sequelae. Arch Dis Child 49:367, 1974

55. Hill AG, Melson L et al: Hemorrhagic periventricular leukomalacia: diagnosis by real time ultrasound and correlation with autopsy findings. Pediatrics 69:282, 1982

56. De Ruck J, Chatta AS, Richardson EP: Pathogenesis and evolution of periventricular leukomalacia in infancy. Arch Neurol 27:229, 1972

57. Shuman RM, Selednik LJ: Periventricular leukomalacia. Arch Neurol 37:231, 1980

58. Fawer CL, Calame A, Perentes E, Anderegg A: Periventricular leukomalacia: a correlation study between real-time ultrasound and autopsy findings. Neuroradiology 27:292, 1985

59. Barkovich JA, Jackson DE: MRI assessment of normal and abnormal brain myelination. MRI Decisions, May/June: 17, 1989

60. Volpe JJ: Perinatal hypoxic-ischemic brain injury. Pediatr Clin North Am 23:383, 1976

61. Volpe JJ: Neurological disorders. In Avery GB (ed): Neonatology: Pathophysiology and Management of the Newborn. JB Lippincott, Philadelphia, 1975

62. Leech RW: Anoxic-ischemic encephalopathy in the human neonatal period: the significance of brain stem involvement. Arch Neurol 34:109, 1977

63. Lucey JF, Hibbard E, Behrman RE et al: Kernicterus in asphyxiated newborn rhesus monkeys. Exp Neurol 9:43, 1964

64. Volpe JJ: Observing the infant in the early hours after asphyxia. In Gluck L (ed): Intrauterine Asphyxia and the Developing Fetal Brain. Year Book Medical Publishers, London, 1978

65. Magilner AD, Wertheimer IS: Preliminary results of a computed tomography study of neonatal brain hypoxia-ischemia. J Comput Assist Tomogr 4:457, 1980

66. Flodmark O, Becker LE, Harwood-Nash DC et al: Correlation between computed tomography and autopsy in premature and full-term neonates that have suffered perinatal asphyxia. Radiology 137:93, 1980

67. Di Chiro G, Arimitsu T, Pellock JM et al: Periventricular leukomalacia related to neonatal anoxia: recognition by computed tomography. J Comput Assist Tomogr 2:352, 1978

68. Hirabayashi S, Ketahara T, Hishida T: Computed tomography in perinatal hypoxic and hypoglycemic encephalopathy with emphasis on follow-up studies. J Comput Assist Tomogr 4:451, 1980

69. Flodmark O, Fitz CR, Harwood-Nash DC: CT diagnosis and short-term prognosis of intracranial hemorrhage and hypoxic-ischemic brain damage in neonates. J Comput Assist Tomogr 4:775, 1980

70. Diebler C, Dulac O: Pediatric Neurology and Neuroradiology: Cerebral and Cranial Disease. p. 139. Springer Verlag, New York, 1986

Radiology of the Premature Infant Chest

Rodrigo Dominguez

5

The care of premature and high-risk neonates has become an expensive and sophisticated part of medicine. It has evolved also into another intensive care subspecialty and it is mostly found in large, tertiary care hospitals where a team of pediatric neonatologists works hand-in-hand with highly skilled pediatric nurses, respiratory therapists, and round-the-clock laboratory and other ancillary services, attended by specialists such as pediatric surgeons, ophthalmologists, and radiologists. Generally, this special intensive care suite is near the delivery room so that immediate appropriate management of the newborn at high risk can be practiced. Practically every patient in an intensive care unit, including the neonatology unit, is in critical condition and requires mechanical ventilation. These patients also may have one or more lines, catheters, or tubes inserted and therefore need daily routine portable chest and abdominal radiographs for adjustment of these life-sustaining devices and for assessment of their possible complications, as well as of the frequent changes these patients can in consequence experience in their lungs and abdominal organs (Fig. 5-1). Sudden deterioration in the clinical condition of a patient may require additional radiographs.

The pulmonary pathology found in the premature neonate is the result of either an acute or a chronic insult to immature lungs. Prematurity is associated with a deficit in alveolar surfactant and increased pulmonary vascular permeability, leading to early interstitial edema, and facilitating in this manner pulmonary hypoxia.[1] Assisted ventilatory support and oxygen administration can then promote superimposed pulmonary oxygen toxicity, barotrauma, adult respiratory distress syndrome, and chronic lung changes. The difficult adjustment of IV fluids and hyperalimentation in the premature body promotes further pulmonary edema and worsening of the hypoxic status. These factors will favor the patency or recanalization of the ductus arteriosus with an increasing amount of additional blood volume loaded into the lungs.

All of this will prolong the need for assisted ventilatory support and oxygen administration, which may lead into chronic lung disease or what is called in neonatology bronchopulmonary dysplasia (BPD). The radiologic interpretation of these subtle and easily changeable pulmonary findings is the core of the present chapter.

With the abnormal pattern of wealth distribution in American society, with its poor prenatal care in many instances, and with the paradoxical improvements in medical and research breakthroughs, the population of high-risk prematures in the neonatal intensive care unit (NICU) has evolved. In consequence, nowadays we deal mostly with extremely premature and very low-birthweight infants or infants small for their gestational age, or those cases of newborns with intrauterine growth retardation. Most of these "micro-premies" are under 1500 g birthweight and usually present pulmonary surfactant deficiency after birth or hyaline membrane disease (HMD), but some do not.

Premature infants without pulmonary surfactant deficiency or HMD can present a normal or a grayish pulmonary appearance on a chest radiograph de-

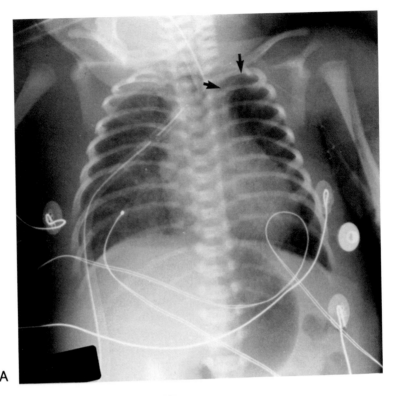

A

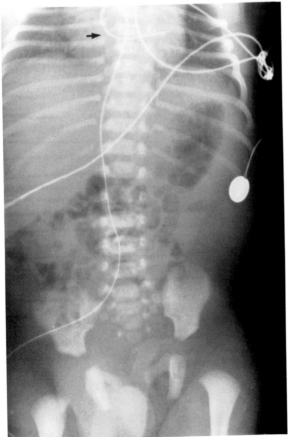

B

Fig. 5-1. **(A)** Central venous line (CVL) placed in the left arm; the tip of the line runs along the left side of the mediastinum (arrows). This infant has a right-sided aortic arch, the mirror image of normal anatomy; the CVL was properly placed at the superior vena cava. **(B)** Placement of an umbilical venous line. The tip of the line has curled inside the right atrium and passed across the foramen ovale into the left atrial chamber (arrow). *(Figure continues.)*

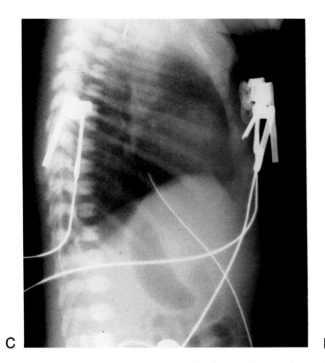
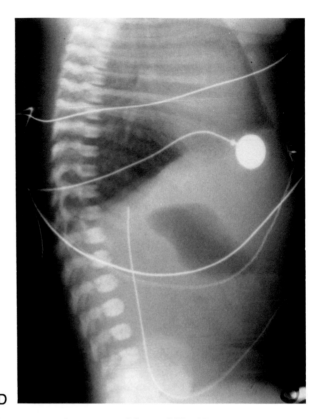

C D

Fig. 5-1 *(Continued).* **(C&D)** When in doubt about the correct placement of the umbilical line, a lateral projection helps to establish its venous **(C)** or arterial **(D)** anatomic location.

pending on the degree of lung inflation. These small-for-gestational-age premature infants may have been stressed sufficiently in utero to stimulate endogenous steroid production, or may have received steroids through maternal administration a few days before delivery, so that their lungs acquired functional, but not yet anatomic, maturity.[2] Still other premature infants, for unknown reasons or after artificial surfactant administration, have enough surfactant to produce radiographically clear lungs, even though they are anatomically immature[3] (Fig. 5-2A). This is not usually a problem per se since the functional activity of surfactant is already present.[4] Both surfactant activity and sufficient alveolar surface area are necessary for the available capillary beds to provide adequate gas exchange. Adequate size of the alveoli and the required alveolus-capillary distance for proper oxygen diffusion set the limits of viability, which can approach 500 g of birthweight or approximately 23 to 26 weeks of gestational age.[5-7] Pathologically, since there is proportionally more interstitial tissue than air spaces as a result of incomplete alveolar growth, the chest radiograph will demon-

strate a set of subtle pulmonary findings ranging from gray, hazy lungs to a mild granularity in the background of the lung fields (sometimes misdiagnosed as HMD) (Fig. 5-2A); a prominent hilar configuration with increased central interstitial markings suggesting wetness, congestion, or early edema may sometimes be present (Fig. 5-2C) or the lung fields may even be completely clear.[3] In any case, these lungs have normal air capacity and lack other radiographic criteria suggestive of pulmonary pathology (Fig. 5-2A&B).

These findings are distinct from the air bronchograms and microatelectatic densities seen in HMD (Fig. 5-2D), or the predominantly interstitial and fluffy perihilar butterfly configuration and unsharp intrapulmonary vascular structures that are the most common hallmarks of vascular congestion with pulmonary edema due to capillary damage seen in older premature infants suffering from patent ductus arteriosus (PDA) (Fig. 5-8C) and in early stages of BPD.[8] Alveolar disease (aspiration, hemorrhage, or pneumonitis) usually presents with irregularly distributed infiltrates accompanied by lung hyperinflation (Fig. 5-3A).

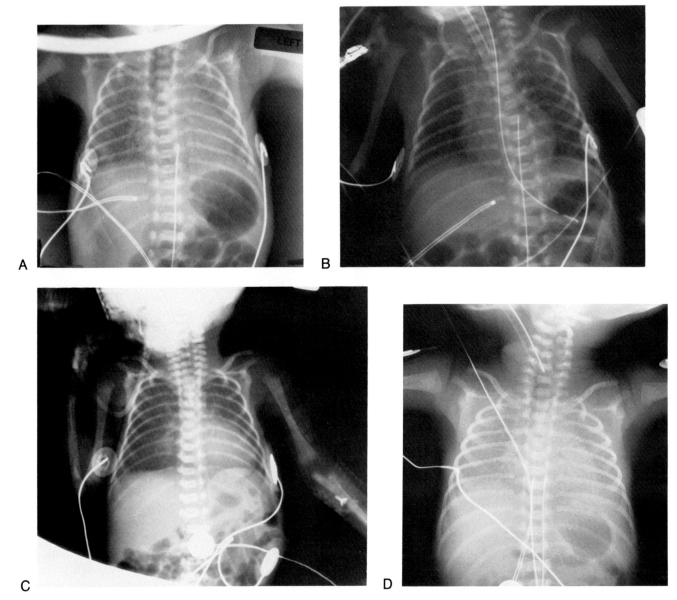

Fig. 5-2. **(A)** Anatomic pulmonary immaturity in a 27 weeks' gestation premature newborn at 1 day of life with no respiratory distress, fair lung inflation, a central air bronchogram (this is a normal finding in neonatology because of the increased translucency of the mediastinal structures at this age), and overall grayness along the pulmonary fields. **(B)** Same infant 24 hours later, after endotracheal intubation for apnea spells. Notice the better inflation of the lungs, providing a darker or normal pulmonary appearance. **(C)** Same infant at 1 week of age, no longer intubated. Notice the haziness at the hilar regions suggestive of some wetness and typical of the increased vascular permeability of the lungs at this premature stage. **(D)** *Hyaline membrane disease* in another premature infant of similar gestational age for purposes of comparison with the anatomically immature lungs of the infant in Figure A, B, and C. Notice the decreased pulmonary inflation, the typical granularity of the lung fields, and the extension toward the periphery of the air bronchograms.

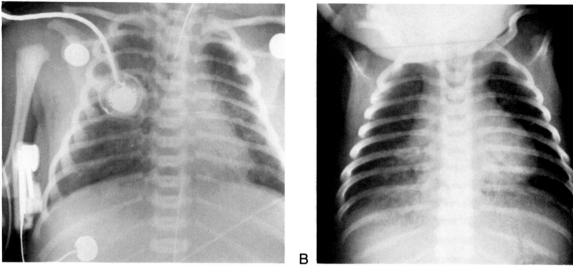

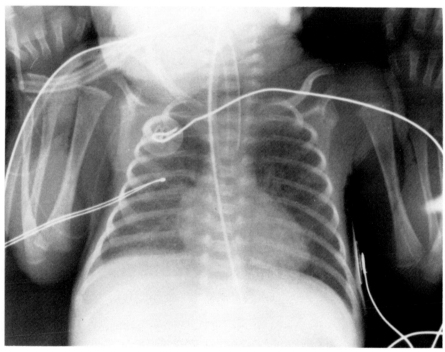

Fig. 5-3. (A) Alveolar-interstitial mixed pattern in a premature newborn infant suffering from *Esche-richia coli* sepsis. Notice the irregular distribution of the abnormalities (which have also an interstitial streaky and/or reticular mixed appearance) and the increased pulmonary inflation. **(B)** Interstitial pattern in a premature newborn who developed cardiopulmonary failure at 4 days of life; cardiac ultrasound demonstrated the presence of total anomalous venous return below the diaphragm. **(C)** Compare with a 26 weeks' gestation premature infant with clear, anatomically immature lungs at 5 days of life, but intubated at low pressures. The grayness of the lungs can be attributed to the decreased degree of pulmonary inflation. *(Figure continues.)*

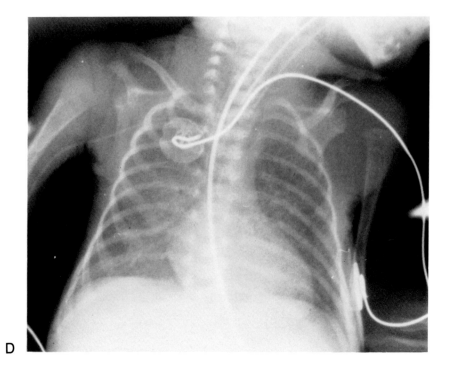

D

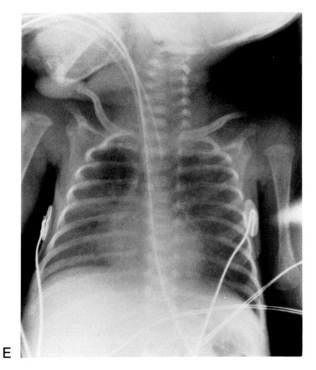

E

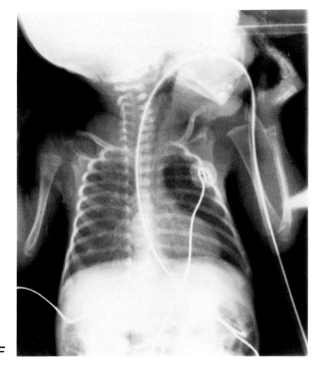

F

Fig. 5-3 *(Continued).* **(D)** Same infant as in Figure C 2 days later. Notice the lungs becoming grayer and the increasing fuzziness of the hilar structures. The infant has had an excessive administration of fluids during the previous day, and the pulmonary findings probably represent mild pulmonary edema. **(E)** Same patient at 10 days of life; the infant displays perihilar subsegmental atelectasis (notice the fluffy perihilar contours) caused by persistant endotracheal intubation. **(F)** After 2 weeks of intermittant endotracheal intubation, the infant is now finally extubated and his lungs are clear.

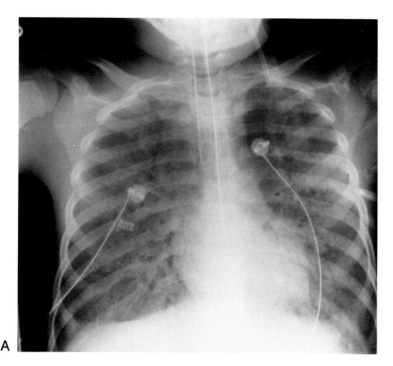

A

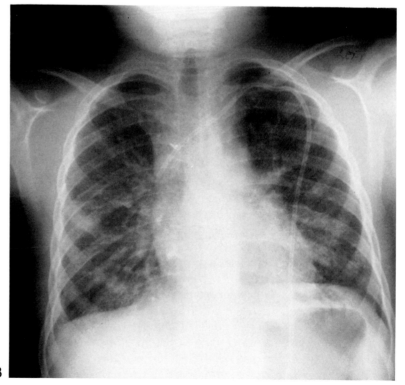

B

Fig. 5-4. **(A)** A 7-year-old child with adult respiratory distress syndrome after severe aspirative pneumonitis. Notice the complex, diffuse alveolar and interstitial pattern that ARDS adopts in the lungs of this particular patient. **(B)** Same child as in Figure A 4 months later; his protracted recovery with the need of significant oxygen administration evolved into residual pulmonary fibrosis (as confirmed by the lung biopsy), with mild interstitial pulmonary markings seen in the chest radiograph. *(Figure continues.)*

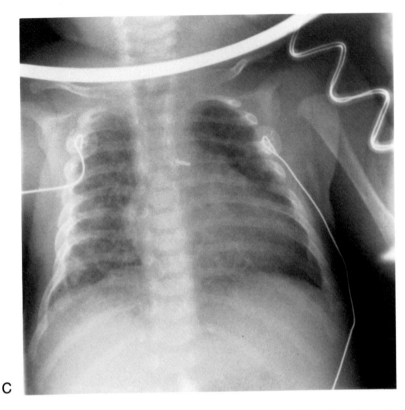

C

Fig. 5-4 *(Continued).* **(C)** A 3-month-old premature infant suffering from *bronchopulmonary dysplasia;* compare this image with that in Figure B. Notice the similarities of chronic fibrosis in the infant and in the older child.

The roentgenographic descriptions of pulmonary pathology in adults do not apply to neonates in the same manner. The primary effect of any pulmonary insult in infancy takes place preferentially on the smaller airways, not on the alveoli. The conductance (the reciprocal of resistance) of the peripheral airways is equal at this early age to that of the central airways, and in consequence any edema, mucus, or inflammatory debris and effects of prolonged intubation can markedly narrow or occlude bronchioles, causing air trapping with hyperinflation and subsegmental atelectasis. The collateral pathway of ventilation (the pores of Kohn and canals of Lambert) are less developed, thus allowing easy formation of atelectasis, and there are also relatively more mucous glands in the infant's airways, promoting plugging of secretions and uneven pulmonary aeration. These special anatomic conditions influence not only the degree of pulmonary inflation but also the roentgenographic appearance of alveolar or interstitial changes, which often are mixed and difficult to separate or categorize[9] (Fig. 5-3).

The premature infant in significant respiratory distress will routinely have aspiration of the airway, intubation, and mechanical ventilation soon after birth. Under these circumstances, the interpretation of the radiographic features should take into account iatrogenic factors that can improve or change the course of these neonatal pulmonary insults: adult respiratory distress syndrome (ARDS), oxygen toxicity, barotrauma, and, last but not least, chronic lung changes (BPD). ARDS, whatever its triggering factor may be, tends to produce edema and, at times, nonspecific alveolar infiltrates[10,11] (Fig. 5-4). Oxygen toxicity and ARDS lead to fibrosis and emphysema, conforming to the radiographic picture of BPD. The spectrum of findings in barotrauma includes alveolar rupture leading to pulmonary interstitital emphysema (PIE) (Fig. 5-5C) and other air leakage complications: pneumothorax, pneumomediastinum, pneumoretroperitoneum, and air in subcutaneous soft tissues and in potential spaces like the pulmonary ligament, the infra-azygous recess, or between the parietal pleura and the chest wall.[12-14] The true location of

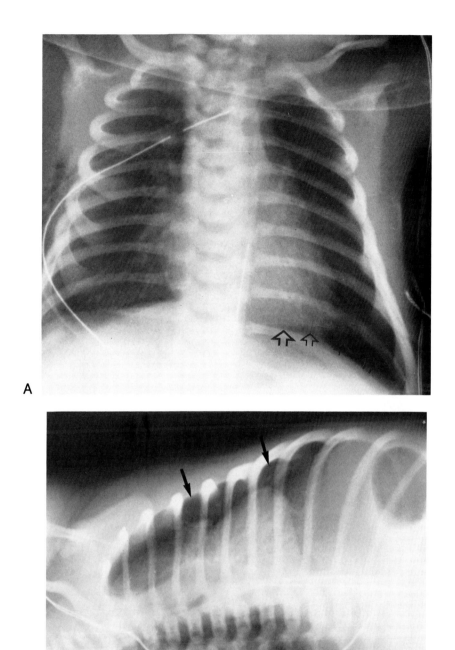

A

B

Fig. 5-5. Examples of barotrauma. **(A)** Collection of air at the base of the left lung (open arrows) and treated right-sided pneumothorax, after rupture of the distal airways by assisted ventilation with positive pressure. **(B)** The right lateral decubitus view fails to demonstrate free passage of air under the left thoracic wall; instead the air remains located at the same place as in Figure A, thus ruling out a left pneumothorax and confirming the air leakage into the potential space between the left parietal pleura and the diaphragm. Notice the pulmonary vascular markings reaching just below the left thoracic wall (arrows). *(Figure continues.)*

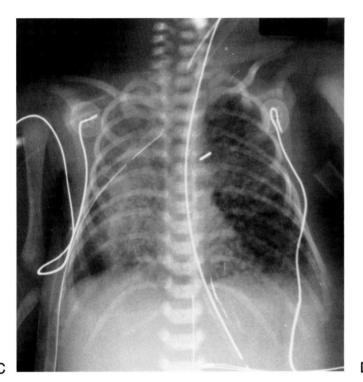

C

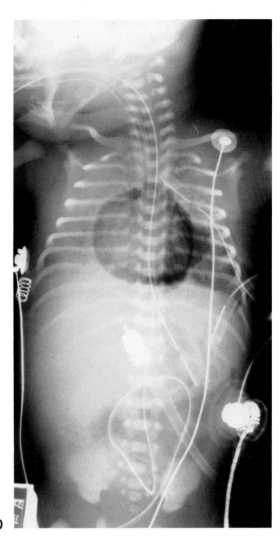

D

Fig. 5-5 *(Continued).* **(C)** *Pulmonary interstitial emphysema* in another case with barotrauma; notice the abnormally formed lucent tubular structures, which lack the normal branching distribution of the bronchial tree. Some of these lucent lines are larger at the periphery than in the central, hilar region. **(D)** *Lethal pneumopericardium.* This premature infant with severe respiratory distress and assisted ventilation developed sudden cardiac tamponade with pneumopericardium and died after the film was obtained, before any decompression could be attempted.

the air can best be determined by portable cross-table lateral or lateral decubitus radiographic examinations (Fig. 5-5). PIE can be diagnosed more easily when the abnormal linear lucencies in the lungs lack the fanning out configuration or branching distribution of the bronchial tree.[15]

The radiographic pattern of BPD is discussed later in this chapter. Diffuse PIE can simulate a radiographic picture of BPD (i.e., cystic honeycombing of the lungs). Diffuse consolidation and edema may be present after the PIE resolves, a process that may lead to early chronic lung disease.[16]

THE FIRST CHEST RADIOGRAPH

The evaluation of the first chest roentgenogram is very important after delivery of the premature infant at high risk and the infant's admission to the NICU;

however, it is the sequential interpretation of that very first roentgenogram and the several others to follow that gives meaning to the diagnostic interpretation. The real value of the first radiograph lies in screening a normal chest from those with any unusual findings and identifying the presence and proper location of tubes and lines. The position of the mandible (usually included in the chest radiograph) will, indirectly, show the degree of flexion, extension, or rotation of the infant's neck and so will tell more

accurately the real location of the endotracheal tube and its proximity to the bronchi or the hypopharynx.[17] The unusual findings to look for would include; odd size and configuration of the cardiothymic silhouette, abnormal pulmonary densities, an increased or decreased lung inflation, presence of air outside the normal pulmonary structures, and abnormal shape of the thoracic cage (Fig. 5-6).

The increased pulmonary air capacity will be an expression of tachypnea or distress of any etiology

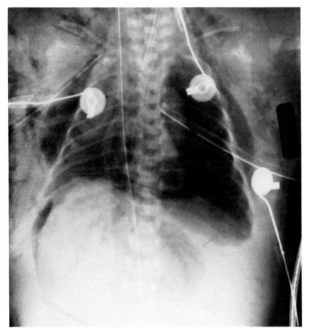

A

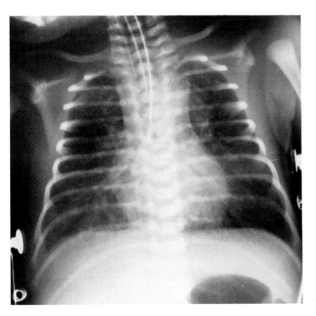

B

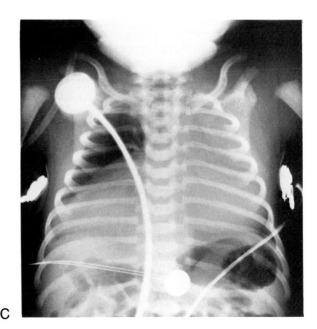

C

Fig. 5-6. **(A)** *Abnormal (bell-shaped) thoracic cage in a severe form of pulmonary hypoplasia.* This premature infant was born with extreme respiratory distress requiring very high positive-pressure assisted ventilation and died a few hours later. Notice the narrow chest cavity secondary to the poor pulmonary expansion in spite of diffuse air leak (there is air also in the hepatic veins and inside the cardiac chambers). **(B)** *Abnormal pulmonary densities.* The lungs are well inflated but too many markings are still noted around a normal-sized heart, and the main pulmonary arteries are not prominent. The abnormalities in this case represent congested pulmonary veins and interstitial edema in total anomalous pulmonary venous return below the diaphragm. **(C)** *Mediastinal mass.* Partial herniation of the liver through an anterior midline defect producing leftward cardiothymic deviation. *(Figure continues.)*

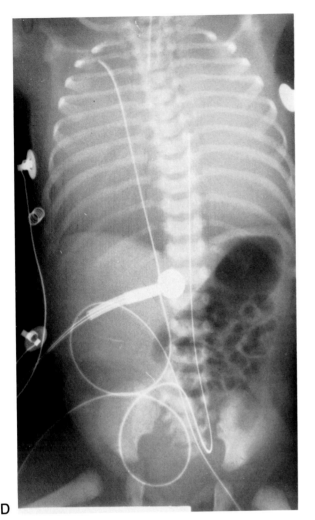

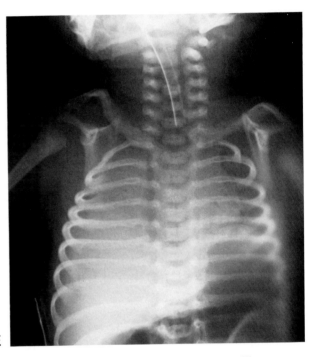

Fig. 5-6 *(Continued).* **(D)** *Huge cardiomegaly.* Congenital pulmonary artery atresia with severe dilatation of the right cardiac chambers. Notice the heart occupying the entire thoracic cavity, with downward displacement of the diaphragms and no identifiable pulmonary parenchyma; severe pulmonary hypoplasia was found at necropsy. **(E)** *Abnormally decreased pulmonary inflation (white-out lungs) and tracheal atresia.* This premature infant died after birth in spite of attempted tracheostomy and intubation. Notice the abnormal pulmonary parenchyma with some air in an irregularly distributed and very hypoplastic bronchial tree. *(Figure continues.)*

except HMD. If this capacity is decreased, alveolar collapse secondary to surfactant deficiency and/or severe neurologic deterioration with central nervous system (CNS) depression is usually present (Fig. 5-7A). The presence on the first chest roentgenogram of irregular (mixed alveolar and interstitial) pulmonary densities, usually perihilar in distribution and accompanied by normal or increased lung inflation,

can represent anything from severely retained fetal lung fluid (as seen in transient tachypnea of the newborn) to neonatal pneumonitis, aspiration, hemorrhage, or even edema (Fig. 5-7D). Since knowledge of the prenatal history, circumstances surrounding the delivery, oxygen requirements, and ventilatory pressures may be very helpful in interpreting the radiologic data, communication with the clinician is essential.

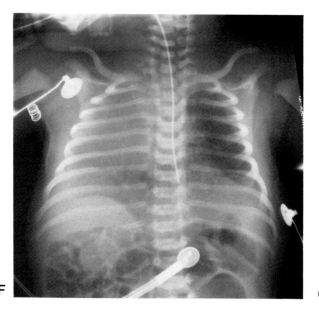
F

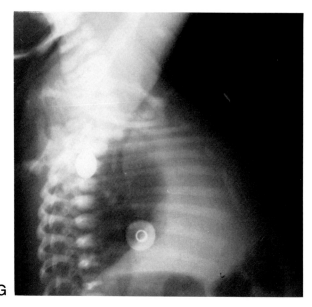
G

Fig. 5-6 *(Continued).* **(F&G)** *Lack of normal features of the cardiopulmonary silhouette in right pulmonary hypoplasia.* Anteroposterior **(F)** and lateral **(G)** views of the chest in an asymptomatic premature infant. Notice the least hypolucent right lung with the cardiothymic silhouette hidden behind it in the right hemithorax. The lateral projection demonstrates a retrosternal oblique line, blended with the anterior mediastinum and representing an accessory right hemidiaphragm.

CARDIOMEGALY

The cardiothoracic ratio considered within the normal limits in infants, on portable supine roentgenograms, can be as much as 0.65.[18] Hypoinflation, lordosis, and rotation will many times distort the cardiac silhouette. The heart size should always be seen in the context of the perihilar vascular markings, and the knowledge of such basic clinical data as the presence of cyanosis and/or heart murmur. One should also remember that during the fist few days of life the pulmonary arterial pressure is high, as a consequence of the physiologic right-to-left cardiopulmonary shunt present in the intrauterine fetal circulation. The extrauterine persistence of this high pulmonary vascular pressure (persistent fetal circulation syndrome) does not have any characteristic roentgenologic pattern.[19] If an intracardiac septal defect is present, pulmonary blood flow will remain normal to decreased until the pulmonary pressure comes down to normal values (usually 4 to 7 postpartum days) and the shunt reverses (Figs. 5-8 and 5-9).

The diagnostic approach to cardiac anomalies (on the roentgenograms and/or in combination with car-diac ultrasound) is dealt with in Chapter 6, but one should always keep in the differential diagnosis the various cardiac-related conditions, other than congenital anomalies (Fig. 5-6D), producing either congestive heart failure and/or an increased size of the cardiothymic silhouette (Table 5-1).

NEONATAL ACUTE PULMONARY INJURY

Most of the premature infants in the NICU suffer from neonatal acute pulmonary injury (NAPI), usually caused by surfactant deficiency or HMD. Other less common pulmonary insults are those secondary to meconium aspiration, neonatal pneumonitis, congenital anomalies such as hydrops fetalis with pulmonary and generalized edema, pulmonary hypoplasia, tracheoesophageal fistulas with or without esophageal atresia and aspiration, severe congenital heart disease, persistent fetal circulation, diaphragmatic hernia and gastroschisis (which can increase the abdominal pressure after surgical reduction of the extrophic gut and affect the respiratory functional ca-

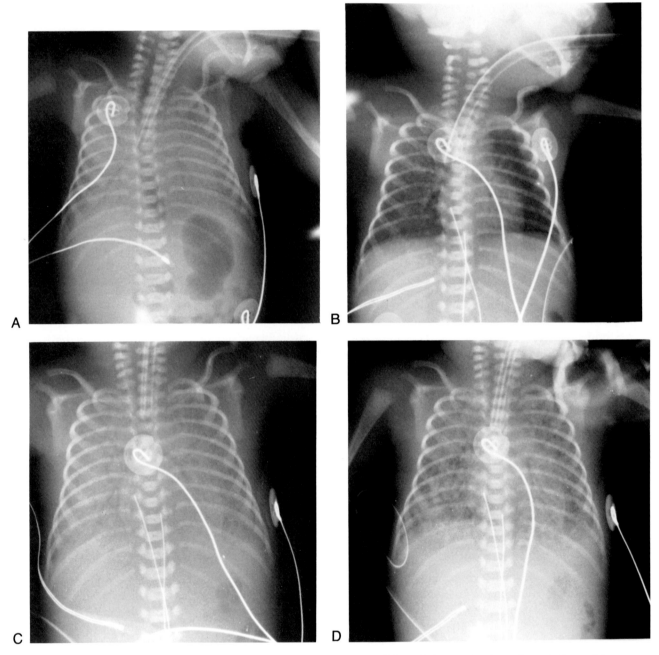

Fig. 5-7. (A) *Hyaline membrane disease.* Extremely immature (25 weeks' gestation) newborn infant with severe respiratory distress. Notice the hypoaerated chest with microgranular densities through out the lung fields, which have acquired a ground glass appearance. Air bronchograms are seen reaching the periphery of the lungs. **(B)** *Pulmonary anatomic immaturity.* Same infant 24 hours later and after administration of artificial surfactant. Observe the marked improvement of the pulmonary findings; only mild grayness of the lung fields is now noted. **(C)** *Severe pulmonary edema.* Same premature infant at 5 days of life; the lungs are now hyperexpanded (compare with Figure A, when the infant was suffering from HMD) but they are whited out because of the presence of alveolar and interstitial fluid; air bronchograms have reappeared. **(D)** *Pulmonary hemorrage* further complicates the prognosis of the same premature infant. At 1 week of life, blood was found in his endotracheal tube and his lungs have adopted a diffuse, predominantly alveolar type of infiltrate.

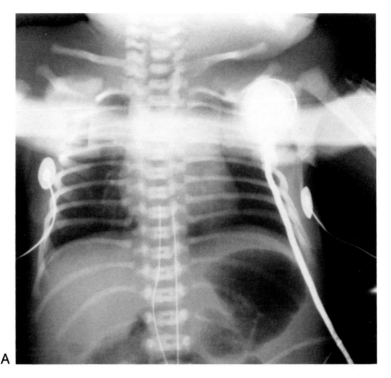

A

Fig. 5-8. *Patent ductus arteriosus in a near-term premature infant.* Chest roentgenograms taken at 1, 4, 7, and 15 days of life show the transition from normal appearance of the heart and lungs **(A)** to cardiomegaly **(B)**, congestion, edema, and increased size of the pulmonary vessels **(C)**, and recovery **(D)** after surgical ligation of the ductus arteriosus. *(Figure continues.)*

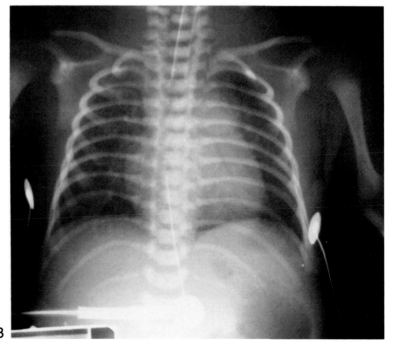

B

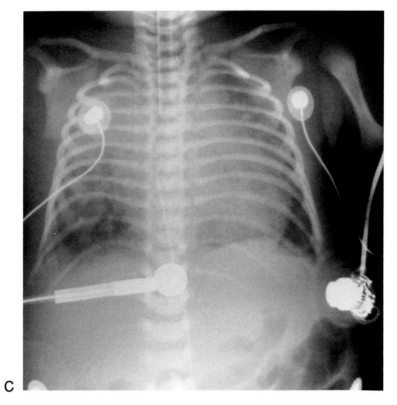

C

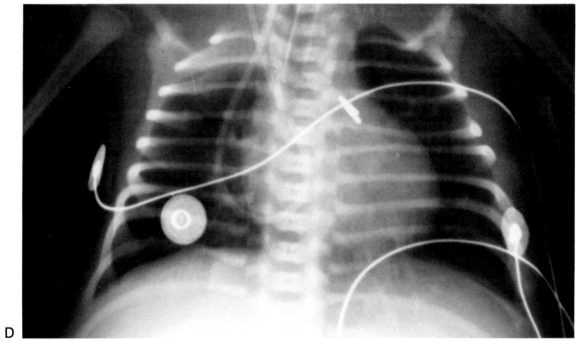

D

Fig. 5-8 *(Continued).* **(C&D)**

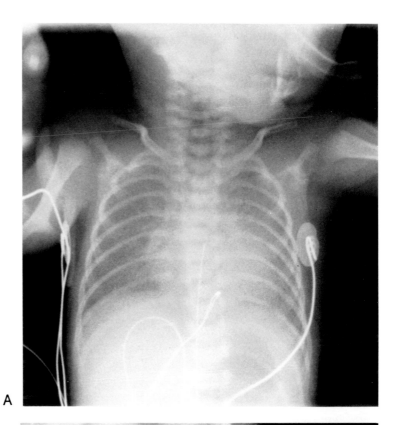

A

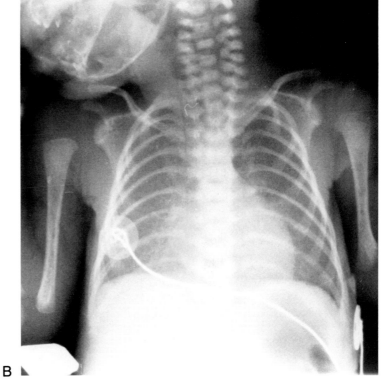

B

Fig. 5-9. *Patent ductus arteriosus in a micropremature infant.* **(A)** A 4-day-old micropremie with sudden haziness of the otherwise normally infiltrated lung fields and moderate cardiomegaly. The left-to-right shunt is expressed in this population of premature infants by passive congestion and interstitial edema, instead of increased pulmonary blood flow (see Fig. 5-8C) typically seen in full-term infants suffering from this complication. **(B)** Same infant after treatment with diuretics and disappearance of the heart murmur 3 days later.

TABLE 5-1.   Causes of Neonatal Cardiomegaly Other Than Congenital Heart Anomalies

Hypervolemia and pulmonary edema and/or congenital heart failure (CHF)
   Cardiac ischemia secondary to brain asphyxia
   Hypertrophic subaortic stenosis
   Cardiomyopathy
   Intracardiac myxoma
   Infant of diabetic mother (IDM)
   PDA
   Hydrops fetalis
   Arteriovenous malformation (AVM)
     –brain
     –liver
   Polycythemia
   Erythrocythemia
   Blood transfusions
Mediastinal masses simulating cardiomegaly
   –Teratomas
   –Liver herniation through an anterior defect of the diaphragm

pacity),[19] and other thoracic congenital anomalies. Any of these conditions can trigger ARDS and the chain of events depicted in Figure 5-10, which may result in BPD.

Hyaline Membrane Disease

Pulmonary HMD is the most common cause of respiratory distress in the newborn premature infant.[20] The condition is yet without a definite etiology, but it is the lack of the surface tension reducing substance (surfactant) that seems to be the most important factor.[21] The smaller and younger the premature infant the more frequent and severe this condition seems to be. The surfactant agent, a lipoprotein, is believed to be produced by the alveolar cells and is essential for initial and sustained alveolar distension.[22] Its absence leads to increased alveolar surface tension, lessened alveolar distensibility, and persistent collapse or atelectasis of the alveoli. This and the predisposition to

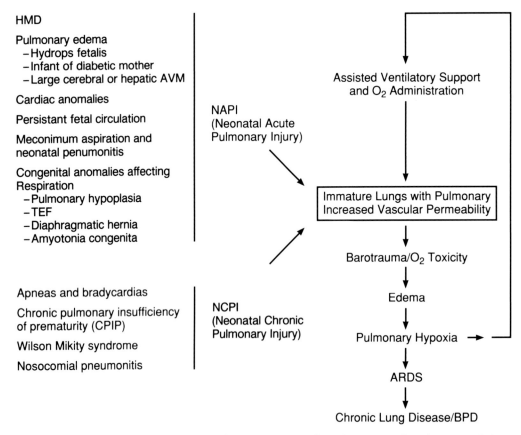

Fig. 5-10. The chain of events resulting from acute or chronic neonatal pulmonary injury that culminates in BPD.

increased pulmonary vascular permeability in the premature lungs lead to more hypoxia and aggravate the problem of decreased surfactant production.

The resultant acidosis also leads to a spasm of the peripheral pulmonary vessels and thus to decreased perfusion of the pulmonary alveolar capillaries. This leads to further hypoxia and more acidosis. The complications of severe hypoxia (intracranial hemorrhage, disseminated intravascular coagulation, pulmonary hemorrhage, and congestive heart failure)[23] may lead to the death of the infant, but oxygen administration, mechanical ventilation, and the administration of artificial surfactant directly into the bronchial tree may hasten the recovery from these conditions. In the usual case, the clinical findings of respiratory distress are apparent by 3 to 6 hours of life and consist of progressive tachypnea, grunting, nasal flaring, and intercostal and sternal retractions. Acidosis also is present and hypoxemia and hypercapnia are pronounced. Histologically, in HMD the alveoli are uniformly collapsed but the end terminal bronchioli are very distended. These latter structures also are rimmed by a layer of fibrine or so-called hyaline membrane.[24] It is this hyaline membrane for which the condition was orignally named, but it should be remembered that its presence is not specific for the disease. Indeed, it can be seen with other conditions such as aspiration pneumonitis, and, in fact, it is generally accepted that the membranes are the result rather than the cause of the hyaline membrane disease. The classic radiographic findings in hyaline membrane disease consist of marked underaeration of the lungs leading to a small pulmonary air capacity and a granular, ground glass appearance of the lung fields with presence of air bronchograms (the distended secondary and tertiary airways) (Fig. 5-7A).

The administration of exogenous surfactant via endotracheal instillation has been shown to be efficacious by clinical improvement within minutes to hours[25] (Fig. 5-11). Once this acute pulmonary insult subsides, the extreme anatomic immaturity of these lungs remains, with a high risk for persistent pulmonary capillary permeability and edema, apnea and bradycardia spells, and alveolar hemorrhage (Fig. 5-7D) as well as for secondary pulmonary insults caused by supported ventilation and oxygenation.

The administration of surfactant has a strong impact on the severity of HMD; the decrease in morbidity after its administration has improved the survival of these premature infants and reduced the incidence of intracranial hemorrhage, barotrauma, and BPD. Recently published data on controlled groups of premature infants have been able to document a significant decrease in the incidence of severe HMD hours after surfactant administration, with a significant concomitant increase in the incidence of mild disease.[25] It is encouraging that most of the surfactant recipients now require minimal ventilatory support, equivalent to that of those ventilated preterm neonates without parenchymal lung disease (anatomic pulmonary immaturity only) (Fig. 5-11). The radiographic findings after surfactant administration are those of a fast-clearing, hazy, granular pattern and a reversal of the pulmonary hypoinflation typical of HMD. In a matter of hours the premature lungs will expand, at times leaving a mildly hazy pulmonary background (anatomic pulmonary immaturity) (Fig. 5-2A) and at times rendering a normal pulmonary radiolucency.

In some instances the extreme immaturity may not allow enough surfactant buildup after its external administration, with the consequent persistence of respiratory distress and a white-out (severe edema) radiographic appearance of the lungs (Fig. 5-7C). The high-pressure assisted ventilation required may then lead to barotrauma or uncontrollable pulmonary edema and/or hemorrhage, which may result in death during the ensuing days. Suboptimal response in some of the surfactant recipients may be related to some degree of early lung injury due to surfactant deficiency but occurring before surfactant therapy, or to increased alveolar capillary permeability and secondary surfactant inactivation by the proteins that leak into the alveolar space.[26]

Pathophysiologic causes of HMD other than surfactant deficiency should be also kept in mind. Recent clinical and experimental evidence suggests that some of these factors affecting the response to this surfactant can be eliminated by administering surfactant at birth or soon after birth, by increasing the dosage, and/or by using a multiple-dose strategy.[27]

Pulmonary Edema

In general terms, increased pulmonary permeability is present in lung injuries leading to respiratory failure. The mechanism of this increase is poorly understood.[28] It has been demonstrated that the total protein plasma concentration increases with decreasing gestational age, thus placing the more premature infant at even higher risk of developing severe pul-

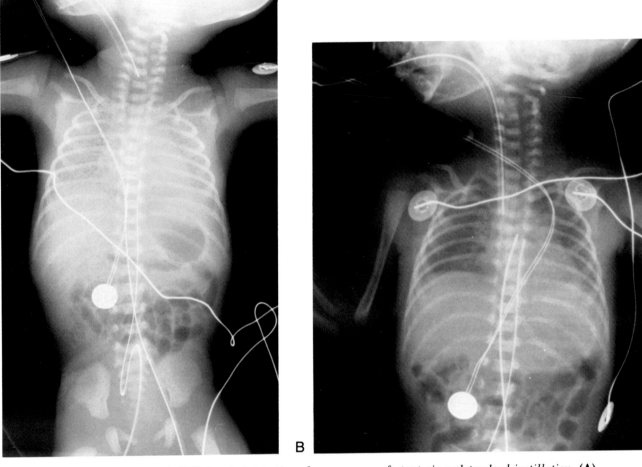

A

B

Fig. 5-11. *Treatment of HMD by administration of exogenous surfactant via endotracheal instillation.* **(A)** Micropremature with HMD at 2 hours of life. **(B)** Same patient 6 hours after surfactant installation presents clear, grayish lungs (now representing anatomic immaturity only).

monary edema[29] (Fig. 5-12). Increased alveolar surface tension with surfactant deficiency (HMD) results in a more negative interstitial pressure, which also promotes pulmonary edema.[28]

Toward the end of the first week of life after a treated NAPI, if clinical improvement is not seen, pulmonary permeability will remain high, and there will be evidence of neutrophil sequestration and activation within the lung. White blood cells, presumably neutrophils, are now believed to play an important role in the pathogenesis of increased permeability pulmonary edema.[30] There is a definitive smaller number of protease inhibitors in plasma in micropremies, thus putting them at a higher risk for persistent

edema secondary to neutrophil-mediated lung injury.[31]

The association between high fluid intake and the subsequent occurrence of clinically significant PDA and BPD provides a further relationship between lung water content and pulmonary dysfunction in the premature infant.[28] A PDA is traditionally thought to be significant only when there is clinical evidence of pulmonary dysfunction that is otherwise inadequately explained, or when overt left heart overload has occurred. This increased pulmonary blood flow is sufficient to produce pulmonary edema in the premature lungs (Figs. 5-8 and 5-9). Certain congenital heart diseases will lead to edema following the same

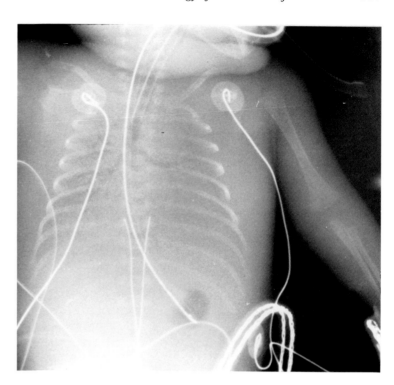

Fig. 5-12. *Hydrops fetalis.* Premature infant delivered with functional (HMD) and anatomic pulmonary immaturity, diffuse edema of the subcutaneous soft tissues, poliserositis, and superimposed pulmonary edema.

or similar physiopathologic mechanisms. The increased pulmonary permeability in these premature infants after acute pulmonary injury enhances the significance of the increased pulmonary blood flow from a PDA, before overt cardiac failure occurs.

Hydrops Fetalis

However clear or obscure the cause for this entity may be, the management of a premature or a high-risk hydropic neonate is complicated even more by an increased total lung water, thus compounding the treatment of pulmonary immaturity or HMD with the addition of pulmonary edema (Fig. 5-12).

Neonatal Pneumonitis

Most neonatal pneumonias result from ascending infection via the vagina following prematurely ruptured membranes.[32] A septic newborn with the focus of infection in the lungs is at a high morbidity and mortality risk[33]; consequently an early diagnosis of pneumonia becomes very important. In this setting the portable radiograph of the chest can be a handy tool in the diagnosis. It is worth emphasizing the clinical similarities between HMD and neonatal pneumonitis at the beginning of life; however, the roentgen-

ographic appearance usually changes, especially if it persists in the following days. Most bacterial penumonitis will present a persistent pattern of alveolar and/or interstitial densities that are irregularly defined and mostly asymmetric[9] and the pulmonary air capacity is usually increased[32] (Fig. 5-3A), although this factor must be measured carefully since almost all high-risk and sick premature infants are intubated and under assisted mechanical ventilation.

Group B streptococcal pneumonitis has even been described with a pulmonary pattern undistinguishable from that of HMD[34] (Fig. 5-13), and at times they both can be superimposed. Blood-borne pneumonitis is much less common and usually presents with a miliary interstitial and/or alveolar pattern, but without hyperinflation as seen in certain cases of congenital tuberculosis, syphilis (Fig. 5-14), or certain strains of viral pneumonitis. This pattern may simulate cystic honeycomb pattern and be misdiagnosed as Wilson-Mikity syndrome. Viral pneumonitis caused by herpes simplex can be transmitted to the fetus with intact fetal membranes before delivery or during the second stage of labor and usually needs 1 to 2 weeks of incubation to manifest its necrotizing alveolitis; in consequence the clinical symptomatology of viremia and pneumonia may not be obvious until the end of the

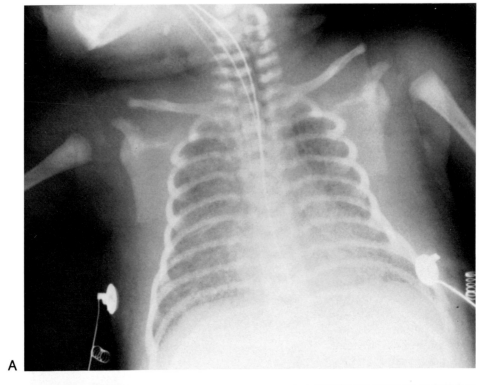

A

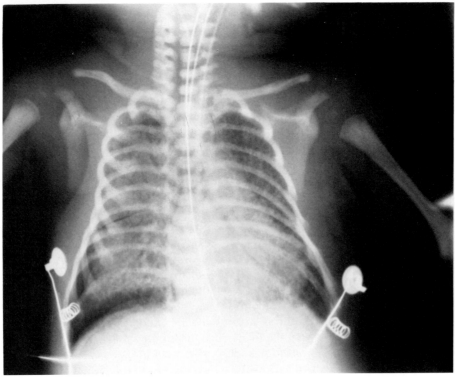

B

Fig. 5-13. *Group B streptococcal pneumonitis.* **(A)** Full-term neonate with severe respiratory distress and a roentgenographic lung pattern similar to that seen in HMD, although with pneumonitis the lungs are hyperinflated. **(B)** Same infant with superimposed stiffed lungs and air leak (right pneumothorax) 3 days later; the infant has developed ARDS.

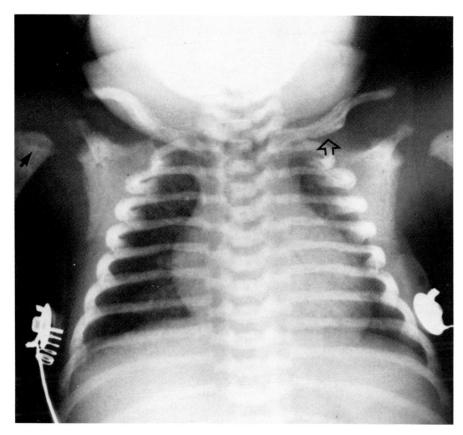

Fig. 5-14. *Neonatal syphilitic pneumonitis* Three-day-old premature infant with abnormal bone changes: irregular metaphyseal ends of the long bones (arrow), thickened cortical bone at the clavicles (open arrow), and lytic lesions in the scapulae. The lungs present a mild interstitial, nonspecific pattern with normal aeration.

first week of life. Radiologically these pneumonias will exhibit sequential increasing interstitial infiltrates leading to diffuse alveolar disease in a matter of a few days and without air trapping[35] (Fig. 5-15).

NEONATAL CHRONIC PULMONARY INJURY

Adult Respiratory Distress Syndrome

Although the initiating insult differs, neonatal HMD and ARDS share many similar pathophysiologic characteristics and mechanisms of lung injury, with the surfactant deficiency as the trigger factor in neonatal HMD.[28] Residual pulmonary dysfunction and/or pulmonary fibrosis after supportive treatment may result in the adult, and BPD in the neonate (Fig. 5-4).

Oxygen Toxicity

The effect of excessive oxygen in the lungs, or hyperoxia, will consist of damage in the endothelial pulmonary cells, promoting interstitial and alveolar edema and cell metaplasia and also affecting the collagen cells of the interstitial space. This damage to interstitial space cells is accompanied by the production of fibrosis and emphysematous bullae,[36] thus promoting the development of BPD.

Wilson-Mikity Syndrome and Chronic Pulmonary Insufficiency of the Premature Infant

The diagnoses of Wilson-Mikity syndrome and chronic pulmonary insufficiency of the premature infant (CPIP) are reserved for micropremies who do not require assisted ventilation in the first days of life

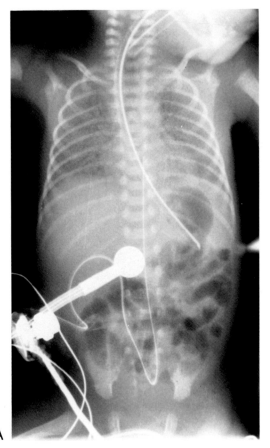
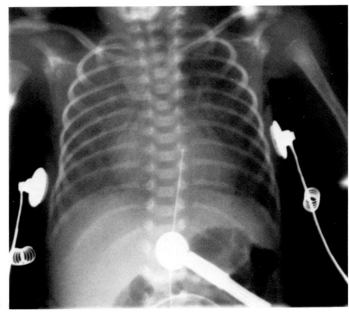

Fig. 5-15. *Neonatal herpes simplex pneumonia.* **(A)** On admission after delivery this, 30 weeks' gestation micropremature infant presented with moderate respiratory distress syndrome (RDS). The roengenographic picture was compatible with mild HMD and the infant was placed on a respirator with assisted ventilation. **(B)** Same infant at 4 days of life; RDS persisted but the roentgenographic picture of HMD has disappeared. *(Figure continues.)*

but who subsequently develop respiratory distress of undetermined etiology[37] (Fig. 5-16). Respiratory distress here is secondary to atelectasis and overly distended areas of lung and it may progress, requiring assisted ventilation. Radiologic findings may range from the lucent or gray lungs seen in anatomic pulmonary immaturity to perihilar interstitial subsegmental atelectasis and/or congestion, or even to cystic changes that are indistinguishable from BPD. Most likely, CPIP and Wilson-Mikity syndrome represent extremes of the same diseases wherein CPIP is the milder of the two forms. Both the inability to radiographically distinguish between Wilson-Mikity

syndrome and BPD and the aggressive use of assisted ventilation in micropremies during the first hours of life have markedly restricted the diagnosis of Wilson-Mikity syndrome in nurseries today.

Bronchopulmonary Dysplasia

The classical clinicoradiologic description of BPD by Northway and coworkers[38] more than 20 years ago included three chronologic stages of pulmonary changes leading to a final fourth stage of chronic lung disease by the end of the first month of life, and characterized by severe morphologic and functional

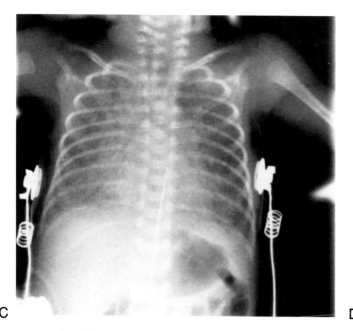

C

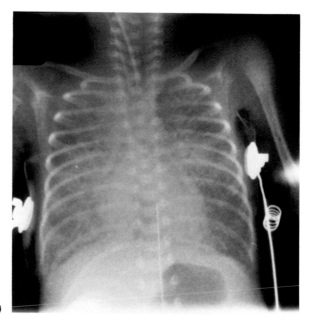

D

Fig. 5-15 *(Continued)*. **(C&D)** Same patient at 5 **(C)** and 6 **(D)** days of life showing a worsening of the roentgenographic pattern of the lungs, which has now become a mixture of interstitial and alveolar patterns. No mucocutaneous lesions were present but maternal history for herpes simplex type II was confirmed 3 days after delivery. The virus was cultured by standard cell culture techniques and the infant was treated with Acyclovir and recovered uneventfully.

lung damage and a radiographic picture of pulmonary hyperinflation and cystic lucent areas with fibrotic strands (Fig. 5-17). This description was based on a different and more near-term newborn population than the micropremies commonly dealt with today. In recent years the classical form of BPD has become less common and the time for its appearance more elusive because of the awareness of this iatrogenic condition and the pulmonary therapeutic innovations in the NICU. In many of these very small preterm infants, classical BPD has been replaced by a milder form of chronic lung damage[39] for which radiographic criteria are not yet fully established (Fig. 5-18).

Edwards and coworkers have established combined clinical, pathologic, and roentgenographic scoring systems for assessing BPD.[40] These systems have limitations before 3 weeks of age because of their inability to differentiate early BPD from resolving HMD. Currently the infants who develop early roentgenographic lung changes by the third or fourth weeks of

life are treated with steroids. As a result both the radiographic and clinical courses of BPD are modified, with a substantial improvement in a matter of days[41] (Fig. 5-19).

It is apparent that any definition of chronic lung disease in the premature infant should be based on its postnatal course. It has been demonstrated that the need for supplemental oxygen at 1 month of life becomes an increasingly poor predictor of BPD and subsequent pulmonary outcome as the gestational age at birth decreases, and that the need for oxygen at a corrected gestational age of 36 weeks is a better predictor of pulmonary outcome for infants less than 30 weeks of gestational age at birth.[42]

It seems also reasonable to assign the roentgenographic impression of BPD to those infants with a respiratory disorder that begins with acute lung injury, whatever the triggering factor may be, requiring prolonged assisted ventilation for any reason and defined by standarized clinical and chronologic criteria.

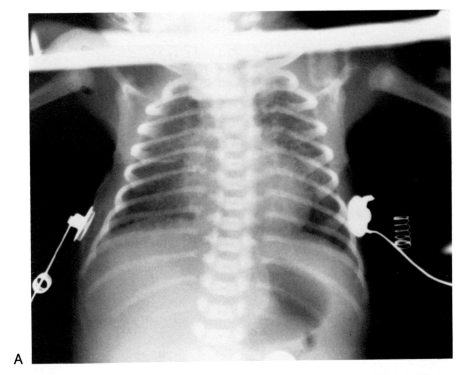

A

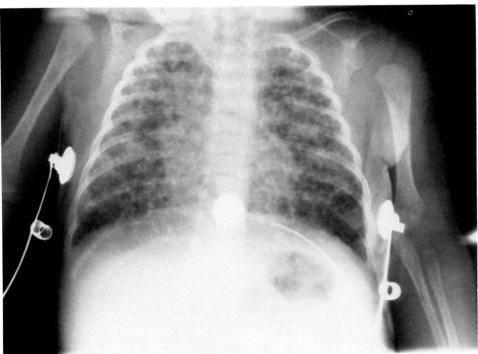

B

Fig. 5-16. *Chronic pulmonary insufficiency of prematurity and Wilson-Mikity syndrome.* **(A)** Eight-day-old micropremature infant placed under an oxygen tent for moderate respiratory distress of recent onset; the chest roentgenogram shows normal to grayish pulmonary background typical of anatomic pulmonary immaturity. The infant spent only 24 hours under oxygen exposure. **(B)** Same infant at 40 days of life with a typical honeycomb pulmonary pattern; viral cultures were negative. This roentgenographic appearance improved dramatically and the infant went home at 90 days of life with no further pulmonary abnormalities.

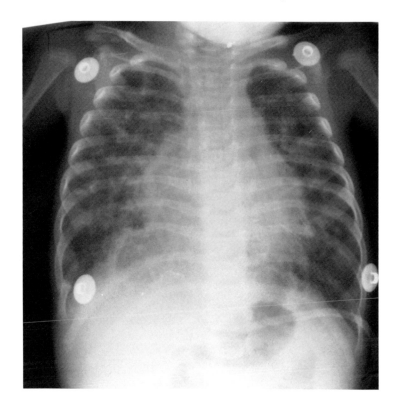

Fig. 5-17. *Bronchopulmonary dysplasia* in a 75-day-old infant born at 26 weeks' gestation with severe HMD. A stormy follow-up kept him under assisted ventilatory therapy and high oxygen for a protracted period. The infant developed chronic lung changes wth fibrosis and emphysematous pulmonary bases and developed pulmonary hypertension with right ventricular hypertrophy.

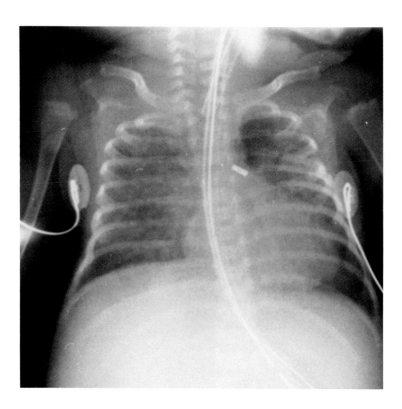

Fig. 5-18. Mild BPD in a 4-week-old micropremature infant with intubation and oxygen exposure since birth. Notice the metallic clip for closure of the ductus arteriosus and the fine interstitial pulmonary pattern without obvious emphysema.

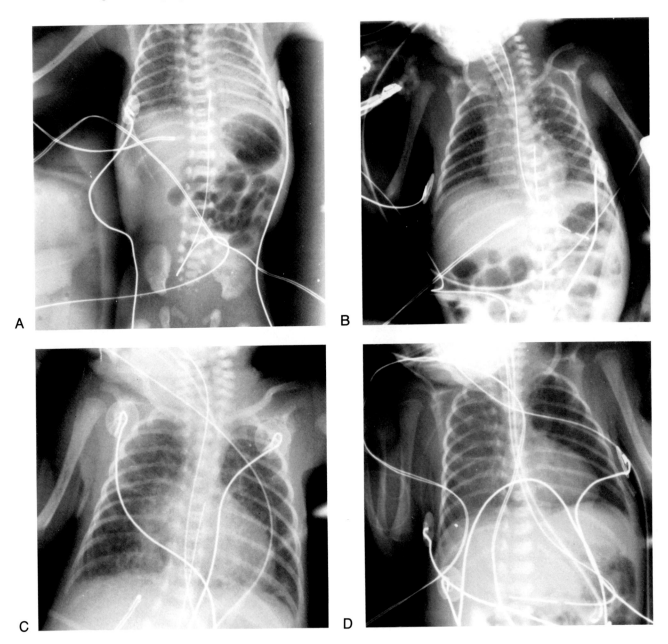

Fig. 5-19. HMD, artificial surfactant administration, mild BPD, and treatment with steroiods.**(A)** A 27 weeks' gestation premature infant with infant respiratory distress syndrome and HMD at first day of life. **(B)** Same infant at 2 days of life and after administration of exogenous surfactant instillation, showing dramatic clinical improvement. **(C)** The same infant at 25 days of life; he had required assisted ventilation since after birth and extubation attempts were unsuccesful at this time (mild BPD). **(D)** Same patient at 1 month of life following a short course of steroid administration. The chest roentgenogram has become normal; he was extubated 2 days later and further oxygen was never required.

This would include even protracted treatment for apnea and bradycardia.

REFERENCES

1. De Sa DJ: Pulmonary fluid content in infants with respiratory distress. J Pathol 97:469, 1969
2. Reid L: Bronchopulmonary dysplasia pathology. J Pediatr 95:836, 1979
3. Edwards DK, Jacob J, Gluck L: The immature lung: radiographic appearance, course, and complications. AJR 135:659, 1980
4. Jacob J, Knapp RA, Merrit TA et al: Immature lung syndrome, abstracted. Pediatr Res 12:527, 1978
5. Cowett RM: Introduction. p. 1. In Cowelt RM, Hay WW (ed): The Micropremies: The Next Frontier. Ross Laboratories, Columbus, OH, 1990
6. Mack M, Fanaroff AA: How small is too small: considerations in evaluating the outcome of the tiny infant. Clin Perinatol 15:733, 1988
7. Nwaesei GC, Young DC, Byrne JM et al: Preterm birth at 23 to 26 weeks' gestation; is active obstetric management justified? Am J Obstet Gynecol 157:890, 1987
8. Thibeault DW, Gregory GA: Neonatal Pulmonary Care. p 251. Addison-Wesley Publishing Company, Reading, MA, 1979
9. Griscom NT, Wohl MEB, Kirkpatrick JA: Lower respiratory infections: how infants differ from adults. Radiol Clin North Am 16:367, 1978
10. Reed JC: Chest Radiology — Plain Film Patterns and Differential Diagnosis. p. 135. Year Book Medical Publishers, Chicago, 1987
11. Amstrong P, Wilson A, Dee P: Imaging of Diseases of the Chest. p. 389. Year Book Medical Publishers, Chicago, 1990
12. Ivey HH, Kattwinkel J, Alford BA: Subvisceral pleural air in neonates with respiratory distress. Am J Dis Child 135:544, 1981
13. Bowen A, Quattroman FL: Infraazygous pneumomediastinum in the newborn. AJR 135:1017, 1980
14. Volberg FL, Everett C, Brill P: Radiologic features of inferior pulmonary ligament air collection in neonates with respiratory distress. Radiology 130:357, 1979
15. Felman AH: Radiology of the Pediatric Chest. Clinical and Pathological Correlation. McGraw-Hill, New York, 1987
16. Merril TA, Northway WM, Boynton BR: Bronchopulmonary Dysplasia: Contemporary Issues in Fetal and Neonatal Medicine. p. 1193. Blackwell Scientific Publications, London, 1988
17. Donn SM, Kuhns LR: Mechanism of endotracheal tube movement with change of head position in the neonate. Pediatr Radiol 9:37, 1980
18. Edwards DR, Higgins CB, Gilpin EA: The cardiothoracic ratio in newborn infants. AJR 136:907, 1981
19. Swischuk L: Radiology of the Newborn and Young Infant. p. 102. Williams & Wilkins, Baltimore, 1984
20. Rudolph AJ, Smith CA: Idiopathic respiratory distress syndrome of the newborn. J Pediatr 57:905, 1960
21. Robert MF, Neff RK, Hubbell JP et al: Association between maternal diabetes and the respiratory distress syndrome in the newborn. N Engl J Med 294:357, 1976
22. Avery ME, Clements JA: Pulmonary surfactant and atelectasis. Physiol Physicians 1:1, 1963
23. Margolis CZ, Orzalesi MM, Schwartz AD: Disseminated intravascular coagulation in the respiratory distress syndrome. Am J Dis Child 125:324, 1973
24. Gregg RH, Berstein J: Pulmonary hyaline membranes and the respiratory distress syndrome. Am J Dis Child 102:871, 1961
25. Fujiwara T, Konishi M, Chida S et al: Surfactant replacement therapy in preterm neonates with respiratory distress syndrome. Pediatrics 86:753, 1990
26. Ikegami M, Jacobs M, Jobe A: Surfactant function in respiratory distress syndrome. J Pediatr 102:443, 1983
27. Shapiro DL: Comments on dosage and timing of surfactant administration. p. 117. In Jobe A, Taeusch HW (eds): Surfactant Treatment of Lung Disease. Report of the 96th Ross Conference on Pediatric Research. Ross Laboratories, Columbus, OH, 1988
28. O'Brodovich H: Pulmonary edema in unresolved neonatal acute lung injury. p. 69. In: Bronchopulmonary Dysplasia and Related Chronic Respiratory Disorders. Report of the 90th Ross Conference on Pediatric Research. Ross Laboratories, Columbus, OH, 1986
29. Markarian M, Jackson JJ, Bannon AE: Serial serum total protein values in premature infants with or without the respiratory distress syndrome. J Pediatr 69:1096, 1966
30. Tate RM, Repine JE: Neutrophils and the adult respiratory distress syndrome. Am Rev Respir Dis 128:552, 1983
31. Andrew M, Massicote-Nolan PM, Karpatkin M: Plasma protease inhibitors in premature infants: influence of gestational age, post natal age and health status. Proc Soc Exp Biol Med 173:495, 1983
32. Wesenberg RL: The Newborn Chest. p. 72. Harper & Row, New York, 1973
33. Stahlmann MT: p. 292. In Kendig EL Jr, Chernick V (eds): Disorders of the Respiratory Tract in Children. WB Saunders, Philadelphia, 1977
34. Modanlou HD, Bosu SK, Weller MH: Early onset group B streptococcus neonatal septicemia and res-

piratory distress syndrome: characteristic features of assisted ventilation in the first 24 hours of life. Crit Care Med 8:716, 1980

35. Dominguez, R, Rivero H, Gaisie G et al: Neonatal herpes simplex pneumonia: radiographic findings. Radiology 153:395, 1984

36. Johnson KJ, Fantone JC, Kaplan J et al: *In vivo* damage of rat lungs by oxygen metabolites. J Clin Invest 67:983, 1983

37. Krauss AN, Klain DB, Auld PA: Chronic pulmonary insufficiency of prematurity (CPIP). Pediatrics 55:55, 1975

38. Northway WM, Rosan RC, Porter DY: Radiographic features of pulmonary oxygen toxicity in the newborn bronchopulmonary dysplasia. Radiology 91:49, 1968

39. Herreghan MA, Sosulski R, Baquero JM: Persistent pulmonary abnormalities in newborns: the changing picture of bronchopulmonary dysplasia. Pediatr Radiol 16:180, 1986

40. Edwards DK, Colby TV, Northway WH: Radiographic pathologic correlation in bronchopulmonary dysplasia. J Pediatr 95:834, 1979

41. Blanchard PW, Brown TM, Coates AL: Pharmacotherapy in bronchopulmonary dysplasia. Clin Perinatol 4:881, 1987

42. Sherman A, Dunn M: Abnormal pulmonary outcome in premature infants: prediction from oxygen requirement in the neonate period. Pediatrics 82:521, 1988

Diagnostic Cardiac Imaging in the Premature Infant

Roma Ilkiw

6

Pediatric cardiologists may choose from a variety of imaging modalities for evaluating cardiovascular anatomy and function in the premature infant. Selecting the appropriate diagnostic imaging modality requires a thorough understanding of the clinical problem, the information to be gained, and the limitations and risk-to-benefit ratio of each technique.

Echocardiography is currently the technique of choice for diagnosing and managing structural heart disease in the newborn. Two-dimensional echocardiography offers optimal visualization of cardiovascular structures, and Doppler echocardiography aids in evaluation of the circulatory dynamics of both normal and abnormal structures. Echocardiography offers major advantages over other imaging modalities in terms of spatial and temporal resolution, cost, ease of the study, portability, radiation exposure, and maximum safety for the patient.

Promising new technology offered by magnetic resonance (MR) imaging and positron emission tomography (PET) provides unparalleled capability for evaluating cardiac function and characterizing myocardial disease processes at the cellular and biochemical levels. Before these modalities can be successfully applied in the premature infant, improvements must be made in temporal and spatial resolution necessitated by the smaller size and faster heart rate of the infant. Shortened data acquisition periods will also be required.

THE CHEST ROENTGENOGRAM

A chest roentgenogram is required for the initial evaluation of a newborn with cyanosis or respiratory distress. The chest film is valuable in distinguishing cardiac from noncardiac disease (such as pneumothorax or respiratory distress syndrome) and aids in providing a reliable differential diagnosis when cardiac disease is suspected. It may not be possible, however, to determine the specific cardiac defect on the basis of the plain film alone. A systematic approach to film examination is essential to obtain the maximum amount of information from the roentgenogram.[1] Close attention must be paid to the pulmonary vascular pattern, configuration of the pulmonary artery and aorta, and heart size and shape, as well as the position of the heart and abnormalities of the bony thorax.

Pulmonary Vascular Pattern

Evaluation of the pulmonary arterial vasculature is essential in attempting to classify congenital heart disease radiographically (Table 6-1). Pulmonary arterial vasculature may be normal, increased, or decreased. Assessment of pulmonary vascularity is difficult in an individual of any age; however, this is especially true in the first month of life. The radiographic appearance of the pulmonary vasculature

117

TABLE 6-1.   Roentgenographic Classification of Congenital Heart Disease by Degrees of Pulmonary Arterial Vascularity

Increased Pulmonary Arterial Vascularity	Decreased Pulmonary Arterial Vascularity	Normal Pulmonary Arterial Vascularity or Passive Venous Congestion
Atrial septal defect	Tetralogy of Fallot	Aortic stenosis
Ventricular septal defect	Pulmonary atresia	Coarctation of the aorta
Atrioventricular canal defect	Tricuspid atresia	Mitral stenosis
Patent ductus arteriosus	Ebstein's malformation	Cor triatriatum
Anomalous pulmonary venous return (unobstructed)	Pulmonary hypertension	Total anomalous pulmonary venous return (obstructed)
Truncus arteriosus	Transposition with pulmonary stenosis	Endocardial fibroelastosis
Transposition of the great arteries		Pulmonary valve stenosis
Hypoplastic left heart syndrome		

depends on many technical factors, including exposure time and the degree of lung inflation. The desired degree of exposure is achieved when the thoracic spine is seen through the mediastinal shadow in the frontal projection. In an overpenetrated film, the lung fields appear dark and the pulmonary vasculature appears decreased. An expiratory film crowds and accentuates the vascular markings.

Severe cardiac malformations such as atrioventricular canal defects, truncus arteriosus, or a large ventricular septal defect may be present in conjunction with normal pulmonary vasculature in the first week of life. The high pulmonary vascular resistance of the newborn circulation limits left-to-right shunting, and pulmonary blood flow is not excessive. The age at presentation of these lesions depends on the rate of decrease in pulmonary vascular resistance. The medial muscle layer in the pulmonary arterioles is less developed in the premature infant than in a full-term infant and this may explain a more rapid postnatal fall in pulmonary vascular resistance.[1,2] Clinical and radiographic signs of a left-to-right shunt may become evident as early as the first few days of life in the premature infant. In the full-term infant, the presence of a large communication between the systemic and pulmonary circulation may retard the fall of pulmonary vascular resistance, and findings of pulmonary overcirculation may not appear until the infant is 4 to 6 weeks of age.

Normal pulmonary vascular markings are usually visualized into the middle one-third of the lung fields. Hilar pulmonary arteries are easily identified. The diameter of a pulmonary artery seen "end on" in the middle third of the lung field is normally similar to that of an adjacent bronchus. It is normal for premature infants to have sparse pulmonary vasculature,

probably because of their small size and decreased number of pulmonary vessels compared with those of the full-term infant. Normal pulmonary vasculature is seen in newborns with uncomplicated or mild semilunar valvular stenosis, in patients with coarctation of the aorta in whom the ductus arteriosus is patent, and in individuals with myocardial disease that has not resulted in left-sided heart failure. Nonstructural types of heart disease, such as arrhythmias or asphyxia, may cause cardiomegaly with normal pulmonary vasculature.

Increased pulmonary arterial vascularity results from increased pulmonary blood flow (Fig. 6-1). This pattern is seen in left-to-right shunting at the atrial, ventricular, or great artery level or with truncus arteriosus or transposition of the great arteries. Enlargement of the pulmonary arteries is not apparent radiographically until the pulmonary flow is greater than twice the systemic flow. The pulmonary trunk is prominent. The diameter of an enlarged pulmonary artery is larger than that of an adjacent "end on" bronchus. If the flow is so excessive that congestive heart failure occurs, pulmonary edema may coexist with increased pulmonary vascularity.

Decreased pulmonary vascularity reflects diminished pulmonary blood flow (Fig. 6-2). This pattern is seen with obstructive lesions of the right ventricular outflow tract such as pulmonary atresia, severe pulmonary stenosis, or tetralogy of Fallot. Pulmonary blood flow is also diminished in persistent pulmonary hypertension of the newborn, which is characterized by postnatal persistence or re-emergence of fetal circulatory patterns: right-to-left shunting at the ductal or atrial level. Lung fields appear hyperlucent or dark. Peripheral pulmonary arteries are thin and stringy and extend into the lung periphery only to the

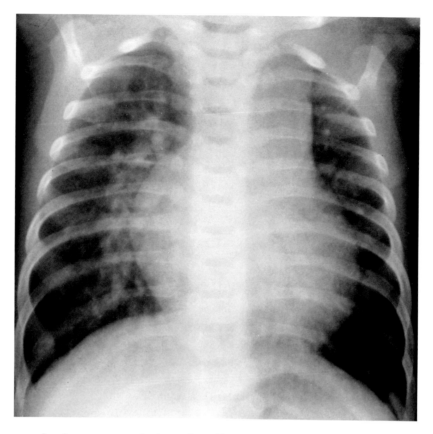

Fig. 6-1. Increased pulmonary vascularity and cardiomegaly as a result of unobstructed total anomalous pulmonary venous return to the coronary sinus. Prominent convexity of right heart border is due to right atrial enlargement.

junction of the inner and middle third. On the lateral film, the pulmonary artery branches are small and the hila appear empty.

It is important to differentiate pulmonary arteries from pulmonary veins on the chest radiogram. Pulmonary arteries radiate from the hila and taper gradually through the middle third of the lung fields. Pulmonary veins are straight in their course and are directed toward the left atrium. Pulmonary veins in the normal state have little influence in the vascular pattern.

Prominent pulmonary vascularity as a result of pulmonary venous hypertension results from left-sided obstructive lesions or left ventricular dysfunction resulting in left ventricular failure. Typical neonatal causes include coarctation of the aorta, hypoplastic left heart syndrome, cor triatriatum, mitral stenosis, pulmonary venous obstruction, endocardial fibroelastosis, and cardiomyopathy. In upright patients there is a redistribution of blood flow from the lower lobe to the upper lobe arteries and veins, a pattern generally not seen in the supine newborn.[3] With the rise in venous pressure, there is transudation of vascular fluid into the perivascular, peribronchial, and interstitial spaces. Individual vessel margins and bronchi in the hilum become indistinct and hazy. Kerley B lines, which are interlobular septa thickened by distended lymphatics and edema, appear as short horizontal lines of increased density in the costophrenic angle. Alveolar pulmonary edema and pleural effusion can occur. Generally, the degree of pulmonary congestion in left-sided obstructive lesions depends on the size of the interatrial communication, which acts to decompress the left atrium and, consequently, the pulmonary veins.

Unequal pulmonary vascularity often is reported with truncus arteriosus and transposition of the great arteries. Unilateral pulmonary atresia or severe stenosis of main pulmonary artery branch may also produce a decreased vascular pattern in the affected lung

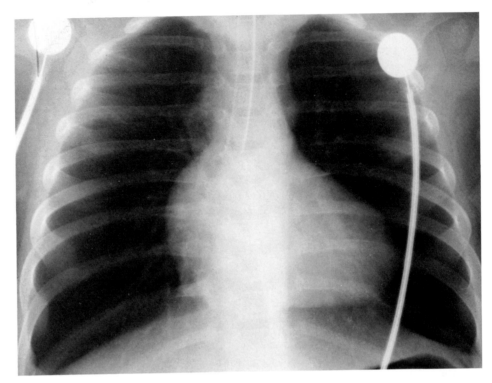

Fig. 6-2. Decreased pulmonary arterial vascularity in a neonate with pulmonary atresia and intact ventricular septal defect. Heart size is normal. Mediastinum is narrow and pulmonary artery segment is concave. The lungs have a hyperlucent apearance. Pulmonary arteries are sparse and thin.

with compensatory increased vascularity in the contralateral lung. The affected lung is usually small. Milder degrees of main pulmonary artery or peripheral branch stenosis are not apparent radiographically. Bronchial compression by a dilated pulmonary artery or left atrium, with resultant emphysema or atelectasis of that lung, produces a discrepancy in pulmonary inflation and apparent vascularity. Similar features are seen with congenital lobar emphysema (Fig. 6-3).

Configuration of Pulmonary Artery and Aorta

Pulmonary Artery

The main pulmonary artery is either normal, dilated (convex), or small (concave). The main pulmonary artery may not be apparent in the normal newborn due to overlying thymic tissue (Fig. 6-4).

Prominence of the main pulmonary artery may be observed with pulmonary valve stenosis due to poststenotic dilation, and in conditions with increased pulmonary blood flow, as in left-to-right shunts or pulmonary insufficiency. Aneurysmal dilatation of the pulmonary artery occurs in association with absence of the pulmonary valve.[4-6] The main pulmonary artery is grossly enlarged and there is frequently dilatation of the branches, more commonly the right. The peripheral pulmonary vessels may also be affected. Bronchial compression by dilated pulmonary vessels may produce air trapping and emphysema in the affected lung. In patients with pulmonary hypertension induced by long-standing increased pulmonary blood flow, proximal pulmonary arteries are prominent with abrupt tapering of the distal two-thirds of the pulmonary arterial tree ("pruned tree" effect).

A small or flat pulmonary artery indicates pulmonary artery underdevelopment or abnormal positioning. Underdevelopment of the pulmonary trunk occurs in most lesions producing right ventricular outflow obstruction (tetralogy of Fallot, pulmonary atresia). Abnormal position of the pulmonary trunk can be obvious in transposition of the great arteries and in most types of truncus arteriosus.

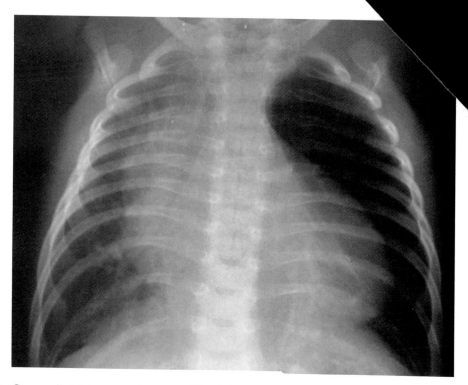

Fig. 6-3. Congenital lobar emphysema. The left lung is hyperlucent with crowding of the lung markings in the medial portion of the left lower lobe. Hyperinflation of the left lung has resulted in shift of the heart to the right.

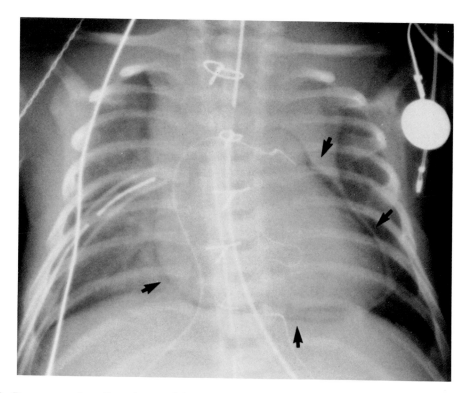

Fig. 6-4. Pneumopericardium (arrows) in a postoperative patient, outlining the cardiac silhouette. The pulmonary artery segment is now distinguishable from thymus.

sualize because
escending aorta
d posteroanter-
ed for size and

ly to decreased
t shunts) or the
nderdeveloped,
, supravalvular
arch. A promi-
ic valve stenosis
(poststenotic dilatation) and conditions that result in increased aortic blood flow, such as great vessel left-to-right shunting (patent ductus arteriosus, aortopulmonary window) and aortic insufficiency. The aorta in the infant form of coarctation of the aorta is normal or small, and the figure-3 sign is absent.

Laterality of the aortic arch is defined by the relationship of the aortic arch to the trachea on the posteroanterior view. A left aortic arch produces a slight deviation of the trachea to the right. A right aortic arch is recognized by a fullness in the right superior mediastinum and by displacement of the trachea to the left (Fig. 6-5). A right aortic arch in the presence of levocardia may be an important distinguishing feature of certain cardiac lesions. Table 6-2 shows the incidence of right aortic arch in various cardiac defects.

Heart Size and Shape

Cardiac enlargement generally indicates underlying cardiac disease, either structural or functional. However, a normal cardiac silhouette does not exclude underlying cardiac pathology. For example, the heart size is typically normal in tetralogy of Fallot and in obstructed total anomalous pulmonary venous return.

Cardiac enlargement in the neonate is defined as a cardiothoracic ratio exceeding 0.58 on a supine film made at a 40-inch focal spot–film distance in adequate inspiration.[7] The cardiothoracic ratio is the ratio of the largest transverse dimension of the heart to the widest intercostal diameter of the chest. Adequate inspiration is assessed by counting the posterior ribs. The diaphragm should be at least at the level

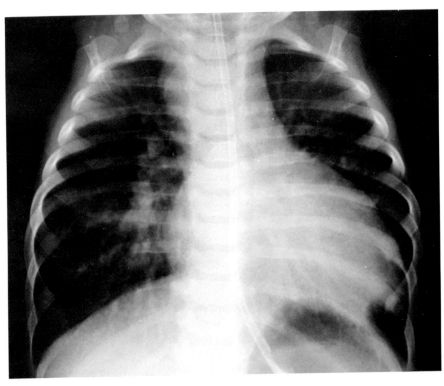

Fig. 6-5. Truncus arteriosus. The heart is enlarged and pulmonary arterial markings are increased. The superior mediastinum is narrow. The trachea is displaced to the left by a right aortic arch.

TABLE 6-2. Incidence of Right Aortic Arch in Congenital Heart Defects

Type of Defect	Incidence (%)
Tetralogy of Fallot	31.0
Truncus arteriosus	31.0
Pulmonary atresia and ventricular septal defect	30.0
Double-outlet right ventricle	20.0
Tricuspid atresia	5.0
Isolated ventricular septal defect	2.3
Complete dextrotransposition of great arteries	2.3

of the ninth rib posteriorly for satisfactory interpretation of chest films. During exhalation, the higher diaphragmatic position gives the heart a more transverse orientation, exaggerating the heart size and compressing the pulmonary vascular markings.

In addition, many technical factors, such as projection and focal spot–film distance, influence the apparent heart size on a thoracic radiogram. For example, the cardiac silhouette appears larger on an anteroposterior (AP) projection than on posteroanterior (PA) projection. Portable roentgenograms cause apparent enlargement, since patients are usually supine, and AP projections are made at a short focal spot–film distance of 40 inches as compared with the standard 6-foot distance for an upright PA view of the thorax.

In the neonate and young child, the thymic silhouette may obscure the heart border, making an interpretation of cardiac size difficult. At times a characteristic notch is visible, separating the lower thymic margin from the heart (the "sail sign") (Fig. 6-6). The thymus may also be identified by its wavy or lobulated margins produced by indentation by the costal cartilages (the "wave sign") and its anterior mediastinal location as seen on an oblique or lateral chest radiograph. Fluoroscopy demonstrates marked variability of thymic size with inspiration and expiration. The thymus regresses in conditions of perinatal stress such as sepsis, asphyxia, and heart disease. The thymus is absent in DiGeorge's syndrome, a developmental abnormality of the third and fourth branchial arch, reulting in thymic hypoplasia, parathyroid hy-

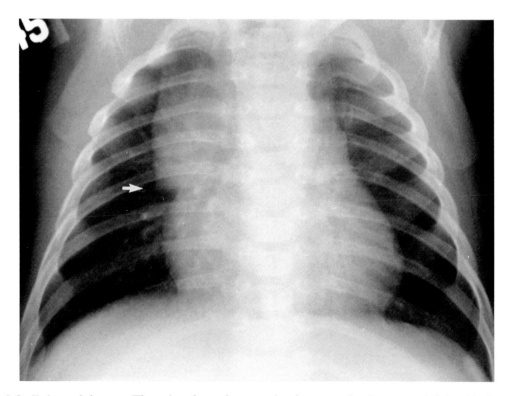

Fig. 6-6. Enlarged thymus. There is a sharp demarcation between the thymus and right-sided cardiac contour (arrow), yielding the typical "sail sign."

poplasia, and conotruncal cardiac defects. Di-George's syndrome should be suspected in infants with truncus arteriosus or interrupted aortic arch with an absent thymic silhouette, persistent hypocalcemia, and immune dysfunction.

The cardiac contour is variable in the neonate since it is greatly influenced by patient position and the angulation of the x-ray beam. A lordotic projection, in which the clavicles are projected above the first rib, is common in neonates. In this projection, the cardiac apex may appear falsely elevated, mimicking right ventricular hypertrophy, and the cardiac contour appears globular. The pulmonary arterial segment is more prominent. Similarly, slight rotation of the patient on the PA view distorts the cardiac shape and contour. The patient is properly positioned when the anterior ends of the clavicles are symmetric and equidistant from the thoracic spine.

The right cardiac border on the PA projection is formed by the superior vena cava (upper one-third) and the right atrium (lower two-thirds). The left cardiac border, running cephalocaudal, is formed by the aortic knob, main pulmonary artery, left atrial appendage, and left ventricle. The right ventricle does not contribute to any of the cardiac borders on this projection. Evaluation of individual cardiac chamber size is difficult and unreliable in infants because of overlying thymic tissue.[8-10] Radiographic findings are much more prominent with chamber dilatation (volume overload) than with chamber hypertrophy (pressure overload). The "coeur en sabot" (boot-shaped heart) or upturned apex occurs in about one-third of patients with tetralogy of Fallot,[11] and an egg-shaped heart with narrow base is more common in newborns with transposition of the great arteries.[12] An abnormal cardiac silhouette is unreliable for establishing an accurate cardiac diagnosis. Abnormalities of cardiac contour are determined by the hemodynamic effects of cardiovascular lesions and are therefore more predictive of a physiologic than an anatomic diagnosis.

An enlarged heart may be the presenting manifestation for a variety of noncardiac conditions. Cardiac enlargement has been reported in term newborn infants who had suffered perinatal asphyxia.[13] The cardiac size in the majority of infants with transient

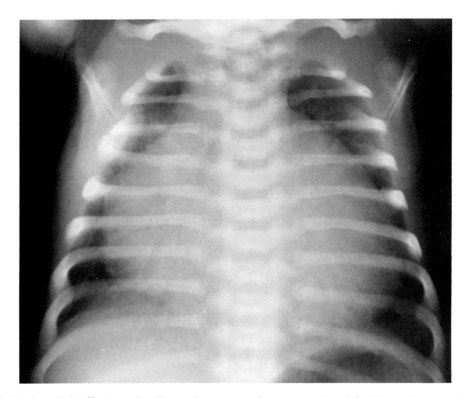

Fig. 6-7. Pericardial effusion. Cardiac enlargement is symmetric, with bilateral convexities and narrow mediastinum.

tachypnea of the newborn is normal or borderline enlarged.[14] Congestive heart failure may result from polycythemia.[15,16] Heart failure from high cardiac output may occur in patients with systemic hemangiomas, arteriovenous malformations such as aneurysm of the vein of Galen, congenital hyperthyroid-

ism,[17,18] or severe anemia, as in the newborn with hemolytic disease or twin-to-twin transfusion.[19] Congenital hypothyroidism may result in cardiomegaly due to congestive heart failure or pericardial effusion.[20]

Nonstructural cardiac disease may result in cardio-

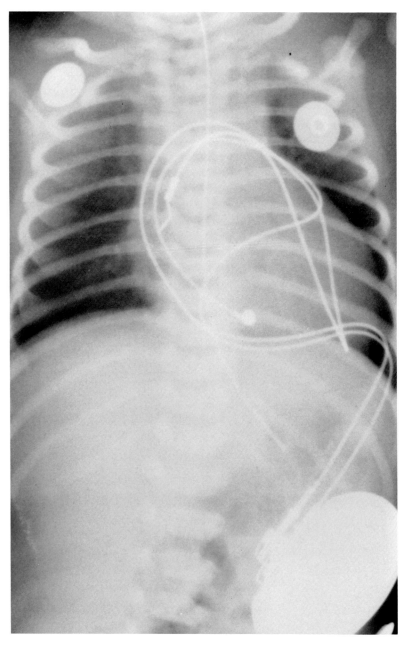

Fig. 6-8. Cardiomegaly and normal pulmonary vascular markings. Pacemaker placement for bradycardia secondary to congenital complete heart block. Patients with bradycardia maintain cardiac output by increasing stroke volume and, therefore, ventricular size.

megaly and abnormal pulmonary vascularity. Myocarditis due to group B coxsackie,[21] rubella,[22] herpes, or enteric cytopathogenic human orphan (ECHO)[23] viruses may cause a devastating illness characterized by cardiomegaly, ventricular failure, and circulatory collapse. Pericardial effusion is a rare cause of cardiomegaly in neonates (Fig. 6-7).[24] It may be infectious or may occur in postoperative cardiac patients as the postpericardiotomy syndrome. Tachyarrhythmias in infants may result in cardiac enlargement and pulmonary vascular congestion.[25] These findings are reversible after successful treatment of the arrhythmias. Infants with bradycardia resulting from complete heart block[26] (Fig. 6-8) may demonstrate mild to moderate cardiomegaly with normal pulmonary vasculature. Cardiac tumors in the newborn infant are an extremely rare cause of cardiomegaly. Rhabdomyoma, the most common cardiac tumor in infancy, is often associated with tuberous sclerosis[27,28] (Fig. 6-9). Other less common cardiac tumors reported in infancy are rhabdomyosarcoma[29] and myxoma.[30] Infants of diabetic mothers may have cardiomegaly in association with macrosomia. Cellular hyperplasia and hypertrophy are thought to be responsible for multiorgan enlargement.[31] In newborns with type II glycogen storage disease, the chest radiograph may reveal moderate to massive cardiomegaly with normal pulmonary vasculature or vascular congestion.[32] Echocardiography may reveal marked thickening of the ventricular wall or significant obstruction of left ventricular outflow.[33]

POSITION ANOMALIES OF THE HEART

Cardiac malposition denotes location of the heart anywhere other than the usual position in the left hemithorax (levocardia). The heart may be right sided (dextrocardia), midline (mesocardia), or extrathoracic (ectopia cordis). Any heart position other than left sided in situs solitus constitutes cardiac malposition. This definition incorporates not only the cardiac position but also the appropriateness of the cardiac position in relation to the position of other organs. For example, a left-sided heart with situs inversus is also an example of cardiac malposition.

True cardiac malposition must be distinguished from shift of the heart within the thorax by extracardiac causes, such as decreased lung volume as in atelectasis, hypoplastic lung, increased lung volume as in lobar emphysema, pleural space abnormalities as in tension pneumothorax, pleural effusion, bronchogenic cyst, diaphragmatic hernia, and thoracic cage abnormalities as in scoliosis.

These conditions result in displacement not only of the heart but all mediastinal structures, including the trachea, aorta, and hilar vessels. The chest radiograph reveals associated findings that are frequently helpful in making this determination. For example, shift of the heart into the right hemithorax due to atelectasis of the right lung is frequently associated with increased density of the right lung, elevation of the right hemidiaphragm, and crowding of the right ribs.

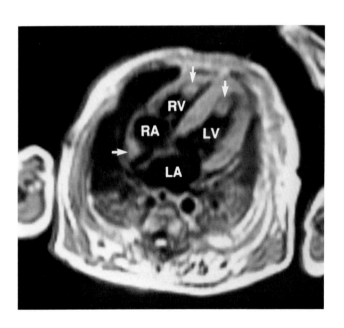

Fig. 6-9. Magnetic resonance imaging showing oblique axial view in a 3-month-old infant with tuberous sclerosis. Intracardiac tumors (arrows) are noted at apex of right (RV) and left (LV) ventricles and in the right atrium (RA). LA, left atrium (Courtesy of Clark L. Carrol, Department of Radiology, Texas Children's Hospital, Houston, Texas.)

There may be compensatory hyperexpansion and overaeration of the left-side lung. Cardiac displacement by extracardiac factors is known as dextroposition, mesoposition, or levoposition, depending on the direction of the shift.

The lungs, liver, spleen, stomach, and atria are usually asymmetric or unpaired organs and the term *situs* is used to define their position relative to the midline or sagittal plane. The location of the morphologic left and right atria may be reasonably determined on the basis of visceroatrial concordance: the types of visceral situs and atrial situs are almost always the same. On the chest radiograph the locations of the stomach bubble (or nasogastric tube course), liver shadow, and air bronchogram usually indicate the atrial locations with accuracy.

There are three types of visceroatrial situs: solitus, inversus, or ambiguus. In situs solitus, which is normal, the liver is on the right and the stomach and spleen are on the left. The morphologic left atrium is posterior and left sided. In situs inversus, the mirror image of normal, the stomach and spleen are on the right, the liver is on the left, and the morphologic left atrium is on the right. In situs ambiguus both the type of visceral situs and the type of atrial situs are anatomically uncertain or indeterminate. The liver may be symmetric and midline and the stomach bubble may be central. There is typically duplication or absence of normally unilateral structures, such as the spleen (asplenia or ploysplenia).

Atria-bronchial concordance is more reliable in predicting atrial situs than is abdominal viscera–atrium concordance. The morphologic right lung has three lobes, and the bronchus to the right upper lobe passes over the right pulmonary artery (eparterial bronchus). The morphologic left lung has two lobes and the left main stem bronchus passes beneath the left pulmonary artery (hyparterial bronchus). Air bronchograms are evident on overpenetrated chest roentgenograms. In newborns, it may be difficult to assess whether a bronchus is eparterial or hyparterial. A more useful feature is that the left main stem bronchus is typically twice as long as the right main stem bronchus.

The most reliable method of atrial localization is by inferior vena cava–right atrium concordance as determined by two-dimensional echocardiography.

The presence of an abnormal visceroatrial relationship has major implications in terms of the likelihood and type of intracardiac abnormalities. In general, if there is discordance between atrial and visceral situs, as in dextrocardia with situs solitus or levocardia with situs inversus, the incidence of complex cardiac anomalies is very high.[34]

Dextrocardia with situs solitus, which may also be termed *dextroversion, dextrorotation, pivotal dextrocardia,* or *isolated dextrocardia,* implies that the dextrocardia is an isolated finding and that all other organs are in their normal position in the body. The condition is almost always associated with intracardiac abnormalities. Conversely, in dextrocardia with situs inversus, or mirror-image dextrocardia, the heart and abdominal organs are on the right side of the body, and the incidence of congenital heart disease is the same as in the general population. Kartagener's syndrome is present in 15 to 25 percent of patients with situs inversus.

Bony Thorax Abnormalities

A higher incidence of abnormalities of the bony thorax occurs in children with congenital heart disease, particularly cyanotic defects, than in the general population. Recognition of abnormalities of the skeletal system are important in the overall prognosis of the child and may assist in the identification of genetically or nongenetically determined syndromes associated with congenital heart disease.

Premature fusion of sternal ossification sites occurs in 15 percent of patients with congenital heart disease, compared with 2 percent of the normal population.[35,36] This deformity results in a pectus carinatum deformity of the sternum, and is more common in patients with cyanotic than in those with acyanotic cardiac anomalies. There is a significant incidence of idiopathic scoliosis in patients with congenital heart disease, especially tetralogy of Fallot and coarctation of the aorta.[37,38] Scoliosis resulting from congenital vertebral abnormalities also occurs with a higher incidence in this population (Fig. 6-10). Unrecognized scoliosis may lead to progressive compromise in cardiorespiratory function. Skeletal maturation may be delayed in patients with congenital heart disease.

Rib notching is a valuable sign in the diagnosis of coarctation of the aorta, although it is usually not seen before age 6 or 7. Most commonly, the fourth to eighth ribs are involved.[39]

Abnormalities of the skeletal system can occur in a variety of genetically determined syndromes that are associated with congenital heart disease.[40] Bone changes described in Down's syndrome are an increased number of ossification centers in the sternum

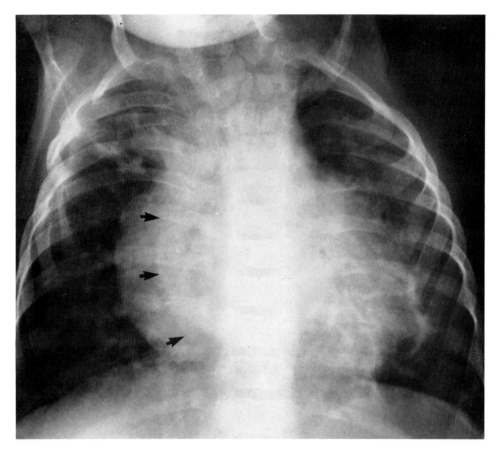

Fig. 6-10. Numerous cervical hemivertebral and rib anomalies in a neonate with tetralogy of Fallot. Placement of a systemic-to-pulmonary artery shunt resulted in pulmonary overcirculation, cardiomegaly, and pulmonary edema. Note the double density shadow of the enlarged left atrium (arrows) superimposed on the right atrium.

(hypersegmentation of the sternum),[41-43] absence of the 12th ribs,[44] and an abnormal configuration of the lumbar vertebrae[45] (Fig. 6-11). When the roentgenographic features of the long bones suggest rubella syndrome, patent ductus arteriosus and peripheral pulmonary branch stenosis are commonly associated cardiac lesions.[46,47]

RADIOGRAPHIC FEATURES OF CONGENITAL HEART DEFECTS

Increased Pulmonary Arterial Markings

Ventricular Septal Defect

The radiographic findings of a patient with ventricular septal defect are not specific for that anatomic malformation, but reflect the size of the left-to-right

shunt and the state of the pulmonary vascular bed (Fig. 6-12). With small defects, the heart size and pulmonary vascularity may be normal.

With moderate-sized defects the cardiac silhouette is enlarged, with a prominent left ventricular contour. The left atrium is usually enlarged. On the PA projection this may be evidenced by displacement upward of the left main stem bronchus. In the lateral projection the left atrium bulges posteriorly, often displacing the esophageal air column. Pulmonary vascular markings are increased, both centrally and peripherally.

Large defects associated with increased blood flow show cardiomegaly with a more globular cardiac silhouette, due to right and left ventricular enlargement, as well as left atrial and, occasionally, right atrial enlargement. Pulmonary vascularity is markedly increased. With large left-to-right shunts and

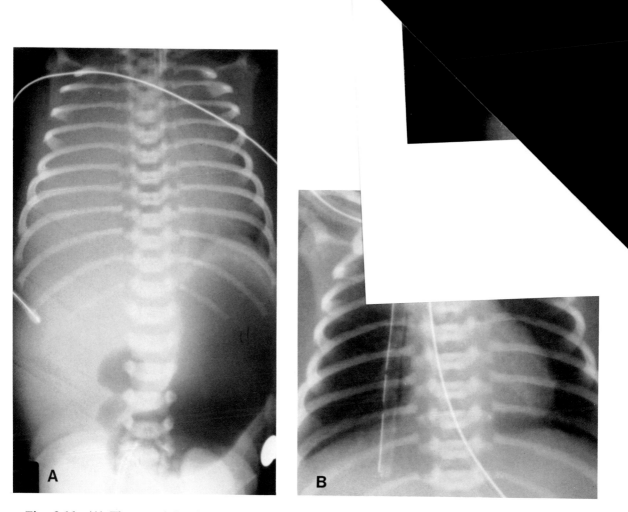

Fig. 6-11. (A) Thoracoabdominal roentgenogram in a 36 weeks' gestation newborn with Down's syndrome demonstrating an opacified thorax, absence of the 12th ribs, and the double bubble sign of duodenal atresia. **(B)** Thoracic roentgenogram in the same patient after chest tube drainage of a right hydrothorax. The heart size and pulmonary vascular markings are normal. Echocardiogram confirmed a structurally normal heart.

congestive heart failure, interstitial edema, alveolar fluid, and Kerley B lines (indicating pulmonary venous engorgement) may be present. The reduced pulmonary compliance and increased respiratory effort are often reflected by chest hyperexpansion and flattening of the diaphragms.

With long-standing pulmonary hypertension, there may be a decrease, or even reversal, in the left-to-right shunt. The heart size is normal or minimally enlarged. Overall pulmonary vascularity is decreased, the main pulmonary artery segment is enlarged, and central hilar pulmonary markings are more prominent than are the peripheral markings ("pruning" of the pulmonary arterial tree).

Atrial Septal Defect

The roentgenographic findings in patients with atrial septal defect depend on the size of the defect and the magnitude of the left-to-right shunt. When defects are small the chest roentgenogram is normal. In case of a large left-to-right shunt there is moderate cardiac enlargement and increased pulmonary arterial vascularity. The right atrium and right ventricle are enlarged. Left atrial enlargement is absent because of the ease with which the atrium decompresses itself through the large atrial communication directly into the right atrium.

Shunting tends to be minimal in the neonate, even

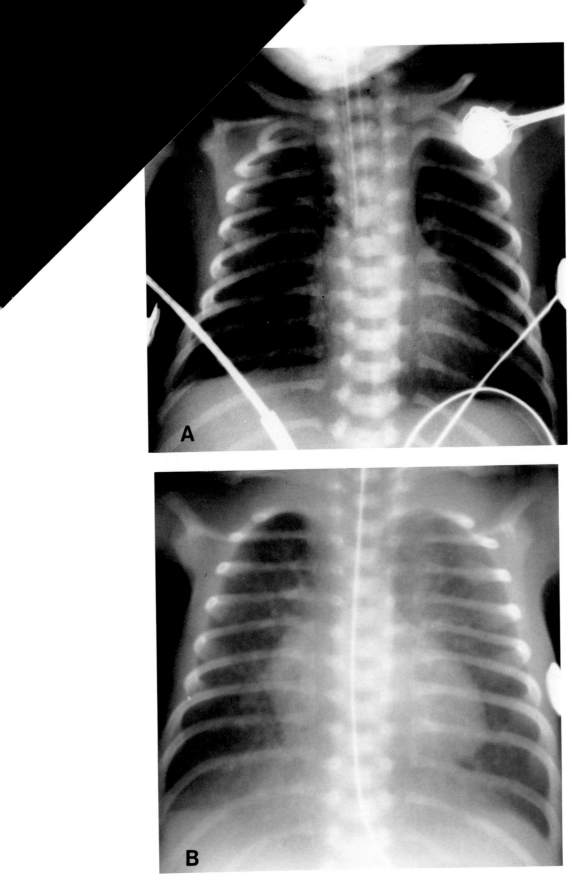

Fig. 6-12. Legend on facing page.

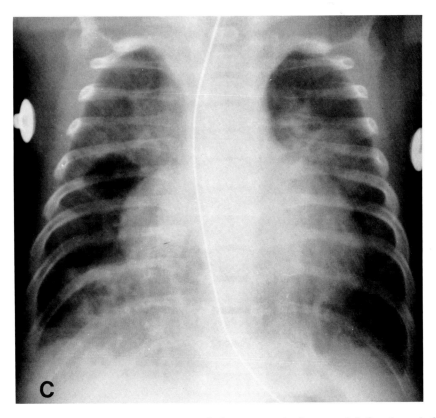

Fig. 6-12. Series of thoracic roentgenograms of a large ventricular septal defect in an infant born at 32 weeks' gestation. **(A)** Immediately after birth, heart size and pulmonary vascularity are normal as a result of elevated pulmonary vascular resistance and minimal shunting through the defect. **(B)** One month later, moderate cardiomegaly is present and pulmonary vascularity is increased. The normal postnatal drop in pulmonary vascular resistance allows a larger left-to-right shunt through the ventricular septal defect. **(C)** At 2 months of age there is progressive cardiomegaly and increased pulmonary vascular markings with patchy, indistinct, fluffy appearance of severe pulmonary edema. The right middle lobe shows increased aeration from air trapping.

when there is a large defect, because of the hemodynamics of the neonatal circulation. The direction and amount of interatrial shunting are determined by the relative pressures in the right and left atria, which, in turn are principally determined by the right and left ventricular diastolic compliance and the ratio of pulmonary to systemic vascular resistance. An increase in interatrial shunting occurs with the postnatal increase in right ventricular compliance that accompanies the normal postnatal drop in pulmonary vascular resistance.

Atrioventricular Canal Defects

The roentgenographic features of atrioventricular canal defects vary, depending on the type and severity of the components of the defect. In complete atrio-

ventricular canal defect the heart size is usually more globular or rounded than it appears in isolated ventricular septal defect because of the combined hemodynamic effects of a left-to-right shunt at the atrial and ventricular levels and atrioventricular valve insufficiency. In the incomplete form of atrioventricular canal defect, the ostium primum atrial septal defect, and cleft mitral valve without significant mitral regurgitation, the roentgenographic findings are indistinguishable from those of an atrial septal defect. If mitral regurgitation is significant the cardiac silhouette is markedly enlarged.

Patent Ductus Arteriosus

There is no correlation between roentgenographic findings and the presence of patent ductus arteriosus in premature infants. Pulmonary vasculature, and often the cardiac silhouette, are obscured by pulmonary parenchymal markings of respiratory distress syndrome. Lung fields may show varying degrees of pulmonary edema. A high index of clinical suspicion and the results of echocardiography are more reliable indicators of a patent ductus arteriosus than are chest roentgenograms.

In infants, the roentgenographic findings vary with the size of the ductus and the amount of left-to-right shunting. The chest radiograph may show increased pulmonary vascularity, as well as left atrial and left ventricular enlargement and a prominent aortic knob along the left upper heart border.

Total Anomalous Pulmonary Venous Connection

Total anomalous pulmonary venous connection (TAPVC) occurs when all pulmonary veins drain into the right atrium or into a venous channel in communication with the right atrium. The heart is enlarged as a result of right atrial and right ventricular en-largement, and pulmonary arterial markings are increased (Fig. 6-1). In the most common anomalous connection, the pulmonary veins drain into the right atrium by way of a common chamber that empties via a left vertical vein into the innominate vein, which then empties into the right superior vena cava. Enlargement of these structures as a result of increased blood flow may produce a characteristic widening of the superior mediastinum in a "snowman" or "figure-8" pattern. The snowman configuration is rare in neonates, what appears to be a snowman configuration in a newborn is most likely caused by a large thymus.

TAPVC below the diaphragm is almost always associated with severe obstruction to pulmonary venous return. Heart size is normal because of obstruction to venous return within the liver. Lung fields demonstrate a diffuse, linear reticular pattern, which represents pulmonary venous engorgement and lymphatic distension (Fig. 6-13). Pulmonary edema with prominent Kerley B lines is present. Ill-defined haziness of

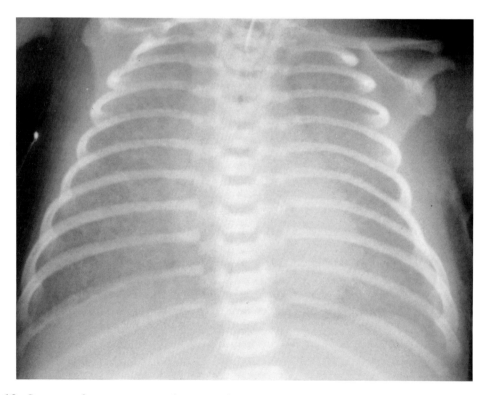

Fig. 6-13. Severe pulmonary venous hypertension as a result of obstructed total anomalous pulmonary venous return below the diaphragm. Heart size is normal. There is diffuse, bilateral, ill-defined haziness of pulmonary edema, indistinguishable from the appearance of respiratory distress syndrome. However, lung volumes are normal and air bronchograms are absent.

both lung fields may obscure the heart border. The overall radiographic appearance may be indistinguishable from that of hyaline membrane disease; however, the presence of normal lung volumes and absence of air bronchograms suggest cardiac rather than pulmonary disease. This entity is distinguished from transient tachypnea of the newborn, which is characterized by cardiac enlargement, fluid in the interlobar fissures, and pleural effusion. A similar roentgenographic pattern is produced by left-sided obstructive lesions such as congenital mitral stenosis, hypoplastic left heart syndrome, pulmonary vein stenosis, pulmonary vein atresia, or cor triatriatum. Echocardiography is particularly helpful in the further evaluation of a newborn with suspected obstructed TAPVC.

The most widely described radiographic finding in partial anomalous pulmonary venous return occurs when the right lung drains anomalously by a single vessel to the inferior vena cava at the level of the diaphragm, with the anomalous vessel resembling a curved scimitar sword. This rare finding, when asso-ciated with malposition of the heart and hypoplasia of the right lung with aberrant arterial supply, is termed *scimitar syndrome.*

Truncus Arteriosus

The heart is enlarged in truncus arteriosus because of right and left ventricular prominence and left atrial dilatation (Fig. 6-5). The pulmonary artery segment is concave and pulmonary arterial markings are usually greatly increased. As congestive heart failure develops, the pulmonary vessels become indistinct and obscured by pulmonary edema. In 30 to 50 percent of patients with truncus arteriosus a right aortic arch occurs, and this is useful radiographic finding in distinguishing truncus arteriosus from transposition of the great arteries.

Transposition of the Great Arteries

There are no distinct roentgenographic features for diagnosing complete transposition of the great arteries (Fig. 6-14). A narrow mediastinum and ab-

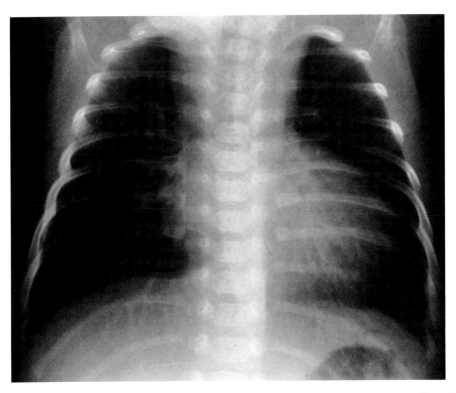

Fig. 6-14. Transposition of the great arteries with intact ventricular septum at 1 day of age. The heart is normal and pulmonary vascularity is at the upper limits of normal. The pulmonary artery segment is concave. The thymus is not atrophic.

sence of a discrete pulmonary segment are due to the AP relation of the great arteries. Cardiomegaly may or may not be seen. The "egg on a string" description (a narrow mediastinal shadow and an ovoid heart shape) occurs in one-third of patients with transposition of the great arteries and an intact ventricular septum. This pattern is nonspecific and occurs in patients with a variety of other congenital heart defects. Pulmonary vascularity is variable, depending on the basic anatomic features that determine the physiology, such as the additional presence of a ventricular septal defect, patent ductus arteriosus, or subpulmonic stenosis.

In the patient with transposition and an intact ventricular septum, the pulmonary vascular markings to the right lung are often increased compared with those to the left since approximately two-thirds of the output of the left ventricle may be directed preferentially to the right lung.[48]

Hypoplastic Left Heart Syndrome

Hypoplastic left heart syndrome is a group of cardiac malformations characterized by varying degrees of underdevelopment of left heart structures. In the most marked cases, severe stenosis or atresia of the mitral and aortic valves is present, and the left ventricle and ascending aorta show marked hypoplasia. The chest radiogram is nonspecific. Cardiomegaly is a feature in 75 to 85 percent of patients. The cardiac silhouette has been described as globular, rounded with a narrow base, or normal with a pulmonary artery bulge.[49] The pattern of pulmonary vascularity is variable, depending on the size of the interatrial communication. Pulmonary vascular markings are increased in the majority of patients because of obligatory left-to-right shunting across a large, nonrestrictive foramen ovale. Marked pulmonary venous hypertension occurs in the presence of a severely restrictive foramen ovale because of the impaired exit of blood from the left side of the heart.

The underdeveloped aorta is often small or nonexistent, but this is difficult to assess in neonates because of the overlying thymus. Furthermore, the pulmonary artery may become so enlarged and highly positioned that it mimics the aortic knob.

Decreased Pulmonary Arterial Markings

Tetralogy of Fallot

In an infant with tetralogy of Fallot the cardiac size and configuration are frequently normal; however,

pulmonary vascular markings are decreased. The chest roentgenogram in older children with tetralogy of Fallot exhibits the classically described "coeur en sabot" (boot-shaped) configuration. It includes an upturned cardiac apex caused by right ventricular hypertrophy (Fig. 6-15) and concavity of the upper left heart border caused by an absence of the main pulmonary artery segment. This configuration may be seen in infants with pulmonary atresia rather than pulmonary stenosis. A right aortic arch is found in approximately 25 to 30 percent of patients with tetralogy of Fallot.

Pulmonary Valve Atresia

Chest roentgenograms in pulmonary valve atresia with an intact ventricular septum vary, depending on the size of the interatrial communication and competence of the tricuspid valve. In cases wherein there is a hypoplastic right ventricle and minimal or no tricuspid insufficiency, the heart size is normal. In cases wherein there is a normal right ventricle or tricuspid insufficiency, the overall heart size is increased and the right atrium is enlarged. The main pulmonary artery may be almost normal, flat, or concave in size. Pulmonary vascularity is reduced or normal, depending on the presence of alternative sources of pulmonary blood flow, such as the patent ductus arteriosus. The aortic arch is left sided; a right aortic arch is more common in cases of pulmonary atresia with a ventricular septal defect.

In contrast, in patients with pulmonary atresia with a ventricular septal defect, the pulmonary arteries are generally small and underdeveloped. Heart size is normal or only mildly increased, and an upturned cardiac apex is often seen. A right aortic arch occurs in approximately 30 percent of patients.

Tricuspid Atresia

The heart is generally enlarged in tricuspid atresia, with a prominent right heart border due to right atrial enlargement. In the majority of patients pulmonary blood flow is diminished and pulmonary vascular markings are decreased. In the remainder of patients pulmonary vascular markings are increased.

Ebstein's Malformation of the Tricuspid Valve

In Ebstein's malformation of the tricuspid valve the septal and posterior leaflets of the tricuspid valve are abnormally displaced toward the ventricular apex.

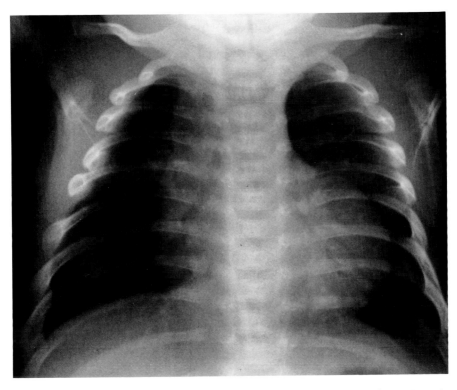

Fig. 6-15. Upturned cardiac apex and decreased pulmonary vascular markings in a 2-month-old infant with pulmonary valve atresia and ventricular septal defect.

The severity of Ebstein's malformation is related to several factors: the amount of displacement of the tricuspid valve, the degree of tricuspid valve incompetence or stenosis, the presence and size of an interatrial communication, and the degree of right ventricular dysfunction. The heart size may vary from near normal to a massive enlargement that is typical of Ebstein's anomaly. A dilated right atrium is responsible for most of the enlarged cardiac silhouette, producing a convex right heart border. A convex left heart border results from an enlarged right ventricular overflow tract. Bilateral convexities produce the characteristic "globular" cardiac silhouette with a narrow base, as seen with pericardial effusion. In the newborn with Ebstein's anomaly, the combination of tricuspid regurgitation and elevated pulmonary vascular resistance can lead to right heart failure and a significant right-to-left shunt. Pulmonary arterial markings are diminished. With the postnatal drop in pulmonary vascular resistance, pulmonary blood flow increases and pulmonary arterial markings are normal.

Normal Pulmonary Arterial Markings

Aortic Valve Stenosis

A normal cardiac silhouette and vasculature are seen in patients with mild stenosis of the aortic valve. The ascending aorta may be normal or may be prominent because of poststenotic dilation. Left ventricular enlargement occurs with cardiac decompensation or associated aortic regurgitation. A dilated left atrium may displace the esophagus posteriorly and to the right. Pulmonary venous distension may result from passive venous congestion.

Coarctation of the Aorta

The chest roentgenogram varies, depending on the degree of patency of the ductus arteriosus, the severity of the obstruction at the coarctation site, and the presence of coexisting cardiac lesions. Ductal closure may precipitate congestive heart failure, resulting in generalized cardiomegaly and passive pulmonary venous congestion (Fig. 6-16). The right and left ven-

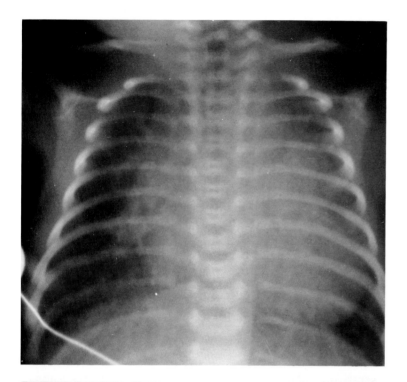

Fig. 6-16. Severe coarctation of the aorta in a neonate. The heart is enlarged. Pulmonary venous congestion is prominent.

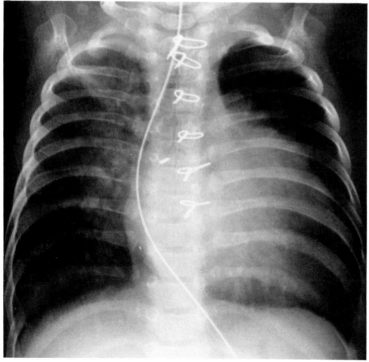

Fig. 6-17. Congenital mitral stenosis. The heart is enlarged. The left atrial appendage is distended and forms a prominent bulge along the left cardiac contour. The esophagus (nasogastric tube) is displaced laterally by an enlarged left atrium. Pulmonary arterial markings are normal but there is an increase in the pulmonary venous pattern. Atelectasis of the left lower lobe with compensatory overinflation of the left upper lobe results from compression of the left main stem bronchus by the enlarged left atrium below and the enlarged left pulmonary artery above.

tricles and left atrium become dilated. Cardiomegaly, pulmonary congestion, and left atrial enlargement are nonspecific radiographic features observed in many other left-sided obstructive lesions and cardiomyopathies occurring in infants.

Rib notching, which is due to erosion or scalloping at the undersurface of the ribs by dilated intercostal vessels, is extremely rare in infancy. The incidence of rib notching increases with age with the development of collateral circulation. The figure-3 sign along the left upper mediastinum in the anteroposterior view produced by pre- and poststenotic dilation of the aorta is absent in symptomatic infants. The aortic arch is usually obscured by the thymic tissue.

Congenital Mitral Stenosis and Cor Triatriatum

Left atrial enlargement occurs in cases of mitral stenosis and cor triatriatum, often displacing the esophagus posteriorly and to the right (Fig. 6-17). The left ventricle size is normal. Passive pulmonary venous congestion is common.

Pulmonary Valve Stenosis

In an infant with pulmonary valve stenosis, the heart size is normal or enlarged. The pulmonary artery segment is often convex because of poststenotic dilation. Pulmonary vascular markings are normal. If there is an associated atrial septal defect with a right-to-left shunt, the pulmonary vascular markings may be diminished.

Vascular Ring

The majority of aortic arch anomalies resulting in a vascular ring can be correctly identified by a combination of chest radiography, barium esophagography, and two-dimensional echocardiography.[50] A vascular ring is defined as complete encirclement of the esophagus and trachea by vascular structures. The vascular structures may be patent or atretic. The presence of symptoms depends on the degree of constriction of the trachea and esophagus by the vascular ring. Symptoms are usually present at birth or develop shortly thereafter. Tracheal compression may result in stridor, respiratory distress, wheezing, or recurrent respiratory infection. Symptoms of esophageal constriction (difficulty in feeding, regurgitation, choking, aspiration pneumonia) are rare. The patient may be asymptomatic.

The most common type of vascular ring is a double

aortic arch. There is persistence of both embryonic aortic arches, resulting in complete right- and left-sided aortic arches.[51,52] The right aortic arch is usually dominant, and the left is often small or atretic. Double aortic arch usually exists as an isolated anomaly; however, it has been reported in association with tetralogy of Fallot and transposition of the great arteries. A vascular ring may also result when a left subclavian artery originates aberrantly from a right aortic arch and a right descending aorta, with a left ductus arteriosus or ligamentum arteriosum completing the ring.

Barium swallow with fluoroscopy is the mainstay of noninvasive diagnosis.[53] Information is obtained from both AP and lateral views (Fig. 6-18). In the AP projection, bilateral indentations of the barium-filled esophagus indicate double aortic arch; an oblique indentation from the left inferior to the right superior is seen in aberrant right subclavian artery. In the lateral projection a large retroesophageal indentation is seen with double aortic arch, with a left aortic arch with a right descending aorta and a right aortic arch with mirror-image branching if a left ductus arteriosus connects the upper descending aorta to the pulmonary artery. A shallow oblique retroesophageal indentation is produced by a left aortic arch with an aberrant right subclavian artery or a right aortic arch with an aberrant left subclavian artery. Anterior indentation of the esophagus is seen with pulmonary artery sling.

Assessment of arch laterality from the plain thoracic roentgenogram may be difficult in the neonate because of the prominent thymus. Two-dimensional echocardiography is useful in establishing the laterality of the aortic arch and descending aorta and in determining the origin of the brachiocephalic vessels from the aorta.[54] An atretic component of a vascular ring is difficult to identify by two-dimensional or Doppler echocardiography since there is no flow in the structure, but it will be apparent by barium swallow because of the its effect of esophageal compression.

If the diagnosis can be confidently established by the above methods, surgery can be performed without angiography.

ECHOCARDIOGRAPHY

Echocardiography has rapidly emerged as the primary diagnostic technique in pediatric cardiology for the evaluation of the newborn with suspected heart

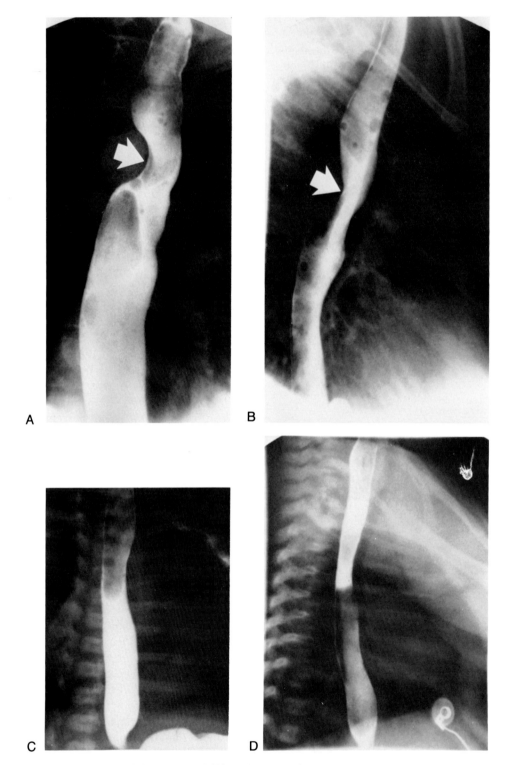

Fig. 6-18. Anteroposterior **(A)** and lateral **(B)** barium esophagrams. Vascular ring consisting of right aortic arch with left descending aorta and ligamentum arteriosus. **(A)** The lateral indentation of the upper esophagus (arrow) and deviation of the trachea and esophagus to the left are produced by a right aortic arch. The large posterior defect (arrow) on the lateral esophagram **(B)** is produced by the transverse arch as it crosses the midline. **(C&D)** Normal anteroposterior **(C)** and lateral **(D)** barium esophagrams.

disease. Transmitted ultrasound waves are reflected from tissue interfaces, and a two-dimensional image is reconstructed from the temporal pattern of the reflected sound energy. Echocardiographic examination consists of obtaining information from several standard echocardiographic windows: subxiphoid, parasternal, apical, and suprasternal notch views. Views are modified as needed to provide the most information. The echocardiographer integrates two-dimensional images of the heart and great vessels obtained in multiple planes to mentally construct a three-dimensional image of the heart. Two-dimensional echocardiography instantaneously provides an accurate, complete, and definitive anatomic diagnosis. Doppler echocardiography provides physiologic information on cardiac function and circulatory dynamics. The technique is noninvasive and risk free and requires relatively inexpensive and portable equipment. Echocardiographic imaging is comparable or superior to angiography. Lesions such as coarctation of the aorta, atrial septal defect, and complete atrioventricular canal may be evaluated adequately without the need for catheterization.[55,56]

Echocardiography is mandatory in the evaluation of the critically ill newborn suspected of having heart disease. Physical examination, chest radiograph, and electrocardiogram may not adequately distinguish cardiac from noncardiac abnormalities when both are present. Echocardiography is indicated as a routine screening test in certain high-risk patients, such as newborns with Down's syndrome, since the incidence of congenital heart defects in these infants is high (50 percent). Many infants with severe defects may be asymptomatic in the immediate postnatal period because of the high pulmonary vascular resistance that is present at birth.

The usefulness of echocardiography is limited when adequate imaging cannot be achieved because of a poor precordial ultrasound window, hyperaeration of the lungs, obesity, or chest wall deformities. Such imaging problems frequently occur in the postoperative patient. These limitations may be overcome by transesophageal echocardiography or may warrant further evaluation by other imaging modalities. Future developments of echocardiography are in the areas of myocardial tissue characterization to detect fibrosis, inflammation, and ischemia, and a three-dimensional reconstruction of echocardiographic images to improve the accuracy of determining ventricular volume and wall motion abnormalities.

Technical Overview

Two-Dimensional Echocardiography

Because of the tremendous anatomic variability and complexity of cardiovascular malformations in neonates, a comprehensive and systematic approach is necessary for accurate cardiovascular diagnosis. The segmental approach includes the determination of visceroatrial situs; description of the presence, position, and alignment of the atria, ventricles, and great arteries; and a systematic assessment of valves, septa, coronary arteries, and systemic and pulmonary veins.[57] By sequentially describing each anatomic segment and noting whether it is normal or abnormal, an accurate, detailed description of cardiac anatomy is possible.

Situs

Proper identification of visceroatrial situs provides the foundation for systematic classification of congenital heart disease with use of the segmental approach. There are four possibilities of visceroatrial situs: solitus (normal), inversus, and right or left atrial isomerism (Fig. 6-19). In situs solitus (normal) the liver, right lung, and morphologic right atrium are to the right, whereas the spleen, stomach, left lung, and morphologic left atrium are to the left.

The most reliable identification of the morphologic right atrium is by means of its connection with the inferior vena cava. Visceroatrial situs is determined from a transverse view of the abdomen at the diaphragm (Fig. 6-20), which shows the relative positions of the inferior vena cava, descending aorta, and spine. In situs solitus (normal) the inferior vena cava lies to the right of the spine and the descending aorta to the left of the spine. In situs inversus the inverse relationship exists. In right atrial isomerism the aorta and the inferior cava lie together on either side of the spine with the cava anterior. In left atrial isomerism there is absence of the renal-to-hepatic segment of the inferior vena cava with azygous continuation, identified as a venous structure that courses behind the aorta and does not enter the heart. Abnormal atrial situs is frequently associated with cardiac malposition, such as dextrocardia.[58] Echocardiography is 100 percent sensitive and 99 percent specific in the detection of abnormal situs.[59]

Atrioventricular Connection

Having established atrial morphology (see above), the echocardiographer proceeds to establish the connection of the atria to the ventricles. The morpho-

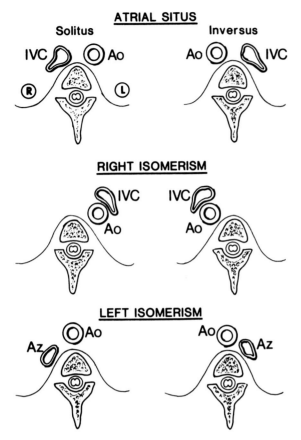

Fig. 6-19. Possible variations of atrial situs diagnosed by the relative portion of the inferior vena cava (IVC), descending aorta (A), and spine. Azygos vein (Az).

logic left ventricle is ovoid in shape, with fine trabeculations and a smooth septal surface. The mitral valve has two papillary muscles that attach to the free wall of the ventricle and a more basal insertion of the valve in the ventricle. The morphologic right ventricle is triangular in shape, with coarse trabeculations, and has a moderator muscle bundle. The tricuspid valve has septal attachments and a more apical insertion in the right ventricle. The appearance of the ventricular outflow tracts may be helpful in determining ventricular morphology. Normally, there is continuity between the mitral valve of the left ventricle and the aortic valve, whereas there is muscle separating the tricuspid and the pulmonary valves in the right ventricular outflow tract.

There are four possibilities for atrioventricular connection (Fig. 6-21): (1) concordant (normal); (2) discordant (ventricular inversion or corrected transposition of the great arteries; (3) univentricular (tricuspid or mitral atresia), double inlet and common inlet; and (4) ambiguos (in the case of two ventricles with atrial isomerism).

Echocardiographic assessment of atrioventricular connections is highly accurate.

Ventriculoarterial Connection

Ventriculoarterial connection is the manner in which the great arteries and semilunar valves connect to the ventricular outflow tracts. There are four pos-

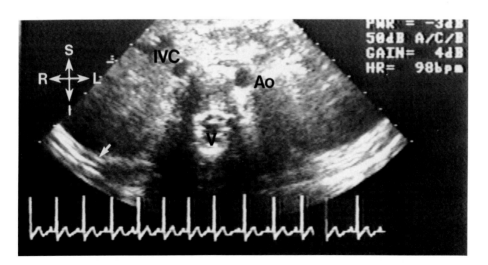

Fig. 6-20. A subxiphoid transverse ultrasound view of the abdomen demonstrating normal visceroatrial situs. The inferior vena cava (IVC) is to the right of the spine (V) and the descending aorta (Ao) is to the left. The soft tissue density is liver. The arrow marks the diaphragm.

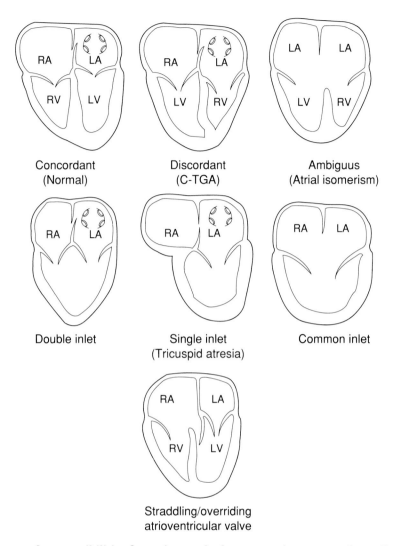

Fig. 6-21. There are four possibilities for atrioventricular connection: concordant, discordant, ambiguos, and univentricular. *Top row:* In concordant atrioventricular connection, the morphologic right atrium (RA) connects normally to the morphologic right ventricle (RV) and the morphologic left atrium (LA) connects to the morphologic left ventricle (LV). In discordant atrioventricular connection, the right atrium connects to the left ventricle, and the left atrium connects to the right ventricle. This relationship is found in corrected transposition of the great arteries. Ambiguus atrioventricular connection occurs when there are bilateral left or right atria in the presence of two ventricles. *Middle row:* Univentricular/atrioventricular connection occurs when all the atrial connection is to one ventricle. Three possibilities exist: double inlet, single inlet (mitral or tricuspid atresia), and common inlet. *Bottom row:* With severe straddling or overriding of an atrioventricular valve, one atrium may drain to more than one ventricle. (From Huhta et al.,[57] with permission.)

sibilities (Fig. 6-22): (1) concordant (normal: morphologic right ventricle connects to the pulmonary valve, and the morphologic left ventricle connects to the aortic valve); (2) discordant (transposition of the great arteries: right ventricle to aorta and left ventri-

cle to pulmonary trunk; (3) double outlet; and (4) single outlet (with aortic or pulmonary atresia or truncus arteriosus).

Echocardiographic assessment of ventriculoarterial connections is highly accurate.[60]

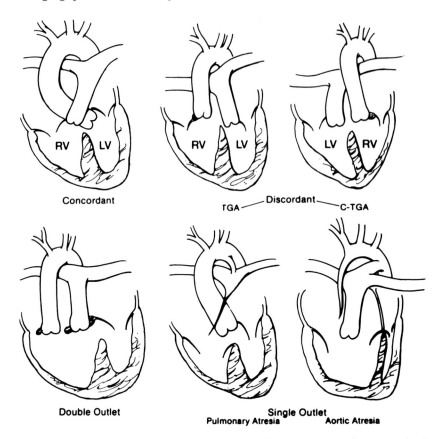

Fig. 6-22. Possible variations in ventriculoarterial connection. In concordant ventriculoarterial connection, the morphologic right ventricle (RV) connects normally to the pulmonary artery, and the morphologic left ventricle (LV) connects to the aorta. Discordant ventriculoarterial connection may occur with transposition such that the right ventricle connects to the aorta and the left ventricle to the pulmonary artery. Both great arteries may arise from a single ventricle, more commonly from the right. Single arterial trunk occurs with truncus arteriosus or with atresia of the pulmonary artery or aorta. (From Huhta et al.,[57] with permission.)

Atrial Septum

Atrial septal defects are more readily detected by echocardiography in neonates than in older children because of optimal ultrasound windows produced by the thin chest wall and shorter distances in a neonate.[61] Pulsed Doppler and Doppler color flow mapping are of value in detecting shunt flow and direction. It may be difficult to differentiate an atrial septal defect secundum from a stretched patent foramen ovale in the premature infant. Serial evaluations may be necessary.

Ventricular Septum

Defects of the ventricular septum are defined by their location in the interventricular system. The ability to detect small muscular ventricular septal defects

has been substantially improved by the use of color Doppler. The peak velocity of flow through the defect can be used to estimate the interventricular pressure difference and to arrive at an estimate of right ventricular pressure.

Atrioventricular Valves

In assessment of the atrioventricular valves, the position, morphology, chordal attachments, and movement of the mitral and tricuspid valves are noted. For example, the valve may be displaced into the ventricle or straddling the interventricular septum. The atrioventricular valve may be common, cleft, dysplastic, hypoplastic, or prolapsing. Valve leaflets may be redundant.

The hemodynamics of atrioventricular valve stenosis or regurgitation are evaluated by color flow Doppler mapping and pulsed or continuous Doppler. The peak velocity in the regurgitant jet is useful for predicting ventricular pressure.

Semilunar Valves

The aortic and pulmonary valves are evaluated to detect valvular obstruction or regurgitation. The valve may be tricuspid, bicuspid, or unicuspid. A thickened, dysplastic valve domes in systole because of limited mobility of the valve leaflets (Fig. 6-23). There may be normal coaptation of valve cusps, and the annulus may be small. The subvalvular area is examined for evidence of obstruction, either muscular or membranous. Supravalvular stenosis may be difficult to demonstrate. Pulsed and continuous-wave Doppler are used to detect and quantify valvular stenosis and regurgitations.

Systemic Veins

The right superior vena cava, inferior vena cava, coronary sinus, hepatic veins, and left superior vena cava (if present) can be identified with a sensitivity of 95 percent.[62]

A left superior vena cava draining into the coronary sinus is a common anatomic variant, occurring in 5 to 10 percent of patients with congenital heart defects and 0.5 percent of the general population. This anomaly is of no physiologic significance, but produces a dilated coronary sinus.[63,64] A left superior vena cava draining into the left atrium or into an unroofed coronary sinus will produce systemic desaturation.

The connection of the inferior vena cava to the right atrium is important for the determination of situs.

Pulmonary Veins

All four pulmonary veins must be confidently identified as entering the left atrium. In TAPVC all four pulmonary veins connect to a structure other than the morphologic left atrium. In the most common form of partial anomalous pulmonary venous connection the right upper pulmonary veins connect to the right superior vena cava, and there is frequently an associated sinus venosus atrial septal defect.

TAPVC can be detected with 85 to 97 percent accuracy, depending on the experience of the echocardiographer. When the diagnosis cannot be confirmed or the connections of all four veins cannot be defined, angiography is indicated.[65] Obstruction to pulmonary venous return can be detected by pulsed Doppler.[66]

Coronary Arteries

In the premature infant, echocardiography is limited to the detection of coronary artery origins. The sensitivity of ultrasound is not adequate to detect anomalies of the coronary circulation unless a coronary artery is enlarged because of a coronary artery fistula. Complete definition of coronary artery anatomy is essential in all infants with transposition of the great arteries before an arterial switch procedure is undertaken. It is also imperative that the coronary anatomy be defined before ventriculotomy is performed in patients with tetralogy of Fallot to deter-

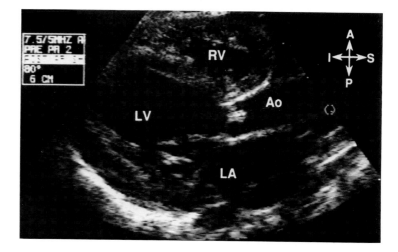

Fig. 6-23. Parasternal long axis echocardiographic image of a thickened and dysplastic aortic valve in a newborn with aortic valve stenosis. Ao, aorta; LA, left atrium; LV, left ventricle; RV, right ventricle.

mine the origin of the left anterior descending artery. Angiography is often necessary in these patients.

Aorta

The entire ascending, transverse, and descending aorta must be examined in a segmental manner. Information is compiled from several tomographic planes, since the aorta does not lie in a single plane.[67]

Laterality of the aortic arch is determined by the direction of the first branch, the innominate artery. A right innominate artery indicates a left arch. Branching of the innominate artery to the left indicates a right arch with mirror-image branching.

Aortic arch anomalies, patent ductus arteriosus, and coarctation of the aorta must be excluded.

Pulmonary Arteries

The main, left, and right pulmonary arteries are imaged segmentally to determine abnormalities of size and origin. In some forms of congenital heart disease, the size of the pulmonary arteries determines the operative procedure. Dilation of pulmonary arteries may occur with pulmonary valve stenosis (post-stenotic dilation), increased pulmonary blood flow (left-to-right shunts), or severe elevation of pulmonary artery pressure (pulmonary hypertension). Absent pulmonary valve syndrome is associated with aneurysmally dilated arteries and pulmonary annular constriction. Small or hypoplastic pulmonary arteries result from decreased pulmonary blood flow, as in cases of right-sided heart obstruction. The right or left pulmonary artery rarely originates from the ascending aorta or from a ductus arteriosus.

Diagnosis of distal pulmonary artery abnormalities requires angiography, or perhaps MR imaging, as does the evaluation of aortopulmonary collateral vessels in patients with a multifocal pulmonary supply.

Noncardiovascular Structures

Movement of the right and left portions of the diaphragm can be visualized simultaneously by echocardiography to exclude paralysis of a hemidiaphragm. Two-dimensional echocardiography may distinguish pericardial from pleural fluid collection and assist in drainage of pericardial and pleural effusions. Imaging of the thymus may distinguish true cardiomegaly from an enlarge d thymus. Two-dimensional echocardiography may identify clots or vegetation that may form in patients with indwelling venous or arterial catheters or assist in the evaluation of patients with positive blood cultures.

Contrast echocardiography is used to reveal shunts and to determine the identity of unusual structures. Contrast material generally consists of normal saline or a solution of albumin that has been agitated to produce stable microbubbles in solution. These microbubbles are large enough to reflect ultrasound, yet small enough to be safe. Systemic venous injection of contrast fills the right heart and is cleared by the lungs. The left heart will be opacified only in the presence of a right-to-left shunt. A left-to-right shunt can be diagnosed by "washout" or early dilution of the contrast material.

An injection of contrast material into the left arm vein can outline the course of a left superior vena cava.

Doppler Echocardiography

Doppler echocardiography is an integral part of a complete echocardiographic examination. The physiologic information provided by Doppler echocardiography complements that provided by two-dimensional echocardiography in that it detects disturbances in blood flow that result from abnormalities of cardiac structure. Doppler echocardiography is used qualitatively to detect atrial and ventricular septal defects, patent ductus arteriosus, shunt site, coarctation, and valvular regurgitation. Doppler-derived calculations are useful in quantifying systemic and pulmonary blood flow, estimating the severity of stenotic lesions, and, in some cases, estimating right ventricular or pulmonary artery pressure. From Doppler echocardiography, inferences can be made about blood velocity and the direction of blood flow based on frequency changes in sound waves reflected from moving structures such as circulating red blood cells.

There are three modes of Doppler interrogation: pulsed Doppler, continuous-wave Doppler, and Doppler color flow mapping. Pulsed Doppler, guided by cross-sectional imaging, allows placement of the Doppler sample volume at the site of interest in the ultrasound image. Pulsed Doppler is used for the detection of flow disturbances, precise localization of abnormal flow, and measurement of flow velocities within the normal range.

Continuous-wave Doppler exceeds the capabilities of the pulsed Doppler system by examining areas with higher flow velocities, such as those associated with a stenotic valve (Fig. 6-24), ventricular septal defect, or patent ductus arteriosus. The lack of spatial resolution is overcome by first using pulsed Doppler to localize the high-velocity jet.

Doppler color flow mapping is a specific form of analysis and presentation of pulsed Doppler information. The velocity and directional information are superimposed in color on the two-dimensional image. The direction of flow is coded by color: red arbitrarily indicates flow toward the transducer and blue indicates flow away from the transducer. The velocity of flow is coded by brightness: higher velocities are displayed as lighter shades of red or blue. Turbulent or nonlaminar blood flow is displayed as yellow or green. Color flow Doppler increases the efficiency of the examination in that it allows rapid detection of areas of disturbed flow by allowing the examiner to view large areas of Doppler information simultaneously. It expedites detection of small ventricular septal defects and patent ductus arteriosus.

M-Mode Echocardiography

M-mode echocardiography displays motion of the heart as a function of time. Newer techniques of two-dimensional and Doppler echocardiography have replaced M-mode echocardiography in the anatomic diagnosis of congenital heart defects. M-mode is of particular value in measuring chamber dimension or wall thickness, in the assessment of left ventricular function (the rate of change in left ventricle dimension over the cardiac cycle) and in studying the motion of cardiac structures as a function of time (such as timing of valve opening and closing).

Echocardiographic Assessment of Cardiac Function

Left ventricular function can be reliably measured by M-mode echocardiography. The shortening fraction is the relative change in left ventricular dimension from diastole to systole measured in the short axis of the left ventricle (Fig. 6-25). The normal range of values is from 28 to 44 percent. Shortening fraction is invalid in the presence of factors that distort the shape of the left ventricle. These factors include right ventricular volume loading, right ventricular systolic hypertension, and left ventricular regional wall motion abnormalities that occur with myocardial ischemia or infarction. Flattening of the septum as seen in normal newborns or the first few days of life invalidates the shortening fraction as an indicator of left ventricular performance in newborns. In these

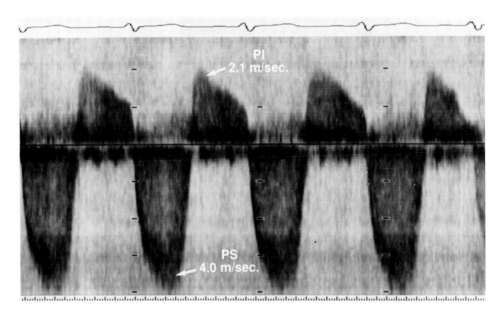

Fig. 6-24. Continuous-wave Doppler recording in the main pulmonary artery in an infant with severe valvular pulmonary stenosis (PS). The peak velocity of pulmonary valve stenosis is 4.0 m/s. This corresponds to a valve gradient of 64 mmHg, according to the Bernouilli equation (pressure drop = 4 times the velocity squared). There is also pulmonary insufficiency (PI) with a peak velocity of 2.1 m/s.

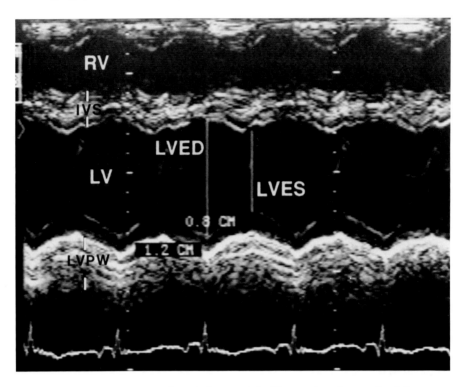

Fig. 6-25. M-mode echocardiogram of the left ventricle illustrating the method for measuring ventricular dimensions and calculating the left ventricular shortening fraction (SF) using the equation SF = (LVED−LVES)/LVED, where LVED = left ventricle end-diastolic dimension and LVES = left ventricular end-systolic dimension. IVS, interventricular septum; LV, left ventricle; LVPW, left ventricular posterior wall. RV, right ventricle.

patients, a qualitative assessment of ventricular function can be made by two-dimensional echocardiography.

The noninvasive measurement of systemic and pulmonary blood flow, pressure gradients across stenotic lesions, right ventricular systolic pressure, pulmonary artery pressure, and stenotic valve areas is particularly appealing in the premature infant. Doppler estimates of cardiac output for the normal fetus [68-70] and for premature and term newborn infants [71,72] have been published. However, those studies do not include simultaneously obtained invasive measures of cardiac output. Use of Doppler estimates is most reliable in serial measurements of cardiac ouptut in the same patient before and after an intervention designed to improve cardiac output, thus minimizing potential errors in measurement of vascular area.

Systemic-to-pulmonary flow ratios (Q_pQ_s) can be derived by comparing the blood flow measured in the pulmonary artery to that measured in the aorta. Such measurements are subject to wide variability, owing to difficulties in accurately measuring the vascular area. [73,74] The technique is invalid in the presence of outflow tract obstruction, semilunar valve regurgitation, or patent ductus arteriosus.

The severity of a stenotic lesion can be noninvasively estimated. The pressure drop across a discrete stenosis can be calculated by using a modification of the Bernouilli equation as follows:

$$P_1P_2 = 4V^2$$

where: P_1P_2 is the pressure drop (in millimeters of mercury) and V is the peak velocity in the Doppler jet (in meters per second). This Doppler method correlates well with catheter-measured gradients in pulmonary stenosis, ventricular septal defect, pulmonary artery bands, surgically created shunts, and patent ductus arteriosus. The Doppler method is less accurate in the estimation of aortic valve stenosis because it measures the instantaneous pressure difference, which may differ from the peak-to-peak velocity pressure difference measured at cardiac catheterization. The Doppler estimation of severity of stenosis is underestimated in the presence of decreased ventricular output.

Pulmonary artery pressure can be inferred from right ventricular systolic pressure in the absence of right ventricular outflow obstruction. Right ventricular systolic pressure can be estimated reasonably accurately in the presence of tricuspid regurgitation or a ventricular septal defect by using the modified Bernouilli equation.

Attempts have been made to estimate pulmonary artery pressure by using the Doppler-derived systolic time intervals. Pulmonary hypertension increases the afterload on the right ventricle, lengthening the pre-ejection period and shortening the ejection time. The ratio of the right ventricular pre-ejection period to the right ventricular ejection time[75] correlates well with catheter-measured pulmonary artery pressures, but they are of poor predictive value in the individual subjects because of wide variability.[76] Right ventricular systolic time intervals obtained from the pulmo-

nary valve echocardiogram were not predictive of pulmonary artery pressure in another study.[77]

Information on ventricular diastolic function and ventricular compliance may be obtained from analysis of Doppler flow velocity waveforms through the atrioventricular valves. Ventricular inflow is characterized by two velocity peaks, a prominent early diastolic filling phase due to ventricular filling (E) followed by a late diastolic filling phase (A) due to atrial systole (Fig. 6-26). The normal fetal pattern includes reversed E/A ratio with higher late diastolic rather than early diastolic peak filling velocities.[78,79] After birth the A/E ratio normalizes, and in adults with advancing age, the pattern reverts to that seen in the fetus.[80]

Transesophageal Echocardiography in Congenital Heart Disease

The precordial approach to transesophageal echocardiography is generally satisfactory in small infants, providing high-quality diagnostic information.

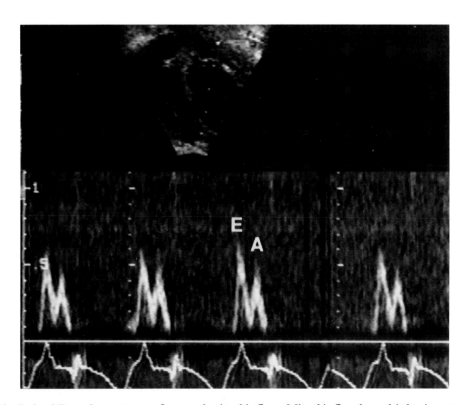

Fig. 6-26. Pulsed Doppler pattern of normal mitral inflow. Mitral inflow has a biphasic pattern with a prominent early filling phase (E) and a less prominent late filling phase that follows atrial contraction (A).

Transesophageal echocardiography is of additional diagnostic value in three specific areas: in the precise morphologic diagnosis of congenital heart disease, in patients with poor precordial window, and in post-surgical follow-up.[81]

It allows a more detailed evaluation of the morphology and function of those cardiac stuctures in closest proximity to the esophagus, namely the systemic and pulmonary veins, the atria, atrial septum, interatrial baffles, and left ventricular outflow tract. Its use in the pediatric population, and particularly the neonatal population, is limited by the size of the currently available esophageal probes and the need for general anesthesia or heavy sedation for studies. The most current published experience in pediatric transesophageal echocardiography comprised 65 infants ages 6 hours to 18 years (mean 32 months) and weighing 2.4 to 30 kg (mean 10.6); 18 patients were younger than 10 days old.[82] Recent miniaturization of probes has allowed transesophageal studies to be safely performed in small premature infants.[83]

At present, transesophageal studies in patients with congenital heart disease are indicated in symptomatic patients with a poor precordial ultrasound window who have suspected abnormalities of either systemic or pulmonary venous return, atrial lesions, abnormalities of the atrioventricular valves, or left ventricular outflow tract obstruction. With the development of smaller-sized transesophageal probes and pediatric-sized biplane probes, the role of transesophageal echocardiography in children with congenital heart disease is likely to increase.[84]

Clinical Overview

In this section some of the more common problems in this age group for which noninvasive assessment is needed are delineated.

Persistent Ductus Arteriosus

Persistent patency of the ductus arteriosus after birth is an important complication of prematurity. The increased pulmonary blood flow and pressure associated with a patent ductus arteriosus may adversely affect the clinical course of the premature infant. Characteristic clinical or radiographic signs of a patent ductus arteriosus may be minimal in the neonate — particularly in the first week of life — and in the newborn with hyaline membrane disease.[85]

Patent ductus arteriosus also occurs in association with other congenital cardiac defects. Similarly, when a major cardiac malformation is present, the signs of the primary defect often mask those of a patent ductus arteriosus, even though the ductus may be playing a significant hemodynamic role.

With the advent of pharmacologic and surgical manipulation of ductal patency, a safe, reliable, noninvasive serial method of assessing ductal patency is essential to the clinical management of these patients. Combined two-dimensional and Doppler echocardiography is the method of choice of diagnosing patent ductus arteriosus. Two-dimensional echocardiography visualizes the ductus, providing information on ductal size and shape. Two-dimensional directed pulsed Doppler, with the Doppler sample placed in the pulmonary end of the ductus, detects ductal patency.

The ductus arteriosus is imaged from the suprasternal or high left parasternal approach (Fig. 6-27). The ductus arteriosus in the normal heart with a left or right arch runs an oblique course from the junction of the main and left pulmonary arteries to insert in the descending aorta just distal to the origin of the left subclavian artery. Ductal morphology is determined in large part by the pattern of blood flow in utero. When there is reduced pulmonary blood flow in utero, such as that seen in patients with severe pulmonary stenosis or atresia, the ductus tends to be more tortuous and arises more cephalad on the aortic arch, forming an acute angle with the descending aorta. This presumably happens because the fetal blood flows from the aorta to the pulmonary artery in utero.[86]

The examiner must be aware of atypical origin of the ductus. The ductus can arise from either the proximal right or left pulmonary artery and can insert at any location on the aortic arch or proximal portions of the brachiocephalic vessels. In the presence of a right aortic arch the ductus arteriosus is usually left sided; however, it may be on the right. Rarely, bilateral ducti are present, commonly associated with interruption of the pulmonary artery confluence. In the setting of an interrupted aortic arch, the main pulmonary artery, ductus, and descending aorta appear as one continuous structure and may be difficult to distinguish from a normal aortic arch. In addition to assessing the ductus arteriosus, a comprehensive echocardiographic examination of the heart and great vessels is essential before medical or surgical ductal closure, to exclude ductal-dependent cardiac lesions in which persistence of the ductus is critical for the survival of the patient.

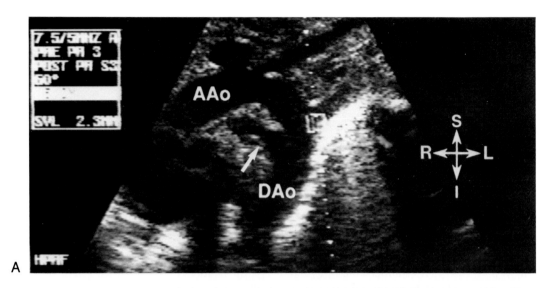

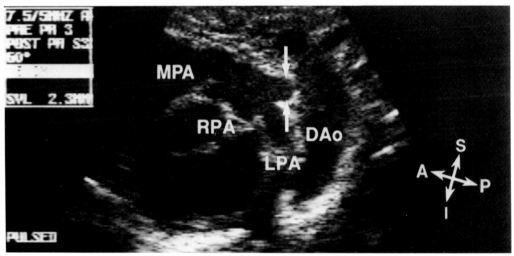

Fig. 6-27. Echocardiographic image of the ductus arteriosus. **(A)** Suprasternal notch view demonstrates the aortic arch, brachiocephalic vessels, and aortic end of the patent ductus arteriosus (arrow). AAo, ascending aorta; DAo, descending aorta. **(B)** High parasternal plane view demonstrates the pulmonary end of the ductus arteriosus (arrows). Note that the ductus is closed at the pulmonary end. DAo, descending aorta; LPA, left pulmonary artery; MPA, main pulmonary artery; RPA, right pulmonary artery.

A ductus may constrict along its entire length or may narrow at one end, usually the pulmonary end. Therefore, it is vital that the examiner visualize the ductus along its entire length; otherwise, an incorrect assessment of patency will be made (Fig. 6–27). Doppler echocardiography confirms ductal patency and the direction of blood flow through the ductus. With Doppler echocardiography, it is possible to detect patency when the ductus is beyond the lateral resolution of the two-dimensional echocardiography.

Analysis of Doppler flow patterns yields important information about the status of the pulmonary vascular bed. Factors that determine the magnitude of the shunt through the ductus are the relative pulmonary and systemic vascular resistances and the diameter of the ductus, which determines the resistance offered to flow.[87] For example, in the presence of elevated pulmonary vascular resistance, ductal shunting is minimal even if the ductus is large. In the presence of normal pulmonary vascular resistance, flow in the ductus is from the aorta to the pulmonary artery (left to right) throughout systole and diastole. This pattern is also seen in patients with ductal-dependent pulmonary blood flow, as in pulmonary atresia or severe pulmonary stenosis. In the presence of elevated pulmonary vascular resistance and/or decreased systemic resistance (hypotension or left heart obstructive lesions), ductal flow is bidirectional.

The recent introduction of color flow mapping (Fig. 6-28) has provided another method for ductal evaluation. Its advantages are increased efficiency and diagnostic accuracy in the detection of the very small ductus arteriosus.

The determination of hemodynamic significance of the ductus arteriosus in the premature infant remains a clinical decision.[88,89] Echocardiography may assist in the evaluation of the ductus by revealing information about the magnitude of the shunt, the size of the ductus, and the pulmonary artery pressure. In premature infants pulmonary edema occurs with only a moderate shunt, perhaps because of decreased pulmonary arterial muscle or developmental differences in the pulmonary parenchyma or interstitium.[90-93] Generally, left ventricular function is normal, al-though the left ventricle and left atrium may be enlarged because of volume overload.

The M-mode measurement of the ratio of the left atrial-to-aortic root diameter (LA/Ao) may be elevated in the presence of a patent ductus, reflecting an enlarged left atrium from volume overload. However, the LA/Ao ratio is neither specific nor sensitive in regard to the diagnosis of a patent ductus arteriosus and should be considered within the context of other clinical and echocardiographic parameters.

Transposition of the Great Arteries

In transposition of the great arteries the morphologic right ventricle gives rise to the aorta and the morphologic left ventricle gives rise to the pulmonary trunk (ventriculoarterial discordance). Two-dimensional echocardiography allows accurate identification of the ventricles by their anatomic characteristics and direct visualization of their respective ventriculoarterial alignments.[94,95]

The ventricles are defined by their morphology.[96] The morphologic left ventricle is ovoid in shape and finely trabeculated, with a smooth septal surface. Its atrioventricular valve has two papillary muscles that attach to the free wall and insert more basally in the ventricle. The morphologic right ventricle is triangular in shape and coarsely trabeculated, with a moderator muscle bundle. Its atrioventricular valve attaches to the septum and inserts in a more apical direction in the ventricle.

The great arteries are identified by their branching patterns. The pulmonary artery bifurcates early into right and left pulmonary arteries, whereas the aorta gives rise to the innominate, left common carotid and left subclavian arteries. Coronary arteries rise from the aorta. The associated lesions that must be evaluated include left ventricular outflow tract obstruction,[97] ventricular septal defect, and patent ductus arteriosus.[97] The coronary artery anatomy must be determined when the patient is being considered as a candidate for the arterial switch operation.[98]

Currently, the echocardiographic diagnosis of simple transposition of the great arteries can be done with the accuracy of cardiac catheterization and angiography, such that performance of balloon atrial septostomy remains the only reason for performing cardiac catheterization in these newborn infants. Furthermore, in the critically ill newborn with simple transposition who is too unstable to be safely transported to the cardiac catheterization laboratory, bal-

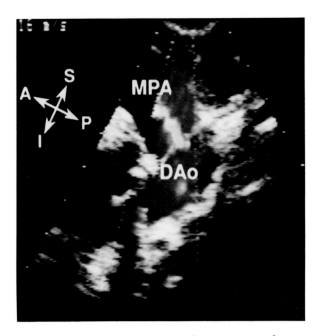

Fig. 6-28. Color flow mapping detects patent ductus arteriosus by turbulent flow (green) in the main pulmonary artery. DAo, descending aorta; MPA, main pulmonary artery.

loon atrial septostomy can be performed in the intensive care unit under echocardiographic guidance (Fig. 6-29).[99,100] Echocardiography will provide a measurement of the adequacy of the interatrial communication created by balloon septostomy.

Persistent Fetal Circulation

Persistent fetal circulation, also known as persistent pulmonary hypertension of the newborn, is a diagnosis of exclusion and altered hemodynamics.

This condition must be distinguished from simple transposition of the great arteries and TAPVC with obstruction.[101] Once structural heart disease has been excluded, the echocardiogram provides useful hemodynamic information in the management of the infant with persistent fetal circulation. Doppler echocardiography reveals right-to-left shunting at the level of the atrial septum and patent ductus arteriosus. The peak velocity of tricuspid regurgitation, as determined by Doppler, is useful for predicting right ventricular pressures.[102] Ventricular dysfunction can

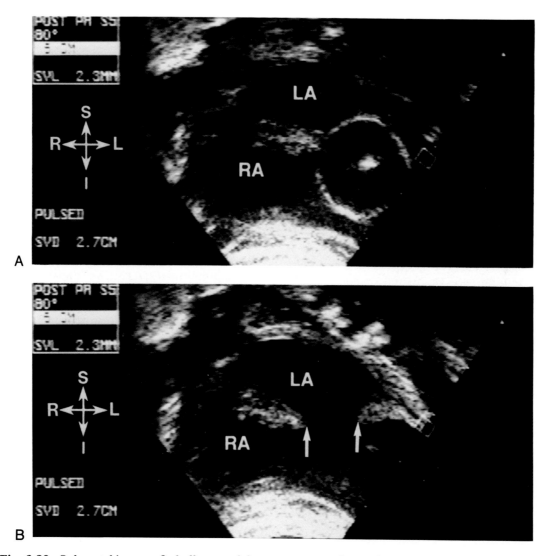

Fig. 6-29. Subcostal image of a balloon atrial septostomy performed under echocardiographic guidance. **(A)** The inflated balloon is rapidly withdrawn from the left atrium (LA) to the right atrium (RA), enlarging the interatrial communication. **(B)** Subcostal image of the atrial septal defect created by balloon atrial septostomy.

be assessed by the shortening fraction and estimation of wall motion.[102] This information can provide a baseline upon which to evaluate the success of therapeutic interventions.[103]

Cor Pulmonale

Cor pulmonale is right ventricular hypertrophy and/or dilation resulting from a disorder that affects either the structure or the function of the lungs. It is a chronic condition that develops over time in response to progressive increases in pulmonary vascular resistance.[104]

Detection of pulmonary hypertension is difficult. There is controversy regarding the value of echocardiography for assessing the presence and severity of pulmonary hypertension. Prolongation of right ventricular systolic time intervals (right ventricular pre-ejection period/right ventricular ejection time) or prolongation of right ventricular isovolumetric contraction time may suggest the presence of pulmonary hypertension.[75,105–108] However, this is not a reliable means of assessment because of wide variability among individuals. A more reliable estimate of right ventricular pressure (and, in the absence of right ventricular outflow tract obstruction, the pulmonary artery pressure) is the systolic pressure gradient across the tricuspid valve, calculated from the peak velocity of the tricuspid regurgitant jet. In patients with a ventricular septal defect or patent ductus arteriosus, the pressure differences across the systemic-to-pulmonary communication can be calculated and subtracted from the systemic arterial pressure (blood pressure) to determine right ventricular or pulmonary artery pressures.

Right ventricular dilatation and increases in right ventricular wall thickness generally reflect advanced disease. Because of hyperaeration of the lungs, patients with these problems are often difficult to image echocardiographically, and the evaluation is often unsatisfactory.

Total Anomalous Pulmonary Venous Return

In cases of TAPVC all four pulmonary veins connect to a structure other than the left atrium. The echocardiographic diagnosis of TAPVC is based on detection of a pulmonary venous confluence posterior to the left atrium and the absence of normal pulmonary venous connection with the left atrium. The site(s) of insertion of the pulmonary venous con-

fluence into the systemic veins must be determined.[109,110]

The entire course of the anomalous pulmonary venous connection may be reconstructed from multiple imaging planes. Right ventricular and right atrial enlargement, deviation of the interatrial septum to the left, and dilated pulmonary arteries are common, albeit nonspecific, features. Dilated portal veins in the subcostal view of the abdomen may suggest infracardiac TAPVC.[110]

Pulsed Doppler can detect obstruction to flow in the anomalous pulmonary venous channels. Flow upstream from an obstruction is nonphasic.[111] At the site of obstruction flow is disturbed, with a peak velocity of greater than 2 m/s occurring in diastole.[112]

TAPVC can be detected with 85 to 97 percent sensitivity, depending on the experience of the examiner.[113]

Coarctation of the Aorta

Coarctation of the aorta is a congenital narrowing of the aorta, either discrete or lengthy, most commonly in the region of insertion of the ductus arteriosus (or ligamentum arteriosus) into the upper thoracic aorta. Coarctation in the neonate typically becomes detectable at 7 to 10 days of age, depending on ductal patency, severity of obstruction at the coarctation site, and the presence of the coexisting cardiac lesions. Lower extremity pulses are diminished or absent; congestive heart failure or cardiogenic shock occurs. The role of echocardiography is to confirm the clinical suspicion of coarctation and to demonstrate the location of the coarctation and thus eliminate the need for cardiac catheterization.

The echocardiographic diagnosis of coarctation depends on the demonstration of a narrowing of the descending aorta just opposite the left subclavian artery caused by posterior ledge, or "shelf." Ancillary evidence of coarctation is elongation of the distance between the left common carotid and left subclavian arteries and decreased pulsatility of the abdominal aorta. With infantile coarctation there is variable diffuse narrowing or hypoplasia of the transverse aortic arch and isthmus. Echocardiography also reveals the presence and hemodynamic significance of associated defects, such as bicuspid aortic valve,[114–116] left ventricular outflow tract,[117,118] subaortic stenosis, valvular aortic stenosis, and mitral valve abnormalities.

Doppler echocardiography confirms the presence of obstruction by the posterior ledge. The typical pattern is that of diastolic "runoff" continuous flow throughout the cardiac cycle caused by the persistent gradient across the coarctation in systole and diastole (Fig. 6-30). Distal to the site of obstruction of the aorta, there is a rapid increase in systolic flow velocity. If the ductus arteriosus is patent, flow is right-to-left to allow blood flow to the descending aorta beyond the obstruction.

Coarctation of the aorta can be difficult to demonstrate because of the difficulty in imaging the aorta throughout its course.[119] Coarctation of the aorta may also be difficult to diagnose in the presence of a patent ductus arteriosus; and in patients with suspected coarctation, serial examinations may be necessary to evaluate the coarctation site coincident with ductal constriction and closure. The certainty with which this diagnosis can be made echocardiographically depends on the quality of the image and on the experience of the echocardiographer.

Hypoplastic Left Hea.

Hypoplastic left heart
varying degrees of underdeve.
cardiac structures. In the most ma.
or atresia of the aortic and mitral valve.
the left atrium, left ventricle, and asce.
show marked underdevelopment. In other c.
the aortic valve is atretic. The left ventricle is .
and thickened, with a slitlike cavity, whereas the l.
atrium is normal or enlarged. Maintenance of the systemic circulation is critically dependent on a patent ductus arteriosus. Hypoplastic left heart syndrome typically presents in the infant's first few days of life and is associated with congestive heart failure, mild cyanosis, and shock due to low cardiac output.

The diagnosis of hypoplastic left heart syndrome can be made by echocardiography alone. The classic features of the syndrome usually include marked hypoplasia of the ascending aorta, an absent or slitlike left ventricle, a small left atrium, and atretic or mark-

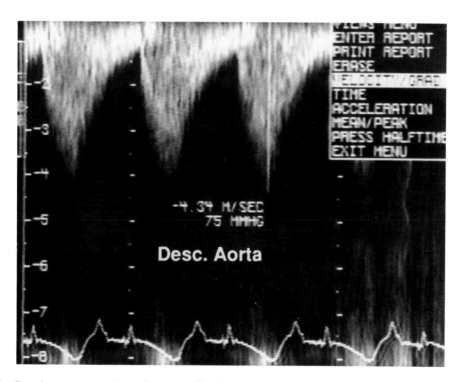

Fig. 6-30. Continuous-wave Doppler recording in coarctation of the aorta. Diastolic runoff (persistence of flow throughout diastole) and high velocity of 4.34 m/s suggest obstruction at the site of coarctation.

The right
...ed. Flow
...since the
...an in the
...ardiogra-
...m patency
...ny restric-
...ovale. Car-
...e palliative
...ial septos-

drome
...ndrome encompasses
...nent of left-sided
...cases, stenosis
...present and
...ing aorta
...es only
...nal
...t

...sis may be a
pathologic condition or a physiologic condition in the
premature infant. There is normally a discrepancy in
size between the main and branch pulmonary arteries
in the newborn because of fetal circulatory patterns.
This should resolve within the first year of life. Peripheral pulmonary stenosis may occur as an isolated
finding or as part of a more complex congenital heart
defect.

Isolated peripheral pulmonary stenosis is associated with maternal rubella syndrome,[120] Williams's
syndrome, tetralogy of Fallot, atrial septal defect, valvular pulmonary stenosis, ventricular septal defect,
and patent ductus arteriosus. The stenosis may involve the main pulmonary artery, right and left
branches, or secondary and tertiary branches and
may be tubular (long segment) or discrete. Although
peripheral pulmonary stenosis is generally a benign
lesion, it may lead to right ventricular failure or may
complicate the repair of associated lesions.

Echocardiography is useful in the demonstration
of significant stenoses of the main or proximal right
and left pulmonary arteries. Distal stenoses, especially involving the secondary and tertiary branches,
are unlikely to be diagnosed by echocardiography,
owing to poor visualization of structures within the
air-filled lung. In such circumstances, angiography or
MR imaging may be indicated.

CARDIAC CATHETERIZATION

Combined two-dimensional and Doppler echocardiography, which can delineate the cardiovascular
anatomy with 95 percent accuracy in the neonatal
period, has decreased the need for cardiac catheterization in this age group. Cardiac catheterization is
indicated in patients in whom noninvasively derived
information is inadequate, inconclusive, or inconsist-
ent with the clinical impression. Angiography remains necessary for imaging of branch pulmonary
arteries and aortopulmonary collateral vessels.

The indications for a diagnostic cardiac catheterization in the neonate are the same as for any age
group and include the following: definition of cardiovascular anatomy, calculations of shunts, quantitation of valvular stenosis or regurgitation, calculation of the pulmonary and systemic vascular
resistance, calculation of valve area, assessment of
myocardial function, and myocardial biopsy. Cardiac
catheterization remains the most reliable and precise
method for obtaining physiologic measurements
such as pressure differences or shunt magnitude.

An increasing number of interventional and therapeutic procedures can be performed during cardiac
catheterization, including balloon or blade septostomy; balloon dilatation of stenotic valves and vessels,
including coarctation of the aorta and branch pulmonary arteries stenosis; transcatheter closure of atrial
and ventricular septal defects and shunts; embolization of abnormal systemic-to-venous or systemic-to-
pulmonary communications; or insertion of vascular
stents to expand stenotic vessels. Most of these procedures can be performed in neonates. These procedures offer a safe and effective alternative to surgical
intervention.

Prospective studies of the complications of cardiac
catheterization have established that cardiac catheterization can be performed in neonates with minimal
morbidity and mortality, even in those weighing less
than 2 kg.[121,122] The morbidity and mortality associated with cardiac catheterization in neonates and
premature infants are directly related to underlying
cardiac defect and the general condition of the patient at the time of catheterization rather than to the
patient's age or size. The major risks of cardiac catheterization are cardiac perforation and tamponade,
blood loss, occlusion of iliofemoral arteries, hypotension after angiography with contrast material, and
transient arrhythmias. Fluids, hematocrit, temperature, and acid-base and ventilatory status must be
strictly monitored. Infants usually are not sedated
before cardiac catheterization because they are especially sensitive to depressant effects of narcotics on
the central nervous, respiratory, and circulatory systems. The use of balloon flotation catheters mini-
mizes the risk of cardiac perforation. Morbidity and
mortality of cardiac catheterization have been reduced in these patients by advances in catheterization

techniques, vascular access, catheter design, and contrast material, and by the information derived from noninvasive sources that modifies or shortens the procedure.

With further technologic refinements and improvements in noninvasive diagnostic imaging modalities, it is possible that in the future cardiac catheterization for congenital heart disease may be reserved solely for therapeutic procedures.

DIGITAL SUBTRACTION ANGIOGRAPHY

Digital subtraction angiography produces a radiographic image by digital conversion of x-ray images. Numerical values are assigned to each section of the image and are stored in a computer. Computer processing and reformatting of the numerical data permits image enhancement, improved contrast resolution, and functional analysis. Imaging and diagnostic accuracy of digital subtraction angiography equals that of conventional cineangiography.[123-125]

Computer-assisted image enhancement allows for the elimination of background structures and optimal visualization of opacified cardiovascular structures. Contrast enhancement allows less contrast media to be used (27.5 to 42 percent of the conventional dose). With intravenous injection of contrast material, opacification of the aorta and pulmonary arteries is satisfactory to detect coarctation of the aorta or branch pulmonary stenosis.[126] However, intracavitary injections remain necessary for satisfactory delineation of intracardiac anatomy. Reducing the total amount of contrast material used in an angiographic study is particularly important in the premature infant, the infant with complex cardiac malformations, and in the critically ill infant with poor ventricular function. Cardiovascular effects of contrast material are dose related,[127] and the total dose of contrast material that can be safely used in such patients may be a limiting factor in obtaining a complete angiographic study. The decrease in radiation exposure with digital subtraction angiography is particularly important in patients in whom repeated angiographic examinations are anticipated. The immediate availability of images for review and analysis[128,129] may shorten or modify cardiac catheterization. These features of digital subtraction angiography may reduce the morbidity associated with conventional cardiac catheterization.

Computer-assisted extraction of numerical data from the images provides quantitative information on circulatory dynamics. Left ventricular ejection function, regional ejection fraction, calculation of cardiac output, and systemic-to-pulmonary blood flow ratios obtained by digital subtraction angiography are comparable to those obtained by cineangiography and thermodilution techniques. Futhermore, the low concentration and small volumes of contrast material used allow the study of ventricular dynamics without significant contrast-related alterations in cardiac function.

Digital subtraction angiography in its current state will not replace conventional cineangiography. The advantage of smaller contrast dose for opacification of intra- or extracardiac structures may be less relevant, owing to the availability of less toxic, nonionic contrast media. Adding the expense of digital subtraction angiography to an already expensive cardiac catheterization laboratory limits the general availability of this technique in pediatric cardiology.

COMPUTED TOMOGRAPHY

Computed tomography (CT) scanning involves computer-assisted reconstruction of a series of sequential tomographic slices of imaged anatomy to provide three-dimensional orientation of cardiac and mediastinal structures. This helps in overcoming the problems associated with overlap from adjacent structures. Furthermore, the single image can be reconstructed and redisplayed in any operator-selected plane.

Because of its excellent soft-tissue contrast resolution and its capability for tissue characterization, CT scanning is particularly useful in the evaluation of mediastinal masses[130] and pleural and pericardial disease (thickening, calcification, and masses),[131,132] and in the characterization of complex parenchymal or chest wall disease.[133] CT may be more sensitive than echocardiography in the imaging of intracardiac tumors and thrombi.[134,135]

CT scanning is of limited use in the anatomic definition of congenital heart defects. Echocardiography, angiography, and MR imaging offer superior imaging. In a series of more than 200 patients with congenital heart disease studied with cine-CT, the diagnostic accuracy was greater than 90 percent.[136]

Present limitations of CT imaging of the heart are primarily technical. Significant image degradation caused by cardiorespiratory motion has been minimized with the development of cardiac gating techniques and faster scanning devices with shorter data acquisition periods. Cardiac gating involves synchronization of the data acquisition period to the cardiac cycle — usually late diastole because it is most often a relatively motionless segment of the cardiac cycle. Furthermore, CT has the disadvantage of radiation exposure, contrast media injection, nonportability, and expense.

A new technology in rapid CT scanning, dynamic cine-CT scanning may be valuable in the functional analysis of cardiac performance. Sequential flow of the injected intravenous contrast is demonstrated through the cardiac chambers. Analysis of time-density curves over regions of interest provides information about blood flow.

A variety of anatomic and physiologic calculations can be made, including ejection fraction, regional ejection fraction, stroke volume, cardiac output, myocardial wall thickness and myocardial mass,[137,138] myocardial perfusion, intracardiac shunt detection and quantitation, volume determinations, and valvular regurgitation.

RADIONUCLIDE STUDIES

Nuclear medicine studies in the field of cardiology provide information on circulatory dynamics such as ventricular function, myocardial and lung perfusion, and shunt detection and quantitation. Radionuclide studies provide limited anatomic information. They are minimally invasive, requiring an intravenous injection of radioisotope. Because injected radiopharmaceuticals do not produce toxic or allergic effects and do not result in hemodynamic or osmotic overload, studies can be performed in small, critically ill patients. The radiation dose to the patient is low. The study may be performed at the patient's bedside by using portable imaging equipment. Radionuclide studies are superior to echocardiography in the assessment of right ventricular function, quantitation of left-to-right shunting, determination of relative lung perfusion, and estimation of myocardial reserve (stress testing).

Two nuclear methods for radionuclide assessment are used: first-pass radionuclide angiocardiography and equilibrium ventriculography. With first-pass radionuclide angiocardiography, a dynamic image of the heart and central vessels is constructed from the sequential passage of an intravenous injection of a small-bolus radionuclide solution through these structures. This provides visualization of venous and right-sided heart structures and is excellent for detection of systemic venous abnormalities such as persistent left superior vena cava, obstructed venous channels, and hemiazygous continuation of the inferior vena cava.[139,140] First-pass angiocardiography is of limited value, however, in defining intracardiac anatomy. In addition, analysis of computer-operated time versus activity for regions of interest permits detection and quantitation of intracardiac shunts and correlates well with pulmonary-to-systemic flow ratios (Q_pQ_s) determined during cardiac catheterization.[141,142] A limitation of this technique is that there is a summation of all left-to-right shunting, and separate sites of shunt cannot be determined. The calculation of shunt flow may be invalid in the presence of valvular regurgitation, large bronchial collateral circulation, multiple cardiac lesions, or severe congestive heart failure and low cardiac output. The disadvantage of this technique is that it requires bolus injection of the radionuclide in a large vein.

Equilibrium ventriculography, also known as multiple-gated acquisition(MUGA scan), allows repetitive sampling of all or selected portions of the cardiac cycle. This technique provides accurate quantitation of left ventricular ejection fraction, ventricular systolic and diastolic function, regional wall motion, and valvular regurgitation. The disadvantage is that the data acquisition period is longer because the radionuclide must remain in the vascular space during image acquisition. Assessments of right and left ventricular ejection fractions by either radionuclide angiocardiography or equilibrium methods are more consistent and sensitive than those obtained from most noninvasive techniques. Normal values for infants are a right ventricular ejection fraction of 0.54 ± 0.09 and a left ventricular ejection fraction of 0.68 ± 0.13.[143] Radionuclide techniques are particularly valuable in the detection of subtle or subclinical ventricular dysfunction, as in asymptomatic children with aortic[144] and/or mitral insufficiency, in patients who have cardiomyopathy, in those who have a single ventricle, and in those who are receiving cardiotoxic drugs (chemotherapeutic or antiarrhythmic agents). Radionuclide techniques also are important in right ventricular evaluation, such as after repair of tetralogy of Fallot or transposition of the great arteries, or in the evaluation of patients with chronic respiratory disease or cor pulmonale.

Myocardial perfusion imaging by use of thallium-201 has been used in children with anomalous or compromised coronary artery flow as in cases involving anomalous coronary arteries,[145] before and after medical or surgical intervention, or in Kawasaki disease. Specificity is low, because abnormalities in myocardial perfusion have also been detected in patients with congestive cardiomyopathy without coronary artery abnormalities.[146] Thallium-201 imaging may be used as a screening test for coronary angiography in the problematic child with a history of severe exercise-induced chest pain and a negative stress electrocardiogram. It is not indicated in the evaluation of routine chest pain because this is a common symptom, which is often benign.

Myocardial infarction may occur in Kawasaki disease or other congenital or acquired coronary artery disease. Infarct-avid myocardial scintigraphy, using technetium-99m pyrophosphate, localizes recent (within 72 hours) myocardial infarction. This may be helpful in situations in which myocardial infarction is difficult to diagnose by conventional means, as in the presence of conduction abnormalities on the surface electrocardiogram or in the postoperative cardiac patient. Its use in children is limited by its low specificity.

Pulmonary blood flow is readily assessed by using technetium-99m–labeled macroaggregated albumin. Radionuclide angiography depicts dynamic blood flow patterns. Static images, obtained once the particles are trapped in the capillary bed, provide precise quantitation of relative blood flow to each lung. This technique is valuable in the diagnosis of pulmonary artery malformations and in determining relative flow to each lung in patients with aortopulmonary collateral vessels or surgically created shunts. The addition of inhaled xenon-133 provides information regarding ventilation-perfusion matching for improved accuracy in diagnosing pulmonary embolism. Caution should be used in the patient with a right-to-left shunt to avoid systemic embolization of injected macroaggregated albumin.

Inflammation of the myocardium or pericardium can be detected with variable success by imaging with gallium-67– or indium-111–labeled white blood cells. This modality demonstrates sensitivity but a lack of specificity in the diagnosis of myocarditis.[147] Positive gallium-67 scans have occurred in patients with postpericardiotomy syndrome.[148,149] These techniques may be appropriate in selected candidates.

MAGNETIC RESONANCE IMAGING

Magnetic resonance (MR) imaging involves the computerized reconstruction of tomographic images produced by the interaction of compositional nuclei of tissues with a strong magnetic field and precisely applied sequences of radiofrequency pulses.[150] The nuclei of certain stable isotopes align themselves in the general direction of an externally applied magnetic field. Once aligned with the external magnetic field, the nuclei may be shifted out of alignment by a short burst of radiofrequency waves. By modification of the characteristics of the magnetic field gradients and radiofrequency pulse, protons can be made to generate radio signals that can be spatially encoded to construct a tomographic image. MR imaging has particular appeal for use in the pediatric patient because it is noninvasive, does not use ionizing radiation, and has no known adverse biologic or genetic effects. Since the MR imaging characteristics of flowing blood are different from those of stationary tissue, there is a natural contrast between intracardiac-intravascular spaces and cardiovascular structures, obviating the need for contrast media.

MR imaging combines high-resolution anatomic imaging with excellent soft tissue contrast and tissue characterization. Initial experience with MR imaging in pediatric cardiology was limited to cardiovascular imaging and documentation of anatomic abnormalities associated with a wide variety of congenital and acquired heart diseases[151–153] (Fig. 6-9). The ease and effectiveness of echocardiography for defining intracardiac anatomy limits the current application of MR imaging to those anatomic areas that may be difficult to image echocardiographically, such as great vessel anatomy, particularly coarctation of the aorta, systemic and pulmonary veins, and right ventricular free wall. MR imaging is also useful in the postoperative patient with poor echocardiographic windows. Furthermore, the resolution of MR is not yet adequate to detect the presence of small defects in the atrial or ventricular septum, nor to detect coronary artery stenosis. Evaluation of cardiac valves is also limited. Three-dimensional image reconstruction can be achieved with MR; the image can be "sliced" in any operator-selected plane.

The disadvantages of MR imaging are a long data acquisition period, which limits its use in very small or acutely ill infants; its nonportability; and the substantial equipment and operational expense that limits its general availability. MR imaging should be used with extreme caution in patients with implanted metallic objects and cardiac pacemakers. It has the potential to displace metallic objects if the magnetic field is strong enough and if they contain sufficient ferromagnetic material. These include intracranial aneurysm clips and heart valves manufactured before 1964. Patients with sternotomy wires and other surgical clips may be routinely studied; however, the wires and clips may cause image artifact. The presence of a cardiac pacemaker is a contraindication to a MR study because it may damage pacemaker electronics and result in pacemaker malfunction.

Functional cardiac evaluation may be performed with dynamic MR imaging. MR data are acquired at multiple points during each cardiac cycle. Separate images reconstructed from data obtained at each point of acquisition during the cardiac cycle are displayed in a sequential or cine-loop format. In the future, flow measurements by MR velocity mapping may permit quantitation of valvular regurgitation, left-to-right shunt flow,[154] and velocity of blood flow through stenotic lesions.

The potential for metabolic imaging of the myocardium is very promising. MR imaging has the capability to measure chemical shifts, for example, in high-energy phosphate and intracellular pH.[155,156] Most of the current work has been in the area of myocardial ischemia or cardiomyopathy. This technique may have tremendous potential in the investigation of the metabolic effects of chronic pressure or volume overload or chronic hypoxia on the myocardium.

Metabolic studies with PET involve the intravenous injection of radionuclides made from biologically active compounds such as oxygen, nitrogen, carbon, and fluorine. Metabolic substrates or metabolites such as glucose, fatty acids, amino acids, ammonia, and water can be tagged with such position-emitting isotopes without modifying their biochemical properties, to study regional blood flow, glucose, and free fatty acid metabolism. PET scanning images consist of cross-sectional emission of tissue or organ concentrations of radiolabeled tracers of blood flow or myocardial metabolism. Measurements can be made of blood flowing through an area of interest, or of mass substrate utilized or metabolized per gram of tissue per time period. Drugs such as calcium antagonists, β blockers, and positive inotropic agents can be labeled with positron-emitting radionuclides to study their myocardial distribution, drug affinity, or receptor concentration. Disadvantages of PET scanning are the expertise and facilities necessary to produce and attach the positron-emitting radionuclides to metabolic substrates, requiring an on-site cyclotron and radiochemistry facilities.

There is currently very little experience with PET scanning in pediatric patients with congenital or acquired heart disease. Initial studies have been in adults with ischemic heart disease or cardiomyopathy. PET scanning has not been widely applied in pediatrics because of limitations of spatial and temporal resolution imposed by small subjects. It is currently available as a research tool. There is great promise for future application of this modality in the study of cardiovascular diseases in the young.

POSITRON EMISSION TOMOGRAPHY

Cardiac positron emission tomography (PET) scanning is not an imaging modality but an in vivo technique for studying myocardial function and disease at a biochemical or cellular level. The detection of myocardial disease at a biochemical or cellular level prior to the development of structural or functional cardiac abnormalities may lead to earlier and more effective therapeutic interventions. As a powerful research tool, PET may characterize the metabolic processes associated with normal cardiac maturation or disease mechanisms or identify metabolic abnormalities associated with cyanotic and noncyanotic congenital heart disease, or pressure or volume overload defects.

REFERENCES

1. Nayey RL: Arterial changes during the perinatal period. Arch Pathol 71:121, 1961
2. Rudolph AM: The pre- and postnatal pulmonary circulation. In: Congenital Diseases of the Heart. Year Book Medical Publishers, Chicago, 1974
3. Simon M, Sasahara AA, Cannilla JE: The radiology of pulmonary hypertension. Semin Roentgenol 2:368, 1967
4. Durnin RE, Willner R, Virmani S et al: Pulmonary hypertension with ventricular septal defect and pulmonary stenosis: tetralogy of Fallot variant. Am J Roentgenol Radium Ther Nucl Med 106:42, 1969
5. Osman MZ, Meng CCL, Girdany BR: Congenital absence of the pulmonary valve: report of eight

cases with review of the literature. Am J Roentgenol Radium Ther Nucl Med 106:58, 1969

6. Lakier JB, Stranger P, Heymann MA et al: Tetralogy of Fallot with absent pulmonary valve: natural history and hemodynamic considerations. Circulation 50:167, 1974

7. Bernard ED, James LS: Radiographic heart size in apparently normal newborn infants: clinical and biochemical correlations. Pediatrics 27:726, 1961

8. Cooley RN, Schreiber MH: Radiology of the Heart and Great Vessels. Williams & Wilkins, Baltimore, 1967

9. Swischuk LE: X-Ray Diagnosis of Congenital Cardiac Disease. Charles C Thomas, Springfield, IL, 1968

10. Swischuk LE: Plain Film Interpretation in Congenital Heart Disease. 1st Ed. Lea & Febiger, Philadelphia, 1970

11. Daves ML: Roentgenology of tetralogy of Fallot. Semin Roentgenol 3:377, 1968

12. Kurlander GJ, Petry EL, Girod DA: Plain film diagnosis of congenital heart disease in the newborn periods. Am J Roentgenol Radium Ther Nucl Med 103:66, 1968

13. Bernard ED, James LS: Failure of the heart after undue asphyxia at birth. Pediatrics 28:545, 1961

14. Kulhn JP, Fletcher BD, Lemos RA: Roentgen findings in transient tachypnea of the newborn. Radiology 92:251, 1969

15. Wallgren E, Barr M, Rudhe V: Hemodynamic studies of induced acute hypo- and hypercythemia in newborn infant. Acta Paediatr 53:1, 1964

16. O'Conner JF, Shapiro JH, Ingall D: Erythrocythemia as a cuase of respiratory distress in newborn: radiologic findings. Radiology 90:933, 1968

17. Farrehi C, Mitchell M, Fawcett DM: Heart failure in congenital thyrotoxicosis. Pediatrics 37:460, 1966

18. Gerald B: Cardiac failure in infancy secondary to thyrotoxicosis. Radiology 91:59, 1968

19. Levy AM, Hanson JS, Tabakin BS: Congestive heart failure in the newborn infant in the absence of primary cardiac disease. Am J Cardiol 26:409, 1970

20. Najjar SS, Nassif ST: Congestive heart failure in infancy due to hypothyroidism. Acta Paediatr 52:319, 1963

21. Van Creveld S, De Jager J: Myocarditis in newborns caused by Coxsackie virus: clinical and pathologic data. Ann Pediatr 187:100, 1956

22. Ainger LE, Lawyer NG, Fitch CW: Neonatal rubella myocarditis. Br Heart J 28:691, 1966

23. Sanders V: Viral myocarditis. Am Heart J 66:707, 1963

24. Valdes-Dapena M, Miller WM: Pericarditis in the newborn. Pediatrics 16:673, 1955

25. Robinson SJ: Treatment of cardiac arrhythmias. Pediatr Clin North Am 11:315, 1964

26. Nakamara FT, Nadas AS: Complete heart block in infants and children. N Engl J Med 270:1261, 1964

27. Kuehl KS, Perry LW, Chandra R, Scott LP III: Left ventricular rhabdomyoma: a rare cause of subaortic stenosis in the newborn. Pediatrics 46:464, 1970

28. Nadas AS, Ellison RC: Cardiac tumors in infancy. Am J Cardiol 21:363, 1968

29. Engle MA, Glenn R: Primary malignant tumor of the heart in infancy: case report and review of the subject. Pediatrics 15:562, 1955

30. Sanyal SK, de Leuchtenberg N, Rojas RH et al: Right atrial myxoma in infancy and childhood. Am J Cardiol 20:263, 1967

31. Naeye RL: Infants of diabetic mothers: a quantitative, morphologic study. Pediatrics 35:980, 1965

32. Rutenberg HD, Steidl RM, Carey LS, Edwards JE: Glycogen storage disease of the heart: hemodynamic and angiographic features in two cases. Am Heart J 67:469, 1964

33. Ehlers KM, Hagstrom JWC, Lukas DS et al: Glycogen storage disease of the myocardium with obstruction to left ventricular outflow. Circulation 25:96, 1962

34. Rose V, Izukawa T, Moes CAF: Syndrome of asplenia and polysplenia: review of cardiac and noncardiac malformations in 60 cases with special reference to diagnosis and prognosis. Br Heart J 37:840, 1975

35. Fisher KC, White RI Jr, Jordan CE et al: Sternal abnormalities in patients with congenital heart disease. Am J Roentgenol Radium Ther Nucl Med 119:530, 1973

36. Gabrielson TO, Ladyman GH: early closure of sternal sutures and congenital heart disease. Am J Roentgenol Radium Ther Nucl Med 89:975, 1963

37. Luke MJ, McDonnelle EJ: Congenital heart disease and sedions. J Pediatr 73:725, 1968

38. Reckles LN, Peterson MA, Biance AJ, Weidman NM: The approach of scoliosis and congenital heart defects. J Bone Joint Surg [Am] 57(suppl):449, 1975

39. Boone ML, Swenson DE, Felson B: Rib notching: its many causes. Am J Roentgenol Radium Ther Nucl Med 91:1075, 1964

40. Poznanski AK, Steln AM, Gall JG: Skeletal abnormalities in genetically determined congenital heart disease. Radiol Clin North Am 9:435, 1971

41. Rowe RD, Uchida IA: Cardiac malformations in mongolism: a prospective study of 184 mongoloid children. Am J Med 31:726, 1961

42. Currarino G, Swason G: Developmental variance of ossification of manubrium sterni in mongolism. Radiology 82:916, 1964

43. Lees RF, Caldicott WJH: Sternal anomalies and congenital heart disease. Am J Roentgenol Radium Ther Nucl Med 124:423, 1975

44. Berberj JW: A new radiographic finding in mongolism. Radiology 86:332, 1966

45. Rabinovitz JG, Moseley JE: Lateral lumbar spine in Down's syndrome: a new roentgen feature. Radiology 83:74, 1964

46. Rabinovitz JG, Wolf BS, Greenberg EI et al: Osseous changes in rubella embryopathy (congenital rubella syndrome). Radiology 85:494, 1965

47. Singleton EB, Rudolph AJ, Rosenberg HS, Singer DB: Roentgenographic manifestations of the rubella syndrome in newborn infants. Am J Roentgenol Radium Ther Nucl Med 97:82, 1966

48. Muster AJ, Paul MH, Van Grodelle A, Conway JJ: Asymmetric distribution of the pulmonary blood flow between the right and left lungs in d-transposition of the great arteries. Am J Cardiol 38:352, 1976

49. Eliot RS, Shone JD, Kanjuh VI et al: Mitral atresia: a study of 32 cases. Am Heart J 70:6, 1965

50. Huhta JC, Gutgesell HP, Nihill MR, Seilheimer DK: Two-dimensional echocardiographic diagnosis of vascular ring in infancy. In Doyle EF (ed): Pediatric Cardiology. Springer-Verlag, New York, 1986

51. Stewart JR, Kincaid OW, Edwards JE: An Atlas of Vascular Rings and Related Malformations of the Aortic Arch System. Charles C Thomas, Springfield, IL, 1964

52. Shuford WH, Sybers RG: The Aortic Arch and Its Malformations with Emphasis on the Angiographic Features. Charles C Thomas, Springfield IL, 1974

53. Berdon WE, Baker DH: Vascular anomalies and the infant lung: rings, slings and other things. Semin Roentgenol 7:39, 1972

54. Huhta JC: Pediatric Imaging/Doppler Ultrasound of the Chest: Extracardiac Diagnosis. Lea & Febiger, Philadelphia, 1986

55. Gutgesell HP, Huhta JC, Latson LA et al: Accuracy of 2-dimensional echocardiography in the diagnosis of congenital heart disease. Am J Cardiol 55:514, 1985

56. Huhta JC, Glasow P, Murphey DJ Jr et al: Surgery without catheterization for congenital heart defects: management of 100 patients. J Am Coll Cardiol 9:823, 1987

57. Huhta JC et al: Segmental analysis of congenital heart disease. Dynamic Cardiovasc Imag J 1:117, 1987

58. Huhta JC, Hagler DJ, Seward JB et al: Two-dimensional echocardiographic assessment of dextrocardia: a segmental approach. Am J Cardiol 50:1351, 1982

59. Huhta JC, Smallborn JF, Macartney FJ: Two-dimensional echocardiographic diagnosis of situs. Br Heart J 48:97, 1982

60. Sanders SP, Bierman FZ, Williams RG: Conotruncal malformations: diagnosis in infancy using subxiphoid 2-dimensional echocardiography. Am J Cardiol 50:1361, 1982

61. Bierman FZ, William RG: Subxiphoid 2-dimensional imaging of the interatrial septum in infants and neonates with congenital heart disease. Circulation 60:80, 1979

62. Huhta JC, Smallhorn JF, Macartney FJ et al: Cross-sectional echocardiographic diagnosis of systemic venous return. Br Heart J 48:388, 1982

63. Cha EM, Khoury GM: Persistent left superior vena cava: radiologic and clinical significance. Radiology 103:375, 1972

64. Fraser RS, Dvorkin J, Rossall RE et al: Left superior vena cava. Am J Med 31:7111, 1961

65. Huhta JC, Gutgesell HP, Nihill MR: Cross-sectional echocardiographic diagnosis of total anomalous pulmonary venous connections. Br Heart J 53:525, 1985

66. Vick GW, Murphy DJ Jr, Ludomirsky A et al: Pulmonary venous and systemic ventricular inflow obstruction in patients with congenital heart disease: detection by combined two-dimensional and Doppler echocardiography. J Am Coll Cardiol 9:580, 1987

67. Tajik AJ, Seword JB, Hagler DJ et al: Two-dimensional real-time ultrasonic imaging of the heart and great vessels: technique, image orientation, structure identification and validation. Mayo Clin Proc 53:271, 1978

68. Alverson DC, Eldridge M, Dillon T et al: Noninvasive pulsed Doppler determination of cardiac output in neonates and children. J Pediatr 101:46, 1982

69. Reed KL, Meijboom EJ, Sahn DJ et al: Cardiac Doppler flow velocities in human fetuses. Circulation 73:41, 1986

70. De Smedt MCH, Visser GHA, Meijboom EJ: Fetal cardiac output estimated by Doppler echocardiography during mid- and late gestation. Am J Cardiol 60:338, 1987

71. Alverson DC, Eldridge MW, Johnson JD et al: Noninvasive measurement of cardiac output in healthy preterm and term newborn infants. Am J Perinatol 1:148, 1984

72. Walther FJ, Siassi B, Ramadan NH et al: Pulsed Doppler determinations of cardiac output in neonates: normal standards for clinical use. Pediatrics 76:829, 1985

73. Cloez JL, Schmidt KG, Birk E, Silverman NH: Determination of pulmonary to systemic blood flow ratios in children by a simplified Doppler echocar-

diographic method. J Am Coll Cardiol 11:825, 1988

74. Barron JV, Sahn DJ, Valdes-Cruz LM et al: Clinical utility of two-dimensional Doppler echocardiographic techniques for estimating pulmonary to systemic blood flow ratios in children with left-to-right shunting atrial septal defect, ventricular septal defect or patent ductus arteriosus. J Am Coll Cardiol 3:169, 1984

75. Kosturakis D, Goldberg SJ, Allen HD, Loeber C: Doppler echocardiographic prediction of pulmonary arterial hypertension in congenital heart disease. Am J Cardiol 53:1110, 1984

76. Goldberg SJ, Allen HD, Marz GR, Flinn CJ: Doppler Echocardiography. 1st ed. Lea & Febiger, Philadelphia, 1985

77. Matsuda M, Sekiguchi T, Sugishita Y et al: Reliability of non-invasive estimates of pulmonary hypertension by pulsed Doppler echocardiography. Br Heart J 56:158, 1986

78. Hata T, Aoki S, Hata K, Kitao M: Intracardiac blood flow velocity waveforms in normal fetuses in utero. Am J Cardiol 59:464, 1987

79. Reed KL, Sahn DJ, Scagnelli S et al: Doppler echocardiographic studies of diastolic function in the human fetal heart: changes during gestation. J Am Coll Cardiol 8:391, 1986

80. Miller TR, Grossman SJ, Schectman KB et al: Left ventricular diastolic filling and its association with age. Am J Cardiol 58:531, 1986

81. Seward JB, Khandheria BK, Oh JK et al: Transesophageal echocardiography: technique, anatomic correlations, implementation, and clinical applications. Mayo Clin Proc 63:649, 1988

82. Ritter SB, Thys D: Transesophageal color flow imaging in infants and children with congenital heart disease, abstracted. Clin Res 38:450A, 1990

83. Sahn DJ, Moises V, Cali G et al: Important roles of transesophageal color Doppler flow mapping studies (TEE) in infants with congenital heart disease, abstracted. J Am Coll Cardiol, suppl. 15:A204, 1990

84. Omoto R, Kyo S, Matsumura M et al: Biplane color Doppler transesophageal echocardiography: its impact on cardiovascular surgery and further technological progress in the probe, a matrix phased-array biplane probe. Echocardiography 6:423, 1989

85. Valdez-Cruz LM, Dudell GG: Specificity and accuracy of echocardiographic and clinical criteria for diagnosis of patent ductus arteriosus in fluid restricted infants. J Pediatr 98:298, 1981

86. Snatos MA, Moll JN, Drumond D et al: Development of the ductus arteriosus in right ventricular outflow tract obstruction. Circulation 62:818, 1980

87. Stevenson JG, Kawabor I, Guntheroth WG: Noninvasive detection of pulmonary hypertension in patent ductus arteriosus by pulsed Doppler echocardiography. Circulation 60:355, 1979

88. Huhta JC, Cohen M, Gutgesell HP: Patency of the ductus arteriosus in normal neonates: two-dimensional echocardiography versus Doppler assessment. J Am Coll Cardiol 4:561, 1984

89. Gentile R, Stevenson G, Dooley T et al: Pulsed Doppler echocardiographic determination of time of ductal closure in normal newborn infants. J Pediatr 98:443, 1981

90. Ellison RC, Peckham GJ, Lang P et al: Evaluation of the preterm infant for patent ductus arteriosus. Pediatrics 71:364, 1983

91. Allen HD, Goldberg SJ, Valdes-Cruz LM et al: Use of echocardiography in newborns with patent ductus arteriosus: a review. Pediatr Cardiol 3:65, 1982

92. Daniels O, Hopman JCW, Stoelinga GBA et al: Doppler flow characteristics in the main pulmonary artery and the LA/Ao ratio before and after ductal closure in healthy newborns. Pediatr Cardiol 3:99, 1982

93. Johnson GL, Breart GL, Gweitz MH et al: Echocardiographic characteristics of premature infants with patent ductus arteriosus. Pediatrics 72:864, 1983

94. Bierman FZ, Williams RG: Prospective diagnosis of d-transposition of the great arteries in neonates by subxiphoid two-dimensional echocardiography. Circulation 60:1496, 1979

95. Daskalopoulos DA, Edwards WD, Driscoll DJ et al: Correlation of two-dimensional echocardiographic and autopsy findings in complete transposition of the great arteries. J Am Coll Card 2:1151, 1983

96. Foate R, Stefanie L, Richards A, Somerville J: Left and right ventricular morphology in complex congenital heart disease defined by two-dimensional echocardiography. Am J Cardiol 49:93, 1982

97. Vitarelli A, D'Addio AP, Gentile R, Burattini M: Echocardiographic evaluation of left ventricular outflow obstruction in complete transposition of the great arteries. Am Heart J 108:531, 1984

98. Pasquin L, Sanders SP, Parness I, Colen SD: Echocardiographic diagnosis of coronary artery anatomy in transposition of the great arteries. Circulation 75:557, 1987

99. Baker EJ, Allan LD, Tynan MJ et al: Balloon atrial septostomy in the neonatal intensive care unit. Br Heart J 51:377, 1984

100. Lin AE, Di Sessa TG, Williams RG et al: Balloon and blade atrial septostomy facilitated by two-di-

mensional echocardiography. Am J Cardiol 57:273, 1986

101. Riggs T, Hirshfeld S, Faranoff A et al: Persistence of fetal circulation: an echocardiographic study. J Pediatr 91:626, 1977

102. Yock PG, Popp RL: Non-invasive estimation of right ventricular systolic pressure by Doppler ultrasound in patients with tricuspid regurgitation. Circulation 70:657, 1984

103. Johnson G, Cunningham MD, Desai NS et al: Echocardiography in hypoxemic neonatal pulmonary disease. J Pediatr 96:716, 1980

104. Rubin LJ: Pulmonary Heart Disease. Martinus Nijhoff, Boston, 1984

105. Riggs T, Hirshfeld S, Borkat G et al: Assessment of the pulmonary vascular bed by echocardiographic right ventricular systolic time intervals. Circulation 57:939, 1978

106. Nanda NC, Gramiak R, Robinson TI, Shah PM: Echocardiographic evaluation of pulmonary hypertension. Circulation 50:575, 1975

107. Hirschfeld S, Meyer R, Schwartz DC et al: The echocardiographic assessment of pulmonary artery pressure and pulmonary vascular resistance. Circulation 52:642, 1975

108. Hatle L, Angelsen BAJ, Tromsdal A: Non-invasive estimation of pulmonary artery systolic pressure with Doppler ultrasound. Br Heart J 45:157, 1981

109. Sahn DJ, Allen HD, Lange LW, Goldberg SJ: Cross-sectional echocardiographic diagnosis of the sites of total anomalous pulmonary venous drainage. Circulation 60:317, 1979

110. Smallhorn JF, Anderson RH, Maratroy FJ et al: Assessment of total anomalous pulmonary venous connection by two-dimensional echocardiography. Br Heart J 46:613, 1981

111. Smallhorn J, Freedom R: Pulsed Doppler echocardiography in the preoperative evaluation of total anomalous pulmonary venous connection. J Am Coll Cardiol 8:1413, 1986

112. Vick GW, Murphy DJ Jr, Ludomirsky A et al: Pulmonary venous and systemic ventricular inflow obstruction in patients with congenital heart disease: detection by combined two-dimensional and Doppler echocardiography. J Am Coll Cardiol 9:580, 1987

113. Huhta JC, Gutgesell HP, Nihill MR: Two-dimensional echocardiographic diagnosis of total anomalous pulmonary venous connection. Br Heart J 53:525, 1985

114. Tawes RL, Berry CL, Aberdeen E: Congenital bicuspid aortic valve associated with coarctation of the aorta in children. Br Heart J 31:127, 1969

115. Brandenburg RO Jr, Tajik AJ, Edwards WD et al: Accuracy of 2-dimensional echocardiographic diagnosis of congenitally bicuspid aortic valve: echocardiographic-anatomic correlation in 115 patients. Am J Cardiol 51:1470, 1983

116. Rosenquist GC: Congenital mitral valve disease associated with coarctation of the aorta. Circulation 49:985, 1974

117. Shone JD, Sellers RD, Anderson RC et al: The developmental complex of "parachute mitral valve," supravalvular ring of left atrium, subaortic stenosis, and coarctation of aorta. Am J Cardiol 11:714, 1963

118. Smallhorn JF, Anderson RH, Macartney FJ: Morphological characterization of ventricular septal defects associated with coarctation of aorta by cross-sectional echocardiography. Br Heart J 49:485, 1983

119. Smallhorn JF, Huhta JG, Adams PA et al: Cross-sectional echocardiographic assessment of coarctation in the sick neonate and infant. Br Heart J 50:349, 1983

120. Venables AW: The syndrome of pulmonary stenosis complicating maternal rubella. Br Heart J 27:49, 1965

121. Cohn HE, Freed MD, Hellenbrand WE, Fyler DC: Complications and mortality associated with cardiac catherization in infants under one year. Pediatr Cardiol 6:123, 1985

122. Porter CJ, Gillette PC, Mullins CE, McNamara DG: Cardiac catheterization in the neonate. J Pediatr 93:97, 1978

123. Levin AR, Goldberg HL, Borer JS et al: Digital angiography in the pediatric patient with congenital heart disease: comparison with standard methods. Circulation 68:374, 1983

124. Moodie DS, Yiannikas J, Gill CC et al: Intravenous digital subtraction angiography in the evaluation of congenital abnormalities of the aortic arch. Am Heart J 104:628, 1982

125. Moodie DS: Assessing cardiac anatomy with digital subtraction angiography. J Am Coll Cardiol 5:485, 1985

126. Buonocore E, Pavlicek W, Modic MT et al: Anatomic and functional imaging of congenital heart disease with digital subtraction angiography. Radiology 147:647, 1983

127. Dawson P: Chemotoxicity of contrast media and clinical adverse effects: a view. Invest Radiol, suppl. 20:S84, 1985

128. Tonkin IL, Fitch SJ, Magill HL: Pediatric digital subtraction angiography: intraarterial and intracardiac applications. Pediatr Radiol 16:126, 1986

129. Leibovic SJ, Fellows KE: Patient radiation exposure during cardiac catheterization. Cardiovasc Intervent Radiol 6:150, 1983

130. Chiles C, Ravin CE: Intrathoracic metastases from

an extrathoracic malignancy: a radiographic approach to patient evaluation. Radiol Clin North Am 23:427, 1985

131. Moncada R, Baker M, Salinas M et al: Diagnostic role of computed tomography in pericardial heart disease: congenital defects, thickening, neoplasms and effusions. Am Heart J 103:263, 1982

132. Glazer GM, Gross BH, Orringer MB et al: Computed tomography of pericardial masses: further observations and comparison with echocardiography. J Comput Assist Tomogr 8:895, 1984

133. Pugatch RD, Faling LJ, Robbins AH et al: Differentiation of pleural and pulmonary lesions using computed tomography. J Comput Assist Tomogr 2:601, 1978

134. Foster CJ, Sekiya T, Love HG et al: Identification of intracardiac thrombus: comparison of computed tomography and cross-sectional echocardiography. Br J Radiol 60:327, 1987

135. Huggins T et al: Left atrial myxoma: computed tomography as a diagnostic modality. J Comput Assist Tomgr 00:253, 1980

136. Eldredge WJ, Flicker S: Evaluation of congenital heart disease using cine-CT. Am J Cardiol Imag 1:38, 1987

137. Lipton MJ: Quantitation of cardiac function by cine-CT. Radiol Clin North Am 23:613, 1985

138. Mcmillian RM, Rees MR, Eldredge WJ et al: Quantitation of shunting at the atrial level using rapid acquisition computed tomography with comparison with cardiac catheterization. J Am Coll Cardiol 7:946, 1986

139. McIlveen BM, Murray IPC, Giles RW et al: Clinical application of radionuclide quantitation of left to right cardiac shunts in children. Am J Cardiol 47:1273, 1981

140. Anderson PAW, Dowger KW, Jones RH: Effects of age on radionuclide angiographic detection and quantitation of left-to-right shunts. Am J Cardiol 53:879, 1984

141. Vick GW, Sutterwhite C, Cassady G et al: Radionuclide angiography in the evaluation of ductal shunts in preterm infants. J Pediatr 101:264, 1982

142. Breitweser JA, Gelfend MJ, Meyer RA et al: Radionuclide angiographic and echocardiographic quantitation of left-to-right shunts in children with ventricular septal defect. Pediatr Cardiol 3:7, 1982

143. Hurwitz RA, Trevs S, Duruc A: Right ventricular and left ventricular ejection fraction in pediatric patients with normal hearts; first pass radionuclide angiocardiography. Am Heart J 107:726, 1983

144. Peter CA, Armstrong BE, Jones RH: Radionuclide measurements of left ventricular function: their use in patients with aortic insufficiency. Arch Surg 115:1348, 1980

145. Finley JP, Howman-Giles R, Gildoy DL et al: Thallium-201 myocardial imaging in anomalous left coronary artery arising from the pulmonary artery: applications before and after medical and surgical treatment. Am J Cardiol 42:675, 1978

146. Gutgesell HP, Pinslky WW, DePuey EG: Thallium-201 myocardial perfusion imaging in infants and children. Circulation 61:596, 1980

147. O'Connell JB, Henkins RE, Robinson JA et al: Gallium-67 imaging in patients with dilated cardiomyopathy and biopsy-proven myocarditis. Circulation 70:58, 1984

148. Bufalino VJ, Robinson JA, Henkin R et al: Gallium-67 scanning: a new diagnostic approach to the post-pericardiotomy syndrome. Am Heart J 106:1138, 1983

149. Greenberg ML, Niebulski HIJ, Vretsky BF et al: Occult purulent pericarditis detected by indium-111 leukocyte imaging. Chest 85:701, 1984

150. Koutcher JA, Burt CT: Principles of nuclear resonance. J Nucl Med 25:101, 1984

151. Kersting-Sommerhoff BA, Piethelm L, Feitel DF et al: Magnetic resonance imaging of congenital heart disease: sensitivity and specificity using receiver operating characteristic curve analysis, Am Heart J 118:155, 1989

152. Chung KJ, Simpson IA, Newman R et al: Cine magnetic imaging for evaluation of congenital heart disease: role in pediatric cardiology compared with echocardiography and angiography. J Pediatr 113:1028, 1988

153. Naylor GL, Firmin DN, Longmore DB: Blood flow imaging by cine magnetic resonance. J Comput Assist Tomgr 10:715, 1986

154. Rees S, Firmin D, Mohiaddin R et al: Application of flow measurements by magnetic resonance velocity mapping to congenital heart disease. Am J Cardiol 64:953, 1989

155. Pernot AC, Ingwall JS, Menasche P et al: Evaluation of high energy phosphate metabolism during cardioplegic arrest and reperfusion: a phosphorus-31 nuclear magnetic resonance study. Circulation 67:1296, 1983

156. Nunally RI, Bottomley PA: 31P NMR studies of myocardial ischemia and its response to drug therapies. J Comput Assist Tomogr 5:296, 1981

Gastrointestinal Radiology in the Premature Infant

Lawrence Robinson
Seiji Kitagawa

7

IMAGING OF THE GASTROINTESTINAL TRACT

Plain Film Evaluation

The gastrointestinal (GI) tract of the premature infant is commonly observed on initial radiographs of the chest. Fetal swallowing and motility of the GI tract in utero have been documented by injection of contrast material into the amniotic fluid. This activity is considered to be an important part in the regulation of the amount of amniotic fluid and also supplies calories to the fetus. The ingested fluid is absorbed into the fetal circulation. Polyhydramnios commonly occurs in fetuses with proximal obstruction or impaired swallowing.

Air enters the GI tract of the newborn infant primarily by swallowing, but also by the respiratory movement of the thorax. Some infants dying shortly after birth have air in the stomach and proximal small bowel but airless lungs. Whether this is due to swallowing or respiratory movement is not known, but it has been shown that air will enter the stomach with inspiratory efforts against a closed glottis when there is relaxation of the superior esophageal sphincter at the pharyngoesophageal junction.[1] Air is present in the stomach immediately after birth, and progresses into the proximal small bowel within 15 min (Fig. 7-1). Normal babies will have air throughout the bowel to the level of the sigmoid colon by 8 to 9 hours of life.[2] It is frequently impossible to distinguish the colon from the small bowel. Delayed passage of bowel gas has been noted in depressed or hypotonic infants.

Normal babies will pass meconium in the first 24 to 36 hours of life. In many premature infants this may be delayed for several days or until feedings are started. Until the meconium is expelled, a granular or soap-bubble appearance can sometimes be seen within the colon. This is considered normal after excluding signs of obstruction and necrotizing enterocolitis. After passage of meconium, however, this ''bubbly'' stool pattern is infrequently seen (in only 3 to 5 percent of normal infants). This lasts until the infant is about 2 weeks old, after which time the bubbly pattern of air mixed with feces is seen in 50 to 60 percent of infants. Thus visualization of the bubbly pattern after meconium is passed and prior to 2 weeks of age may indicate the presence of necrotizing enterocolitis, and close follow-up is necessary.[3]

There is considerable variability in the amount of bowel gas normally present. Typically there are multiple loops of bowel present in a cystic or honeycomb pattern in which no one loop stands out (Fig. 7-2). Resuscitation may increase the amount of bowel gas, and placing the feeding tube to drainage will diminish the gas pattern. The infant lies supine for the usual abdominal radiograph, and air may normally distend the transverse and sigmoid colon, since they lie anteriorly on a mesentery. This pattern is considered normal when the remainder of the bowel appears normal. The sigmoid colon is relatively long and

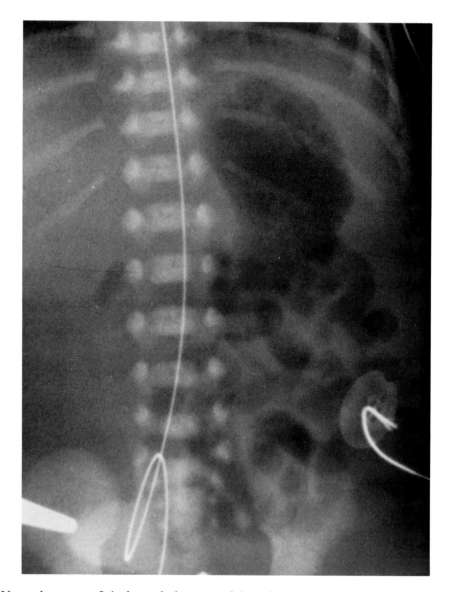

Fig. 7-1. Normal passage of air through the stomach into the jejunum is present on this film at about 15 minutes of age for localization of the umbilical arterial catheter.

redundant in infants, resulting in some variability in position. If there is clinical concern about the presence of obstruction or focal inflammation, a prone or left lateral decubitus view should be obtained (Fig. 7-3). Normally the air will then move into the superior portion of adjacent loops. Air will remain fixed in an obstructed or ischemic noncompliant loop.[4] The left lateral decubitus position is the most sensitive to evaluate free peritoneal air, which will be identified over the right lobe of the liver (see Fig. 7-39).

A gasless abdomen presents a diagnostic dilemma in the sick premature infant. Most commonly this is due to diminished swallowing and orogastric tube drainage or suction. Infants who are pharmacologically paralyzed to improve assisted ventilation will also have a gasless abdomen. Occasionally ascites or bowel ischemia may be present. If there is a clinical suspicion of abdominal pathology, abdominal ultrasound examination is indicated. It can differentiate fluid-filled bowel loops from ascites. Echogenic ma-

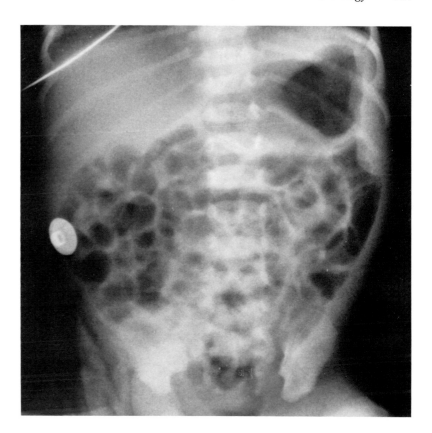

Fig. 7-2. Normal bowel gas pattern. Air is present throughout the bowel and no focal dilated loops are noted.

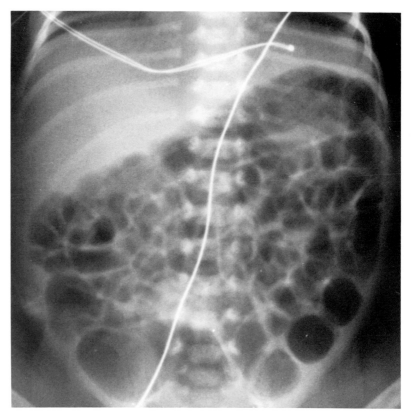

Fig. 7-3. Focal air trapping in the sigmoid colon. The focally dilated loop of bowel in the right lower quadrant and pelvis is the normal sigmoid colon.

terial within the ascitic fluid usually means that there has been a perforation and that surgery may be necessary.[5]

Contrast Examinations

No preparation is usually required for contrast examinations in sick neonates. Feedings should be withheld for only 2 hours prior to an upper GI series. Barium sulfate suspension remains the contrast material of choice for most examinations, except when aspiration into the lungs or perforation is a possibility. The newer low-osmolar, water-soluble contrast materials are ideal in these situations. They are relatively safe when aspirated in small amounts into the trachea,[6] and they are less likely to be diluted or absorbed in the GI tract than are hyperosmolar materials.[7] They remain, however, quite expensive and are used only in select cases. For use in the colon, diluted hyperosmolar water-soluble contrast agents (about 600 mOsm/L) are still quite satisfactory, and may be therapeutic in reducing the obstruction in meconium ileus.

Most contrast procedures are best performed in the radiology department under fluoroscopic control. Prior consideration needs to be given to maintaining the body temperature in premature infants. Some radiology departments have an infant warmer modified for use on the radiography table.[8] Others borrow a portable warmer from the nursery, or use heat lamps or even warmed IV solution bags. The procedure should be performed efficiently and the baby returned to the isolette as quickly as possible. Portable upper GI studies are occasionally useful when the baby is clinically unstable and on a ventilator. Indications for such a study are very limited, such as unexplained perforation. Up to 5 ml/kg of hypo-osmolar water-soluble contrast material is slowly instilled through an orogastric tube over several minutes. This should reduce the possibility of gastroesophageal reflux around the tube. An immediate portable radiograph is taken, and subsequent films are obtained as needed.[9]

MAJOR GASTROINTESTINAL DISORDERS

Many gastrointestinal disorders may affect the premature infant. Those conditions that commonly result in significant morbidity and mortality include the following: necrotizing enterocolitis, intestinal perfo-

ration, gastroschisis, tracheoesophageal fistula, disorders of intestinal motility, and intestinal atresia/stenosis. Disorders occasionally affecting the premature infant are anorectal anomalies and meconium ileus. Hirschsprung's disease is rarely seen in premature infants. These conditions will quite often require immediate surgical intervention. The following sections will discuss the major neonatal gastrointestinal disorders, although some of them are observed usually in full-term infants.

Diaphragm

Diaphragmatic Hernia

The incidence of diaphragmatic hernia is about one in 4,000 births. At 8 to 10 weeks of embryonic life the central tendon of the diaphragm is formed from the septum transversum. Following formation of the lateral and posterior portions of the diaphragm, the last portions to close are the posterolateral triangular pleuroperitoneal canals, or the foramen of Bochdalek, through which the majority (80 to 90 percent) of hernias occur. The left hemidiaphragm closes later than the right and this explains the preponderance of diaphragmatic hernia on the left side (Figs. 7-4 and 7-5). Hernias associated with a retrosternal defect in the foramen of Morgagni occur occasionally (fewer than 2 percent of cases). If there is a defect in the diaphragm while the intestine is rotating counterclockwise, the intestine will enter the chest cavity. The organs involved in the herniation will vary and may include the liver, spleen, stomach, and transverse colon in addition to the small bowel (Fig. 7-6).

In most instances, the neonate with diaphragmatic hernia will require emergency surgery. Rarely, however, a patient will have few symptoms in the neonatal period and present later in life with an unsuspected diaphragmatic hernia. The plain radiographic examination will usually suggest the diagnosis, although occasionally a congenital diaphragmatic hernia may be difficult to distinguish from an eventration of the diaphragm or an adenomatoid malformation of the lung. In such cases contrast studies of the GI tract may be helpful in confirming the diagnosis. Malrotation of the midgut is present in all cases.[10–13]

Eventration

Eventration or weakness of the hemidiaphragm and paralysis are uncommon. These conditions, however, must be differentiated from classic diaphrag-

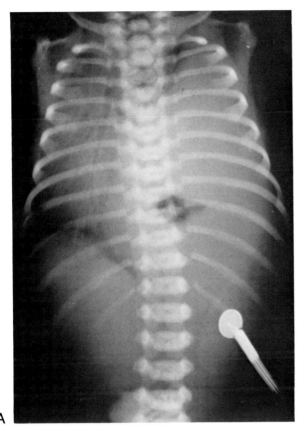 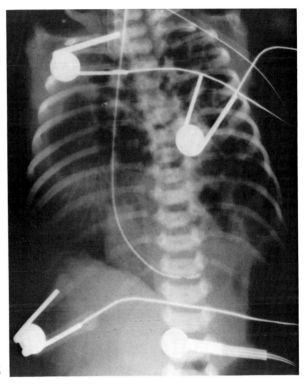

A   B

Fig. 7-4. Left diaphragmatic hernia. The heart and mediastinum are shifted to the right. The abdomen is scaphoid. **(A)** There is no air in the bowel. **(B)** A nasogastric tube has been passed into the stomach and air has been injected, demonstrating the bowel loops in the left chest.

matic hernia, since they are often managed nonsurgically.[14] Ultrasound or fluoroscopy may be utilized to evaluate motion of the diaphragm in order to distinguish the diminished but appropriate motion of eventration from paradoxical motion seen with diaphragmatic paralysis. If the infant requires ventilation, this procedure needs to be delayed until removal from the respirator can be tolerated for a 30- to 60-second period for observation of diaphragmatic motion. In eventration the upward bulge of the diaphram is typically medial and anterior in location (Fig. 7-7).

Abdominal Wall Defects

Gastroschisis/Omphalocele

The anterior abdominal wall is formed from the confluence of cephalic, caudal, and lateral folds between the third and fifth weeks of embryonic devel-

opment. Failure of the lateral folds to fuse in the midline results in an anterior abdominal wall hernia.

The incidence of these abdominal wall defects is about 1:5,000 live births. If there is delayed migration of the intestinal loops back into the abdominal cavity at about the 10th-week of fetal gestation, an omphalocele will occur. It is a congenital hernia involving the umbilicus, and is covered by an avascular sac composed of the fused layers of amnion and peritoneum (Fig. 7-8).

Gastroschisis, however, is a full-thickness, complete abdominal wall defect, usually to the right of the normal umbilicus. The extruded intestine in gastroschisis is never covered by a membrane. Fifty percent of babies with gastroschisis are premature.

The liver and spleen frequently extrude into a large omphalocele, whereas this is never observed in a gastroschisis. Omphalocele patients frequently (60 percent) have other associated anomalies, such as malro-

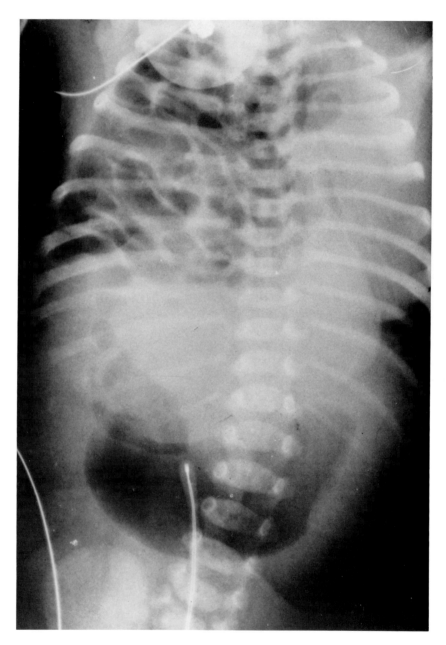

Fig. 7-5. Right diaphragmatic hernia. Bowel is present in the right hemithorax with shift of the heart and mediastinum to the left. The stomach is in the abdomen.

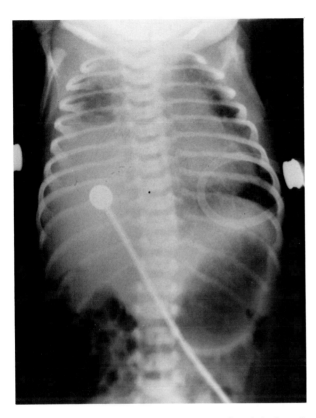

Fig. 7-6. Herniation of the liver into the right hemithorax. The hepatic flexure of the colon is elevated. Abdominal ultrasound confirmed the diagnosis.

tation, diaphragmatic hernia (Fig. 7-9), and renal and cardiovascular defects. These are rarely seen in patients with gastroschisis. In spite of improving surgical techniques, the return to normal function of damaged bowel may take 3 to 6 months. Adhesive intestinal obstruction and malabsorption are frequent complications.[15]

Esophagus

Esophageal Atresia

The incidence of esophageal atresia is 1:3,000 to 1:3,500 live births. The most common form of esophageal atresia includes an associated distal tracheo-esophageal fistula (85 percent). Fifty percent of babies with esophageal atresia also experienced maternal polyhydramnios. An additional finding of esophageal atresia on prenatal ultrasound is a very small stomach or one that cannot be identified.

Prematurity is common in cases of esophageal atresia, resulting in higher mortality.[16] The incidence of associated congenital anomalies is around 50 percent and cardiac, anorectal, urogenital, and skeletal anomalies predominate. This group of anomalies has been termed the VATER (*v*ascular or *v*ertebral, *a*norectal, *t*racheo*e*sophageal and *r*enal or *r*adial) association.[17] The baby's inability to swallow saliva occurs immediately after birth, with episodes of coughing, choking, and cyanosis. Failure to advance a size 8 French radiopaque tube beyond 9 to 11 cm through the nose or mouth is diagnostic. Radiographs of the chest and abdomen should be obtained with the tube in place. When there is a fistula between the distal esophagus and trachea, air is present in the GI tract (Fig. 7-10). Complete absence of air in the GI tract suggests a pure esophageal atresia (Fig. 7-11). Contrast studies are rarely indicated, but early clinical or radiographic evidence of aspiration suggests the possibility of an upper pouch fistula (Fig. 7-12) or H-type fistula (Fig. 7-13). In this case a careful contrast study of the upper esophageal pouch under fluoroscopic control is indicated, utilizing a small catheter (5 or 8 French) with barium or low-osmolar, water-soluble contrast material. Only a small amount should be injected and then aspirated following the study. A fistula, if present, is best visualized in the lateral projection. Rapid sequence spot films and/or videotape recording are essential.[18,19]

Esophageal Stenosis/Web

Esophageal stenosis/web is an extremely rare condition that occurs in 1:25,000 to 1:50,000 live births. Much confusion has occurred because of the difficulty in distinguishing this entity from reflux esophagitis at an early age. When the stenosis is severe, dysphagia for liquid occurs in infancy. Commonly the child will have recurrent respiratory infections, dribbling of saliva, and failure to thrive.

Congenital esophagal stenosis has been described in association with tracheoesophageal anomalies, duodenal atresia, and anorectal anomalies. Stenosis may be associated with tracheobronchial remnants in the lower esophagus. The clinical picture should prompt both radiographic and endoscopic investigation. These studies are complementary in evaluating stenosis and gastroesophageal reflux. The upper GI series can more easily identify duodenal pathology and malrotation.[20,21]

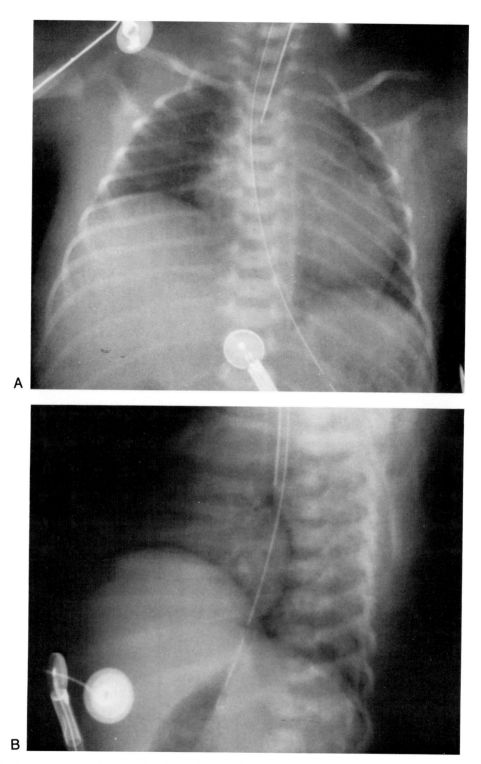

Fig. 7-7. Eventration of the right hemidiaphragm. Anteroposterior **(A)** and lateral **(B)** views show the anterior position of this moderate eventration.

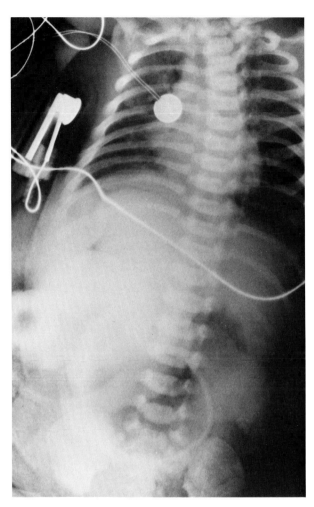

Fig. 7-8. Omphalocele. Bowel loops covered by dressing are located anterior to the abdomen.

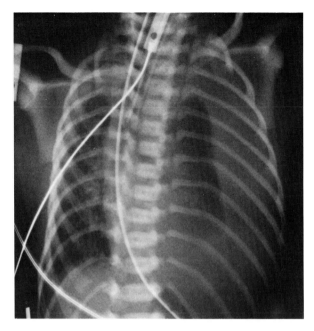

Fig. 7-9. Omphalocele associated with a left diaphragmatic hernia. The bowel loops in the left lateral hemithorax have not yet filled with air.

Disorders of Esophageal Motility

Disorders of both the oral and pharyngeal phases of swallowing may be associated with a variety of neurologic and myopathic conditions. The very premature infant, however, commonly has a weak sucking effort and uncoordinated swallowing. Newborn infants with poorly coordinated or weak pharyngeal contraction have difficulty propelling liquid into the esophagus because of the ineffective peristaltic wave[25] (Fig. 7-15).

Gastroesophageal Reflux

Gastroesophageal reflux (GER) is a common motility disorder in the infant. The premature infant is especially prone to have GER, probably owing to reduced lower esophageal sphincter pressure as a consequence of decreased muscle mass and responsiveness (Fig. 7-16). Delayed gastric emptying may also be responsible for GER in these newborn infants. Apnea and bradycardia have been implicated in these conditions, thought in some cases to be secondary to the aspiration of small amounts of refluxed material in the hypopharynx. A pH probe is the most sensitive method of detecting reflux, but is time consuming.

Esophageal Trauma

Esophageal injury in the newborn may result from excessively vigorous oropharyngeal suction or the passage of a nasogastric tube. Perforation usually occurs in the hypopharynx when a catheter is advanced while the cricopharyngeal muscle is contracted. This will result in a traumatic diverticulum, and in some cases the catheter passes into the superior mediastinum, is deflected to the right by the aortic arch, and enters the right pleural space (Fig. 7-14). Rarely necrotizing enterocolitis and neonatal Boerhaave's syndrome may result in rupture of the esophagus.[22-24]

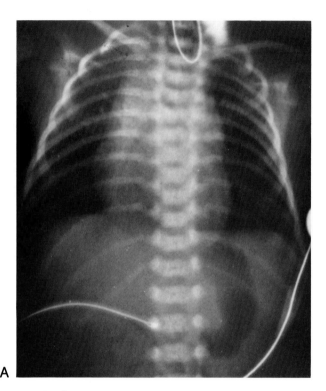
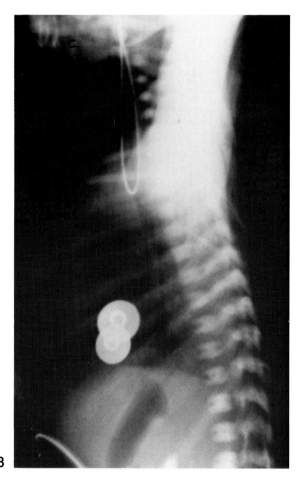

A   B

Fig. 7-10. Esophageal atresia with distal fistula. Anteroposterior **(A)** and lateral **(B)** views show a nasogastric tube coiled in the blind proximal esophageal pouch. Air is present in the stomach, indicating a fistula between the distal esophagus and the carina.

Gastroesophageal scintigraphy is very sensitive and allows quantification of the reflux over 45 to 60 minutes. The standard upper GI series is a crude method with intermittent observation over only 5 to 10 minutes, but does allow an anatomic assessment of the gastroesophageal junction as well as partial obstruction and motility disorders.[26,27]

Stomach

Gastric Perforation

Perforation of the stomach in critically ill neonates is usually attributed to local hypoxia and ischemia, but spontaneous gastric rupture is also described. An increased risk of perforation has been found in mechanically ventilated neonates. A particular risk of GI perforation occurs with use of indomethacin for pharmacologic closure of a patent ductus arteriosis in very low-birthweight infants. Gastric perforation in premature infants may also result from massive necrotizing enterocolitis, stress from sepsis or hypoglycemia, and trauma from tube feedings in premature infants[28–31] (Fig. 7-17).

Antral Diaphragm

An antral diaphragm is a rare anomaly composed of a submucosal web covered by gastric mucosa. Obstruction may be complete or partial. The complete web appears on the plain film as an air-filled stomach with no distal gas. With an incomplete web, careful contrast studies may demonstrate a lucent line across the gastric antrum, often associated with poor antral

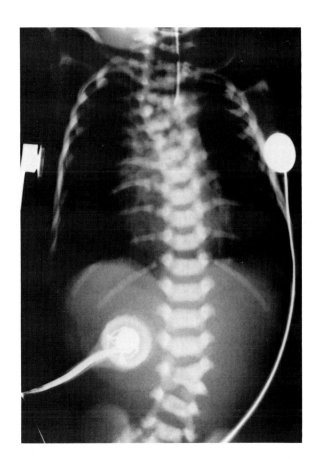

Fig. 7-11. Esophageal atresia without fistula. The tip of the nasogastric tube is in the proximal esophageal pouch. The abdomen is gasless because there is no fistula. Associated vertebral anomalies include hemivertebrae in the upper thoracic and mid-lumbar spine.

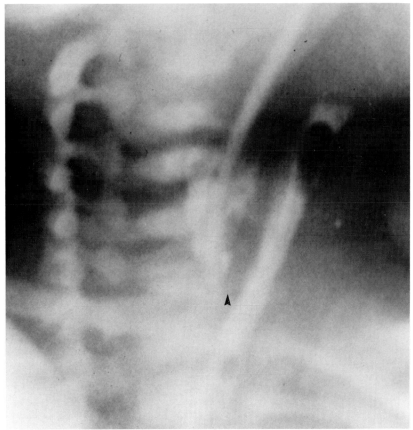

Fig. 7-12. Esophageal atresia with proximal fistula. A small amount of contrast instilled through a 5 French catheter in the proximal esophageal pouch rapidly passes through a small fistula (arrowhead) into the trachea.

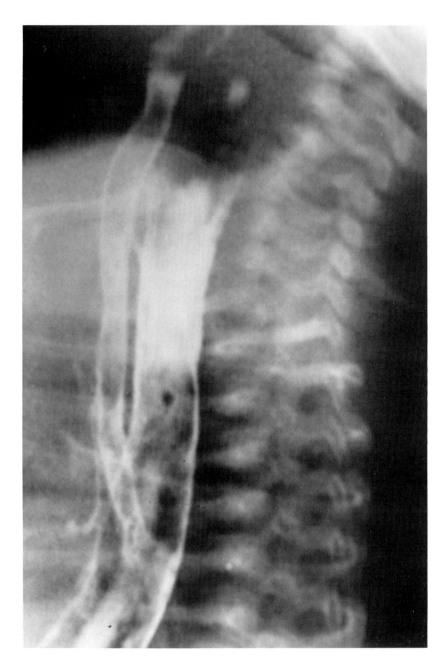

Fig. 7-13. H-type tracheoesophageal fistula. A small amount of barium was swallowed and the fistula was identified passing anteriorly and superiorly from the esophagus to the trachea just below the level of the clavicle. The esophagus distended with air on each inspiration.

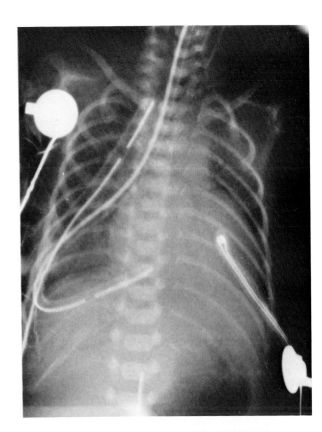

Fig. 7-14. Cricopharyngeal perforation with a nasogastric tube. The course of the feeding tube is posterior to the trachea and enters the right pleural space. A right chest tube has been inserted as a result of the pneumothorax. These patients are treated with antibiotics and chest tube drainage, usually without surgery.

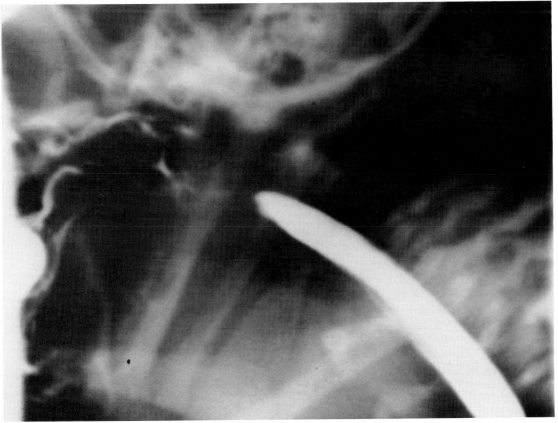

Fig. 7-15. Uncoordinated swallowing results in nasopharyngeal reflux in this premature infant. No aspiration was noted.

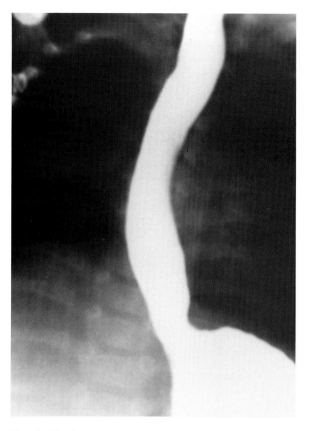

Fig. 7-16. One episode of gastroesophageal reflux associated with regurgitation is seen. The esophagus is dilated in this 3-week-old infant with moderate GER.

filling. Upper endoscopy now plays the major role in diagnosis.[32,33]

Gastric Duplication

Duplication of the stomach is rare, but can present early in the neonatal period. The majority of gastric duplications do not communicate with the lumen of the GI tract unless ulceration of a common wall occurs. A large cyst may present as an abdominal mass. Infants with gastric duplication may present with vomiting, similar to pyloric stenosis, and sometimes may have hematemesis from ulceration of the cyst wall. Diagnosis is made by upper GI series, which demonstrates obstruction and extrinsic compression, or ultrasound, which identifies the cystic mass.[34]

Microgastria

Microgastria, an extremely rare condition, has been described in association with multiple intra-abdominal malformations and skeletal anomalies. Most infants with microgastria present with failure to thrive and symptoms of gastroesophageal reflux. An upper GI series will show a small tubular stomach with a dilated esophagus in most cases.[35]

Duodenum

Duodenal Atresia/Stenosis/Web

Intrinsic duodenal obstruction is the result of atresia in 40 to 60 percent of cases, stenosis in 35 to 40 percent, and web in 5 to 15 percent, and presents as a high intestinal blockage (Fig. 7-18). About 80 percent of atresias are at or distal to the ampulla of Vater and virtually all webs are near the ampulla. The incidence varies between 1:10,000 and 1:20,000 live births. About 30 percent of patients with duodenal atresia also have Down's syndrome. Stenosis is most often due to extrinsic duodenal obstruction, as in annular pancreas, peritoneal band, or preduodenal portal vein[36,37] (Fig. 7-19).

Annular Pancreas

Annular pancreas is the most common cause of external compression on the second part of duodenum, resulting in partial or complete obstruction. Up to 70 percent of infants with annular pancreas have other anomalies. High-grade duodenal obstruction is easily diagnosed by abdominal plain films, which show the typical "double bubble" with little or no small bowel gas. An upper GI study is helpful when there is partial obstruction. Although it may be impossible to distinguish stenosis from annular pancreas, the "wind sock" appearance of a web can sometimes be identified. Duodenal obstruction can be identified on prenatal ultrasound and should be checked for in the presence of polyhydramnios.[38,39]

Small Bowel

Atresion/Stenosis

Atresia and stenosis of the small intestine result from ischemic necrosis of the fetal intestine, often due to intrauterine volvulus, intussusception, or occlusion of a mesenteric artery. Atresia is far more common than stenosis (15:1 ratio) and occurs more frequently in the ileum than the jejunum (Figs. 7-20 through 7-22). Atresias may be multiple or may involve a long segment associated with a mesenteric defect. About half of the cases have an associated major malformation, such as malrotation, Down's syndrome, or cystic fibrosis. Prematurity is common

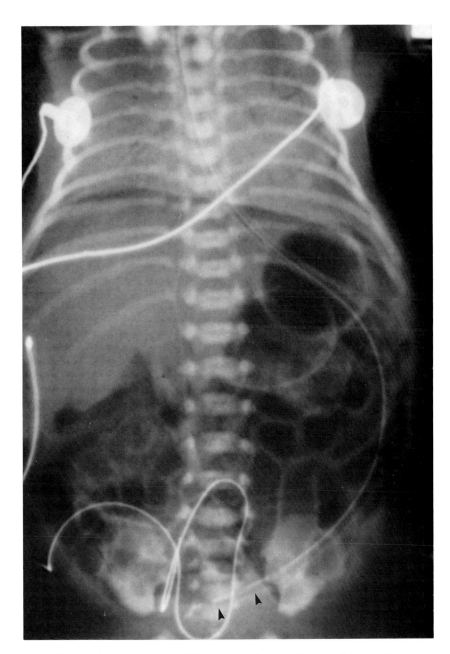

Fig. 7-17. Traumatic gastric perforation. The oragastric tube is passed through the posterior wall of the gastric fundus in this premature infant with hyaline membrane disease. The tip of the tube is in the pelvis (arrowheads). Free air is present over the liver and around loops of bowel. The position of the umbilical arterial catheter is also low, in the right common iliac artery.

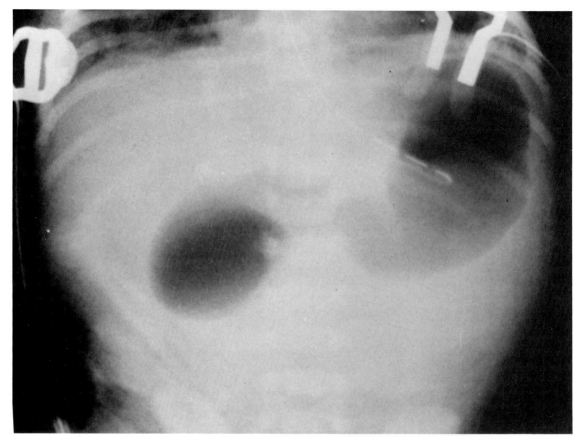

Fig. 7-18. Duodenal atresia. A typical "double bubble" of congenital duodenal obstruction is present. No bowel gas is present distal to the obstruction.

in these babies, occurring in 25 percent of those with ileal atresia, 40 percent of those with jejunal atresia, and 50 percent of those with multiple atresias. Multiple skip areas of involvement are reported in up to 25 percent of cases.

The plain abdominal radiograph shows dilated loops of bowel with air-fluid levels on decubitus views. The number of loops roughly correlates with the level of the obstruction. The size of the colon on barium enema is helpful in excluding long segment or multiple atresias (Fig. 7-23). A short segment duodenal or proximal jejunal atresia will show a normal-caliber colon on barium enema, whereas an ileal atresia will show a microcolon or unused colon. Intestinal secretions provide sufficient volume to distend the colon in the more proximal lesions. Thus when a proximal obstruction is present on plain film and a microcolon is found on barium enema, either long segment atresia, multiple atresias, or meconium ileus will be found

at surgery. A small bowel series is usually contraindicated since the contrast material is difficult to remove and may be aspirated into the lungs if the child vomits.[40-42]

Abnormal Intestinal Fixation and Malrotation

Disorders of intestinal fixation rank as the second most common cause of neonatal intestinal obstruction. Malrotation of the small intestine is due to incomplete movement or rotation of small intestine around the superior mesenteric artery during the 10th week of gestation. There is a male preponderance and it has an incidence of 1:6,000 births. Nonrotation of the midgut is a significant finding in all cases of omphalocele, gastroschisis, and diaphragmatic hernia.

Malrotation or incomplete rotation may produce duodenal obstruction resulting from peritoneal

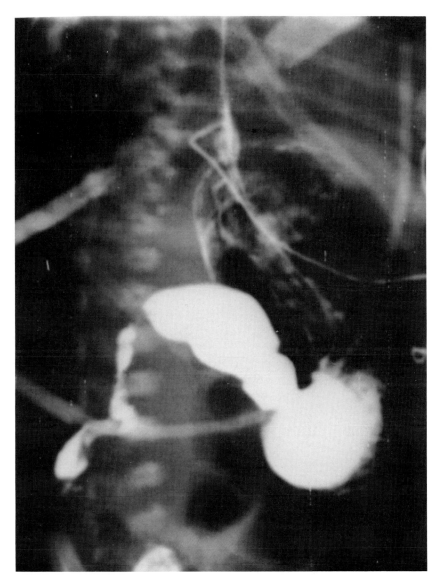

Fig. 7-19. Preduodenal portal vein. The portal vein was found to be anterior to the duodenum in this premature baby with malrotation and obstruction at the apex of the duodenal bulb as a result of stenosis.

bands, volvulus, or internal hernia (Fig. 7-24). Over 50 percent of cases will present in the first week of life with high internal obstruction due to volvulus. However, there are many variations in the clinical picture and age of onset. Obstruction of the duodenum by peritoneal bands will require surgery during the neonatal period in 75 percent of cases. Findings on the plain film with midgut volvulus are quite variable. Dilatation of the stomach and duodenum are frequently present, but the bowel gas pattern may be normal, diminished, or generally distended. When

gastric and duodenal obstruction are present on plain films, a contrast study may not be necessary. Air can be added to the stomach while the baby is in the left lateral decubitus or prone position, distending the duodenum to the level of obstruction. If this is not diagnostic, a small amount of barium can be instilled, following which tapered narrowing in the third or fourth portions of the duodenum is commonly seen. A "corkscrew" appearance to the proximal small bowel is sometimes seen, caused by the twisting of the bowel around the mesentery (Fig. 7-25). A contrast

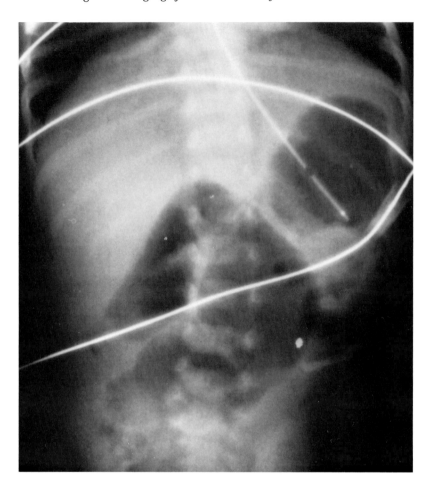

Fig. 7-20. Jejunal stenosis. The stomach, duodenum, and proximal jejunum are dilated. Small amounts of air can be seen in decompressed loops of bowel distal to the obstruction.

enema may be the initial study, especially when there is generalized distension of bowel loops. In this case the cecum will be located under the transverse colon. Occasionally, when there is small bowel obstruction with gangrenous bowel, there will be obstruction at the midportion of the transverse colon.[43,44]

Duplication

Alimentary duplications occur anywhere in the GI tract, but are more common in the distal ileum. Duplications are either spherical and have no communication with normal intestine, or tubular and communicate with the bowel lumen. Except in the duodenum, duplications occur on the mesenteric side of the bowel and share a common blood supply and muscle wall. Small bowel duplications often contain gastric mucosa, which may be demonstrated by technetium-99m nuclear imaging. Complications of duplication include obstruction, intussusception, hemorrhage, perforation, and enteric fistula.[45,46]

Meconium Ileus

Meconium ileus is the third most common cause of neonatal intestinal obstruction and occurs almost exclusively in newborns with cystic fibrosis. Between 10 and 15 percent of patients with cystic fibrosis present with this condition. Twenty percent of these infants are premature. Abnormal mucus production results in thick, tenacious meconium, which becomes inspissated and impacted in the distal ileum.

The plain film findings of uncomplicated meconium ileus are somewhat variable, but there is commonly distension, which may simulate colon obstruction; decreased or absent air-fluid levels due to viscous secretions; and a bubbly pattern of air mixed

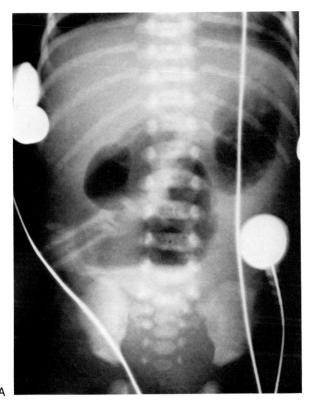

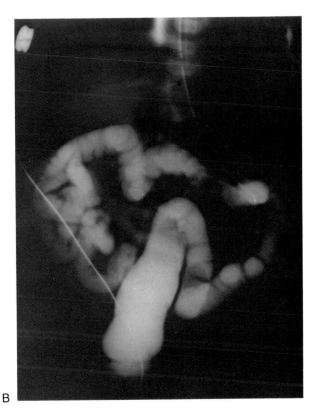

A   B

Fig. 7-21. Jejunal atresia. **(A)** No air is seen distal to the dilated loops of jejunum. **(B)** A normal caliber colon was found on barium enema.

with meconium in dilated loops of ileum. A microcolon or unused colon, due to the distal ileal obstruction(Fig. 7-26), is found on contrast enema. Hypertonic water-soluble contrast may be therapeutic if refluxed into the small bowel by drawing fluid into the bowel (Fig. 7-27). Full-strength meglumine diatrizoate (Gastrografin) is very hyperosmolar (1,900 mOsm/L) and may be irritating to the intestinal mucosa. It should be diluted with water (1:1 or 2:1) prior to use. Routine cystographic contrast media (approximately 600 mOsm/L) may also be used. Administration of intravenous fluids and careful monitoring of the patient are necessary to prevent hypertonic dehydration.

Many cases of meconium ileus are complicated by atresia, stenosis, volvulus, or perforation. Air-fluid levels may be present when the obstruction is in the mid or proximal small bowel. In some series, up to 25 percent of patients with atresia or stenosis have cystic fibrosis. The meconium-filled loops of bowel are prone to volvulus, and gangrenous bowel may

present as a mass or pseudocyst with proximal atresia (Fig. 7-28). Meconium peritonitis is the result of bowel perforation in utero. The meconium causes a chemical peritonitis and formation of thick adhesions and calcifications. Although such calcifications are commonly curvilinear along the margins of the peritoneum, they may be finely nodular or globular and located in the mesentery, the bowel wall, or even the bowel lumen (Fig. 7-29). Occasionally a male infant will have masses with calcification in the scrotum. Prenatal volvulus and meconium peritonitis are not specific for meconium ileus, but cystic fibrosis is confirmed in about 50 percent of cases.[47,48]

Colon

Meconium Plug Syndrome and Small Left Colon Syndrome

Meconium plug syndrome and small left colon syndrome are related disorders of unknown etiology in which normal meconium becomes impacted in the

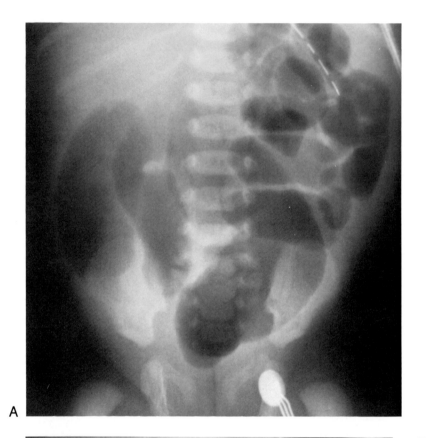

A

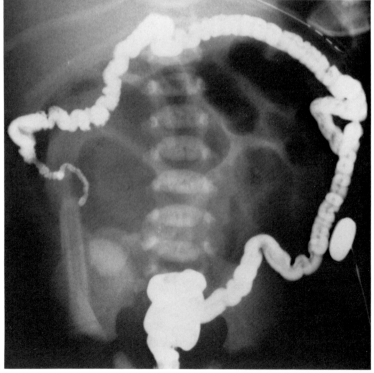

B

Fig. 7-22. Ileal atresia. **(A)** Multiple dilated loops of bowel are present consistent with a low intestinal obstruction. **(B)** An unused colon is noted on barium enema.

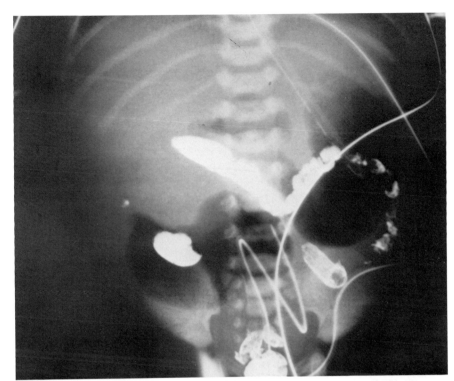

Fig. 7-23. Long segment small bowel atresia. A microcolon was present in this infant with jejunal obstruction. Long segment atresia was found at surgery and short gut syndrome developed postoperatively.

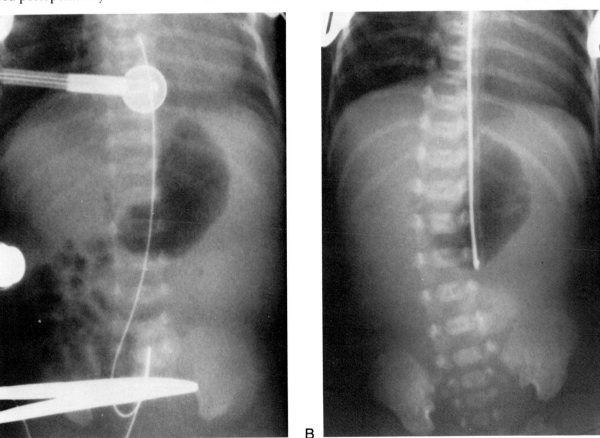

A

B

Fig. 7-24. Malrotation with volvulus. **(A)** Demonstration of abnormal position of proximal jejunum on the radiograph documenting the position of the umbilical arterial catheter. **(B)** On day 3 the baby had vomiting, and there is high intestinal obstruction without duodenal dilatation. *(Figure continues.)*

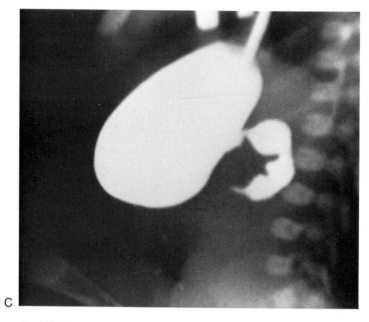

C

Fig. 7-24 *(Continued).* **(C)** The upper GI series demonstrates tapered narrowing and obstruction of the third portion of the duodenum.

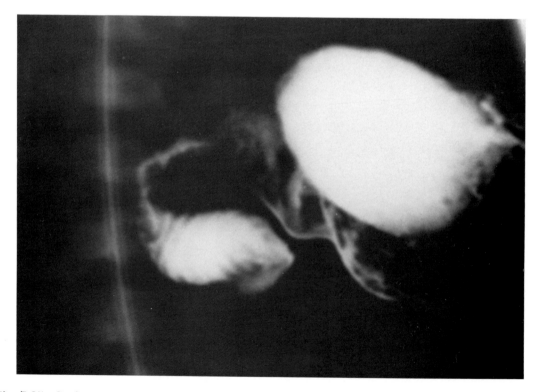

Fig. 7-25. Corkscrew appearance of midgut volvulus. A small amount of contrast passes through the site of obstruction and reverses direction in the configuration of a "Z" or corkscrew.

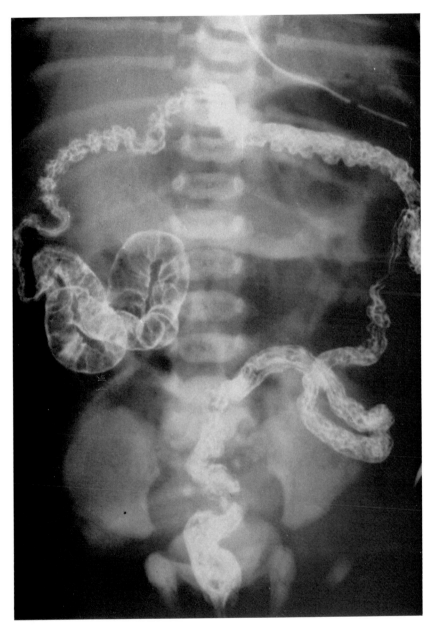

Fig. 7-26. Meconium ileus. A microcolon or unused colon is present on this postevacuation film. The filling defects in the terminal ileum are due to inspissated meconium.

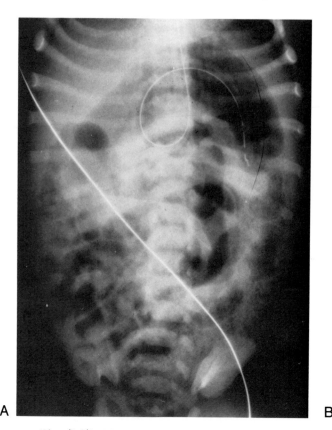
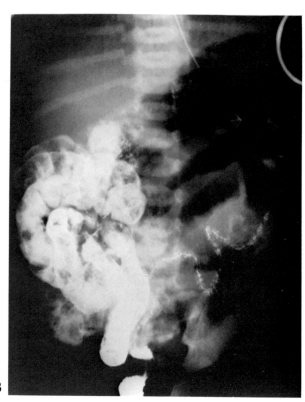

A   B

Fig. 7-27. Meconium ileus. **(A)** No air or fluid levels are noted on the plain erect film, and a soap-bubble appearance is noted in multiple dilated loops of bowel. **(B)** Diluted Gastrografin was refluxed into dilated groups of ileum. *(Figure continues.)*

distal colon. In meconium plug syndrome the obstruction is typically in the sigmoid colon (Fig. 7-30). The site of obstruction is the splenic flexure in small left colon syndrome, and distally there is a small or unused colon (Fig. 7-31). Functional immaturity of the colon is thought to be responsible for the initial inability to expel the meconium. Some of these babies are depressed or hypotonic at birth. Phenothiazines given to the mother have been implicated in others. Small left colon syndrome, in particular, occurs commonly in infants of insulin-deficient diabetic mothers.

It may be very difficult to distinguish meconium plug and small left colon syndrome from Hirschsprung's disease, and rectal biopsy should be performed if the obstruction is not relieved by the enema or if constipation recurs. Up to 40 percent of newborns with findings of meconium plug or small left colon syndrome on barium enema subsequently are proven to have Hirschsprung's disease. Rare compli-

cations of these conditions include pneumatosis intestinalis and perforation of the ileum or colon.[49,50]

Hirschsprung's Disease

Aganglionic megacolon is due to a congenital absence of ganglion cells in both the submucosal (Meissner) and myenteric (Auerbach) plexuses. The aganglionosis extends from the anus proximally without skip areas. Ganglion cells are found at the transition zone, and the proximal colon is normal even though it is dilated. The distal aganglionic area is normal or slightly small in caliber. The incidence of Hirschsprung's disease is 1:5,000 live births and the disease is uncommon in preterm infants. There is a sigmoid or rectal transition in 75 percent of cases, with a 4:1 male preponderance. In 10 to 15 percent of cases the entire colon and terminal ileum are involved, with a male-to-female ratio of 2.5:1. Varying

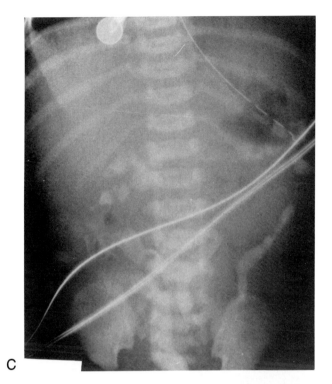

Fig. 7-27 *(Continued).* (C) The obstruction was relieved following three enemas over a 12-hour period.

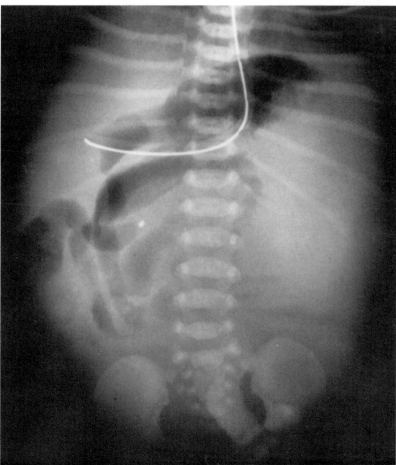

Fig. 7-28. Meconium ileus with volvulus. There is a mid–small bowel obstruction and a left-sided abdominal mass. Inspissated meconium is noted in the dilated segment of small bowel just proximal to the obstruction.

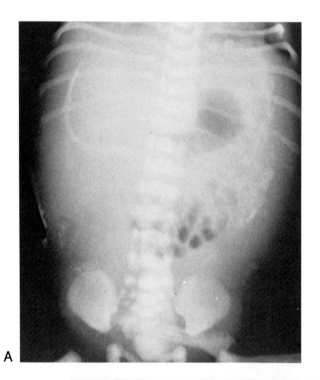

A

Fig. 7-29. Meconium ileus with meconium perito-nitis. **(A)** Perforation of the ileum in utero has re-sulted in speckled and rimlike calcifications within the peritoneum. **(B)** Free intraperitoneal air is noted on the cross-table lateral view.

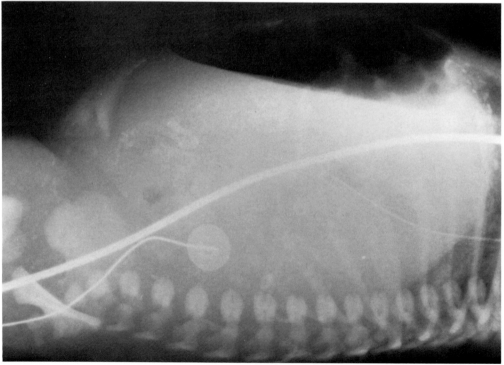

B

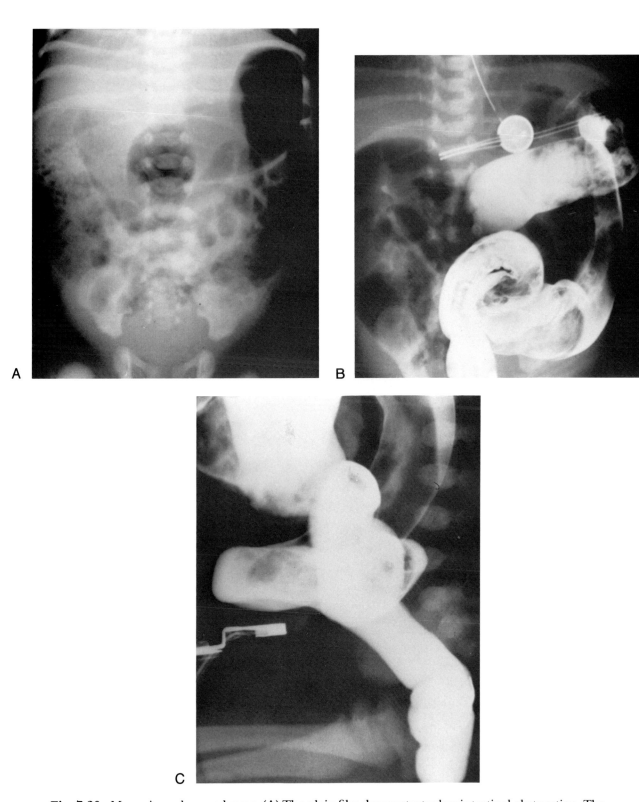

Fig. 7-30. Meconium plug syndrome. **(A)** The plain film demonstrates low intestinal obstruction. The bubbly pattern of intraluminal meconium mixed with air is not specific for meconium ileus. **(B)** The colon was normal in size on the barium enema, and long tubular filling defects representing meconium are present throughout the descending and sigmoid colon. **(C)** A lateral radiograph is important to exclude a transition zone indicating Hirschsprung's disease.

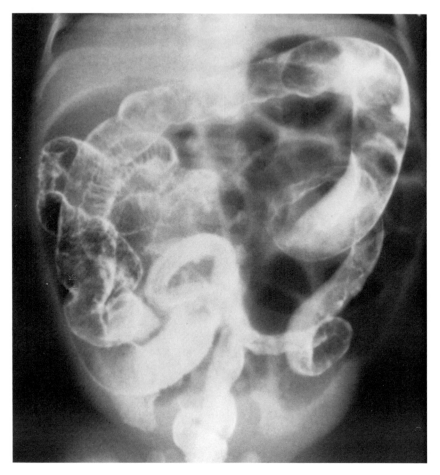

Fig. 7-31. Small left colon syndrome. The colon distal to the anatomic splenic flexure is small or unused in this premature infant of a diabetic mother.

lengths of colon are involved in the remainder. Most cases are diagnosed in the neonatal period, and Hirschsprung's disease accounts for about 20 to 50 percent of all cases of neonatal intestinal obstruction.

The classical presentation includes delayed meconium passage, abdominal distension, and bilious vomiting in the first few days of life. Enterocolitis will occur in 20 to 25 percent of untreated cases, usually in the first 3 months, and occurs more commonly in long segment disease. Mortality with enterocolitis is up to 30 percent and this is the major cause of death in Hirschsprung's disease. Appendiceal perforation is a rare complication.

On plain film examination there is generalized gaseous distension of the bowel, often with air-fluid levels. The barium enema should be performed unprepared with no recent rectal dilatation (by enema,

digital exams, or suppository), which might temporarily dilate the aganglionic portion. For the same reason a flexible catheter without a balloon should be used for the enema. Findings in Hirschsprung's disease include a transition zone between the aganglionic colon and the dilated proximal colon, disordered motility in the aganglionic portion resulting in a "sawtooth" pattern, and delayed evacuation at 24 or 48 hours. A rectosigmoid transition will be best visualized on the lateral view (Fig. 7-32). Since the rectosigmoid curves posteriorly as it descends into the pelvis, it appears foreshortened and a low transition may be missed on the anteroposterior view. It must be emphasized that the transition zone may not be as apparent in the newborn period since the proximal colon has not yet been dilated by formed feces (Fig. 7-33). This zone will not be seen with ultrashort

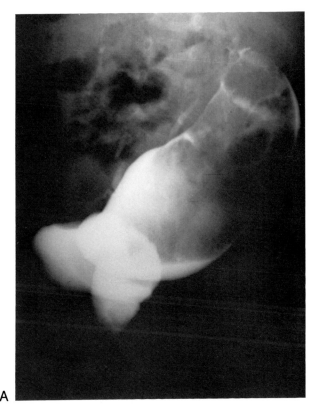
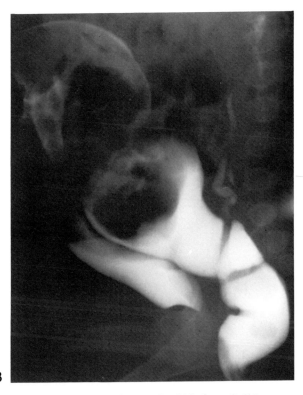

A

B

Fig. 7-32. (A&B) Hirschsprung's disease with rectosigmoid transition in a 3-month-old infant. Solid fecal material dilates the normal colon and makes the transition more apparent in older infants. An excretory urogram was performed just prior to this examination.

segment or long segment involvement (Fig. 7-34). Failure to evacuate barium within 24 hours is very suggestive of Hirschsprung's disease but is not specific. Since up to 25 percent of newborns with this condition have a completely normal barium enema, a rectal biopsy is still indicated if there is a strong clinical suspicion of Hirschsprung's disease.[51-53]

Anorectal Anomalies

Anorectal malformations occur in about 1:5,000 births. Most infants are born full term and with weight appropriate for gestational age. There are basically two main groups based on the location of the rectal pouch: supralevator or high imperforate anus and infralevator or low imperforate anus. High lesions predominate (75 percent). In each group the rectal pouch may end blindly or communicate by a fistula to a nearby viscus or to the perineal surface. Such a fistula is also known as an ectopic anus.

The majority of fistulas occur with high lesions and involve the posterior urethra or bladder base in boys and the vagina in girls. In a female infant a single perineal orifice indicates the presence of a cloacal fistula. Cloacal deformities are difficult to treat and the results of surgery are disappointing, with eventual incontinence in at least 40 percent of treated cases.

Associated anomalies are common, including the vertebral column (28 percent), central nervous system (18 percent), heart (9 percent), and GI tract (9 percent). The coexistent anomalies are often severe and 25 percent occur in low-birthweight infants. Sacral deformities are common and may lead to urinary and bowel incontinence. Imperforate anus occurs commonly in a complex of lumbar, sacral, and lower extremity abnormalities termed the *caudal regression syndrome*. The legs may be hypoplastic and are sometimes fused (sirenomelia or "mermaid" deformity).

The plain film evaluation of the rectal pouch should be delayed until about 24 hours of age to allow

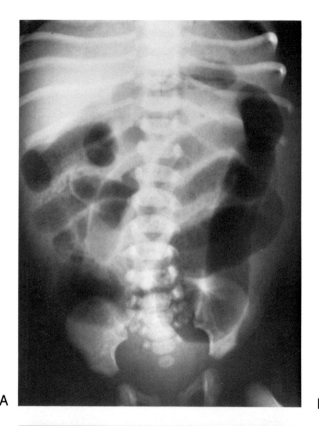

A

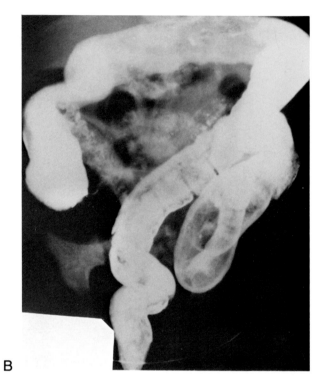

B

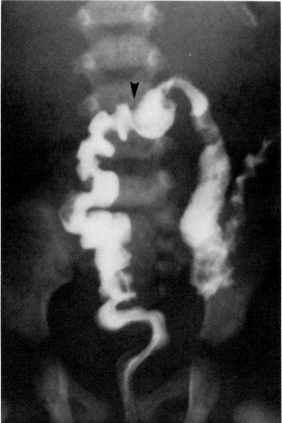

C

Fig. 7-33. Neonatal Hirschsprung's disease without a transition zone. Although there is clearly a low intestinal obstruction on the plain film at 1 day of age **(A)**, the barium enema fails to identify the transition zone **(B)**. There was moderate initial evacuation of the barium. However, retained barium is still present in the sigmoid 3 days later, and a sawtooth pattern of disordered motility is present in the distal sigmoid. (C) The pathologic transition was in the mid–sigmoid colon (arrowhead).

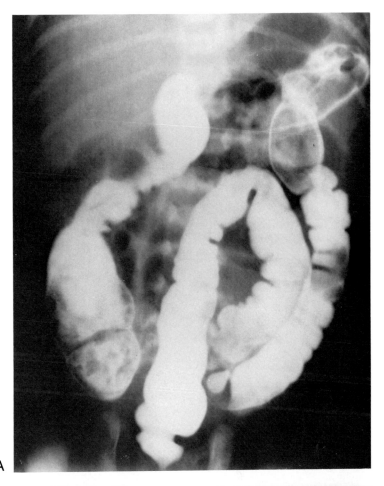

Fig. 7-34. Total colon and aganglionosis. No transition zone is noted on the barium enema **(A)**. The colon is normal in size and length. **(B)** At 48 hours there is moderate residual barium in the colon along with recurrent distension of the small bowel.

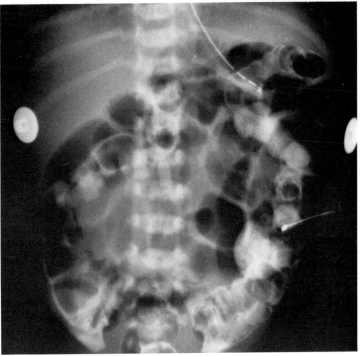

air to proceed distally and distend the rectum. Prone cross-table lateral views have practically replaced the classic upside-down views for this conditon. The rectum is the most superior part of the GI tract when in this position (Fig. 7-35). It should be emphasized that the level of the puborectalus muscle may vary somewhat with crying, and the drawing of a line between the pubis and coccyx may not indicate the exact location of this muscle. More recently ultrasound, computed tomography (CT), and magnetic resonance (MR) imaging have all successfully been used to define the level of the rectal pouch (Fig. 7-36). Evaluation of the spine and urinary tract are also important prior to discharge. Both a voiding cystourethrogram (VCUG) and evaluation of the kidneys by ultrasound are performed. A rectouretheral or rectovesical fistual in boys will be identified on VCUG (Fig. 7-37). If a colostomy is performed the fistula may also be identified by injecting contrast through the distal colos-

tomy. Many high lesions, however, are now being surgically corrected by a primary perineal repair in the neonatal period.

An enlarged, poorly contracting bladder indicates bladder atony. Perineal anesthesia is usually also present with paresis of the levator ani muscle. In this case a permanent colostomy is indicated.[54-58]

Neonatal Necrotizing Enterocolitis

Necrotizing enterocolitis (NEC) is the most common cause of intestinal perforation in the newborn period. Most cases are sporadic and there is significant variation in the incidence between institutions and at different times in the same institution. The etiology is probably multifactorial, but prematurity is present in 90 percent of cases, particularly in babies weighing less than 1500 g. Of the many theories that have been proposed, the most popular is that mesen-

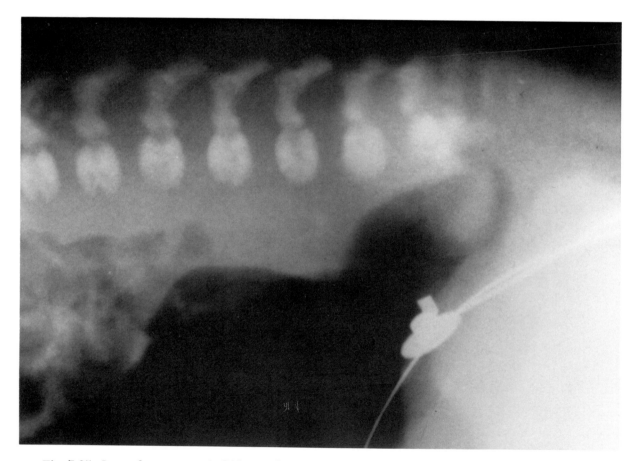

Fig. 7-35. Imperforate anus. At 24 hours the prone cross-table lateral view shows the distal extent of the rectal pouch. Note also the partial sacral agenesis.

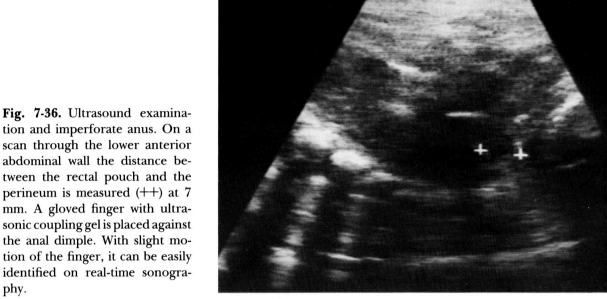

Fig. 7-36. Ultrasound examination and imperforate anus. On a scan through the lower anterior abdominal wall the distance between the rectal pouch and the perineum is measured (++) at 7 mm. A gloved finger with ultrasonic coupling gel is placed against the anal dimple. With slight motion of the finger, it can be easily identified on real-time sonography.

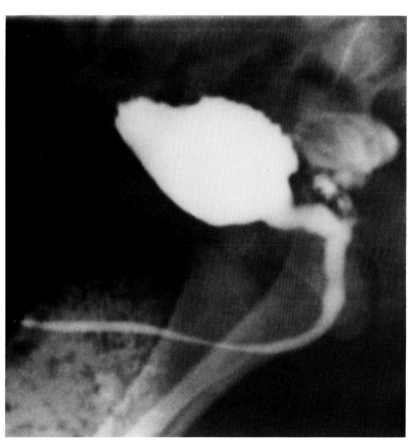

Fig. 7-37. High imperforate anus with rectourethral fistula. The lateral view demonstrates retrograde passage of contrast through the posterior urethral fistula into the rectum.

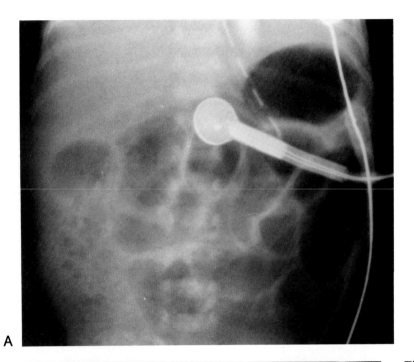

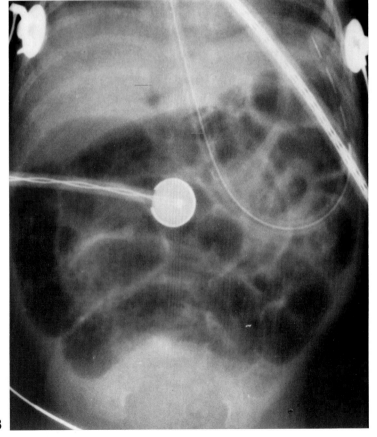

Fig. 7-38. Necrotizing enterocolitis. **(A)** Small bowel dilatation and pneumatosis in the right colon are present. **(B)** Portal venous air in a different patient. Pneumatosis is more difficult to identify with the increased dilatation of the bowel.

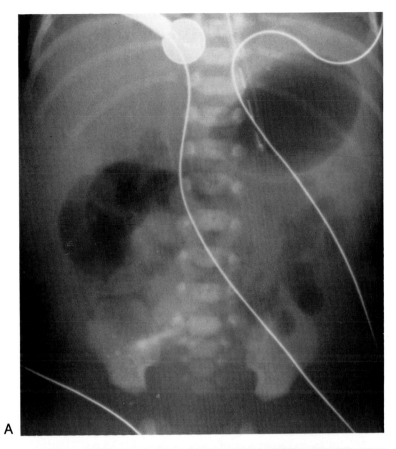

Fig. 7-39. Necrotizing enterocolitis with perforation. Pneumatosis and focal dilatation is noted in the right and mid-abdomen. **(A)** There is a vague suggestion of free peritoneal air over the medial portion of the liver on the supine view. **(B)** Free air is easily identified on the left lateral decubitus.

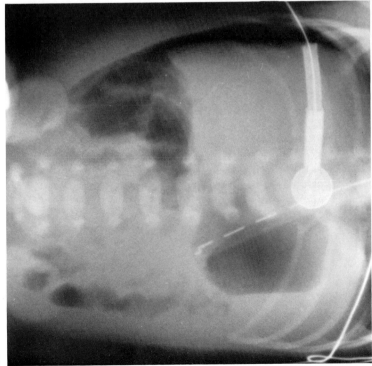

teric vascular ischemia with hypoxia of the intestinal wall leads to a loss of mucosal integrity with subsequent ulceration, necrosis, and hemorrhage. The mucosal epithelium will usually slough, and large air-filled cysts of pneumatosis intestinalis develop within the submucosa and later the serosa. The gas may eventually enter the portal veins. Although the entire colon may be affected, the right colon and terminal ileum are most vulnerable. Bacterial overgrowth and intestinal toxins are also factors in the etiology of NEC. Nutritional factors have been implicated in some cases. Occasionally previously healthy premature or full-term infants develop NEC without identifiable risk factors.

Clinical symptoms range widely from mild abdominal distension with blood-streaked stools to peritonitis, shock, and a fulminant course leading to death. Clinical manifestations may present anytime during the first 6 weeks of life but are uncommon in the first 2 days of life. Any early onset of symptoms, however, tends to be associated with more serious disease.

Plain abdominal radiographs are obtained to evaluate the bowel distension and to look for pneumatosis intestinalis, portal venous gas, and free abdominal gas, which would indicate perforation (Fig. 7-38). Generalized bowel distension alone is the most common early radiographic sign, and pneumatosis may be absent in 10 to 15 percent of cases. Although distension is not specific for NEC, its presence plus clinical suspicion is sufficient to institute medical therapy. Ultrasound examination is especially helpful when there is a gasless abdomen and a clinical suspicion of NEC. Breath hydrogen studies may also be beneficial in diagnosis. Regular follow-up films are obtained following the diagnosis of NEC, as frequently as every six hours in severe cases. Most perforations occur within 72 hours of the onset of symptoms. The left lateral decubitus view is the most sensitive for the detection of free air (Fig. 7-39).

Although sequelae and prognosis in NEC are variable, mortality figures range from 20 to 40 percent. Survivors develop strictures of the small or large intestine in 10 to 25 percent of cases. Strictures usually occur within 60 days of recovery from NEC and most are in the left colon. Some have been reported to resolve spontaneously, but most will require surgical resection or balloon dilatation. Although a routine barium enema prior to discharge has been advocated by some for the detection of strictures, most centers investigate only babies with persistent symptoms following medical management.[59-61]

REFERENCES

1. Singleton E, Wagner M, Dutton R: Congenital abnormalities of the small bowel and intestinal obstruction. In: Radiology of the Alimentary Tract. WB Saunders, Philadelphia, 1977
2. Padolsky ML, Jester AW: The distribution of air in the intestinal tract of infants during the first twelve hours as determined by serial roentgenograms. J Pediatr 45:633, 1954
3. Patriquin HB, Fish C, Bureau M, Black R: Radiologically visible fecal gas pattern in "normal" newborns and young infants. Pediatr Radiol 14:87, 1984
4. Johnson JF, Robinson LH: Localized bowel distention in the newborn: a review of the plain film analysis and differential diagnosis. Pediatr 73:206, 1984
5. Coradello H, Ponhold W, Lubec G, Pollak A: Disappearance of bowel gas in newborn infants on mechanical ventilation. Pediatr Radiol 12:11, 1982
6. McAlister WH, Askin FB: The effect of some contrast agents in the lung: an experimental study in the rat and dog. Am J Roentgenol 140:245, 1983
7. Kuhns LR, Kanellisas C: Use of isotonic water soluble contrast agents for gastrointestinal examinations in infants. Radiology 144:411, 1982
8. Sovis TL, Poland RL: A radiant warmer for fluoroscopic procedures. Radiology 134:540, 1980
9. Cohen MD, Weber TR, Grosfeld JL: Bowel perforation in the newborn: diagnosis with metrizamide. Radiology 150:65, 1984
10. Silverberg M, Daum F: Congenital malformations and surgical emergencies of infancy. p 199. In: Textbook of Pediatric Gastroenterology. 2nd Ed. Year Book Medical Publishers, Chicago, 1988
11. Walker WA, Durie PR, Hamilton JR et al: Hernias. p 494. In: Pediatric Gastrointestinal Disease—Pathophysiology, Diagnosis, Management. BC Decker, Inc, Philadelphia, 1991
12. Anderson KD: Congenital diaphragmatic hernia. p 589. In Welch KJ et al (eds): Pediatric Surgery. 4th Ed. Year Book Medical Publishers, Chicago, 1986
13. Raphaely RD, Downes JJ: Congenital diaphragmatic hernia: prediction of survival. J Pediatr Surg 8:815, 1973
14. Berdon WB, Baker DH, Anoury R: The role of pulmonary hypoplasia in the prognosis of newborn infants with diaphragmatic hernia and eventration. Am J Roentgenol 103:413, 1968
15. Silverberg M, Daum F: Congenital malformations and surgical intestinal emergencies of infancy. p 195. In: Textbook of Pediatric Gastroenterology. 2nd Ed. Year Book Medical Publishers, Inc, Chicago, 1988
16. Rickham PP: Infants with esophageal atresia weighing under three pounds. J Pediatr Surg 16:595, 1981

17. Barnes JC, Smith W: The VATER Association. Radiology 126:445, 1978

18. Spitz L, Kiely E, Brereton RJ: Esophageal atresia: five year experience with 148 cases. J Pediatr Surg 22:103, 1987

19. Hoder TM, Cloud DJ, Lewis E, Pilling FP: Esophageal atresia and tracheoesophageal fistula: a survey of its members by the surgical section of the American Academy of Pediatrics. Pediatrics 34:542, 1981

20. Nihoul Feket C, Debacker A, Lortat-Jacob, S, Pellerin D: Congenital esophageal stenosis: a review of 20 cases. Pediatr Surg Int 2:81, 1987

21. Nishina T, Tsuchida Y, Saito S: Congenital esophageal stenosis due to tracheobronchial remnants and its associated anomalies. J Pediatr Surg 16:190, 1981

22. Shephard R, Raflensperger J, Goldstein R: Pediatric esophageal perforation. J Thorac Cardiovasc Surg 74:261, 1977

23. Clarke TA, Coen RW, Feldman B, Papil L: Esophageal perforations in premature infants. Am J Dis Child 134:367, 1980

24. Molkit D, Schullinger J, Santulli TV: Selective management of iatrogenic esophageal perforation in the newborn. J Pediatr Surg 16:989, 1981

25. Gryboski JD: Suck and swallow in the premature infant. Pediatrics 43:96, 1969

26. Herbst JJ, Minto SD, Book LS: Gastroesophageal reflux causing respiratory distress and apnea in newborn infants. J Pediatr 95:763, 1979

27. Hillemeier AC, Large R, McCallum DW et al: Delayed gastric emptying in infants with GER. J Pediatr 98:190, 1981

28. James EA, Heller RM, White JJ et al: Spontaneous rupture of the stomach in the newborn. Pediatr Res 10:79, 1976

29. Garland JS, Nelson DB, Rice T, Neu J: Increased risk of GI perforation in neonates mechanically ventilated with either face mask or nasal prongs. Pediatrics 76:406, 1985

30. Nagaray HS, Sandhn AS, Cook LN et al: Gastrointestinal perforation following indomethacin therapy in very low birth weight infants. J Pediatr Surg 16:1003, 1981

31. Walker WA, Durie PR, Hamilton JR et al: Stomach. p 452. In: Pediatric Gastrointestinal Disease — Pathophysiology, Diagnosis, Management. BC Decker, Inc, Philadelphia, 1991

32. Tunnel WP, Smith IE: Antral web in infancy. J Pediatr Surg 15:152, 1980

33. Schwartz SE, Rowden DR, Dudgeon DL: Antral mucosal diaphragm. Gastrointest Endosc 24:33, 1977

34. Kreniel RM, Lepoff RB, Izant RJ: Duplication of the stomach. J Pediatr Surg 5:360, 1970

35. Hochberger O, Swoboda W: Congenital microgastria: a follow-up observation over six years. Pediatr Radiol 2:207, 1974

36. Fonkalsrud EW, de Lorimier AA, Hays DM: Congenital atresia and stenosis of the duodenum. Pediatrics 69:43:1979

37. Haller JA, Tepas JJ, Shermeta RL: Intestinal atresia: current concepts of pathogenesis, pathophysiology and operative management. Am Surg 49:385, 1983

38. Free EA, Gerald B: Duodenal obstruction in the newborn due to annular pancreas. Am J Roentgenol 103:321, 1968

39. Whelan TJ, Hamilton GB: Annular pancreas. Ann Surg 146:252, 1957

40. Grosfeld JL: Jejuno-ileal atresia and stenosis. In Welch KJ, Randolph JG, Ravitch MM et al (eds): Pediatric Surgery. Year Book Medical Publishers, Chicago, 1986

41. Louw JH: Jejunal atresia and stenosis. J Pediatr Surg 1:8, 1966

42. Rescoria FJ, Grosfeld JL: Intestinal atresia and stenosis surgery. 98:688, 1985

43. Stewart DR, Colodny AL, Daggett WC: Malrotation of the bowel in infants and children. Surgery 79:716, 1976.

44. Howell CG, Vozza F, Shaw S et al: Malrotation, malnutrition and ischemic bowel disease. J Pediatr Surg 17:469, 1982

45. Hocking M, Young DE: Duplications of alimentary tract. Br J Surg 92:96, 1981

46. Idstad ST, Tollerad DJ, Weiss RG, Ryan DP et al: Duplications of alimentary tract. Ann Surg 208:184, 1988

47. Holsclaw DS, Eckstein HB, Niton HH: Meconium ileus: a twenty year review of 107 cases. Am J Dis Child 109:101, 1965

48. Careskey JM, Grosfeld JL, Weber TR: Giant cystic meconium peritonitis. J Pediatr Surg 17:482, 1982

49. Philippart AI, Reed JO, Georgeson KE: Neonatal small left colon syndrome. J Pediatr Surg 10:733, 1975

50. Clatworthy HW, Howard WHR, Lloyd J: Meconium plug syndrome. Surgery 39:131, 1956

51. Martin CW, Torres AM: Hirschsprung's disease. Surg Clin North Am 65:1171, 1985

52. Swenson O, Davidson FX: Similarities of mechanical intestinal obstruction and aganglionic megacolon in the newborn infant. N Engl J Med 262:64, 1960

53. Kekonaki M, Rapola J, Lourimo I: Diagnosis of Hirschsprung's disease. Acta Pediatr Scand 68:893, 1979

54. Templeton JM, O'Neil JA: Anorectal malformations. p 1022. In Welch KJ et al (eds): Pediatric Surgery. Year Book Medical Publishers, Chicago, 1986

55. Stephens FD, Smith ED: Anorectal Malformation in

Children. Year Book Medical Publishers, Chicago, 1971

56. Kiesewetter WB, Chang JHT: Imperforate anus. Prog Pediatr Surg 10:111, 1977

57. Schuster SR, Teole RC: An analysis of ultrasound scanning as a guide in determination of high and low imperforate anus. J Pediatr Surg 14:798, 1979

58. Ikawa H, Yokoyama H, Sanbonmatsn T et al: The use of computerized tomography to evaluate anorectal anomalies. J Pediatr Surg 20:640, 1985

59. Berdon WE, Grossman H, Baker DH et al: NEC in the premature infant. Radiology 83:879, 1964

60. Kliegman RM, Fannoroff AA: Necrotizing enterocolitis. N Engl J Med 310:1093, 1984

61. Walsh MC, Kliegman RM: NEC treatment based on staging criteria. Pediatr Clin North Am 33:179, 1986

Abdominal Ultrasonography of the Premature Infant

8

Ignacio Pastor
Rodrigo Dominguez

Real-time duplex Doppler ultrasound is a very popular diagnostic modality in the radiology community for the well-known advantages of portability and lack of ionizing radiation. Clinicians, on the other hand, prefer the clearer and more comprehensive anatomic images of computed tomography (CT) scans and magnetic resonance (MR) images to understand the conditions affecting their patients. The relatively localized, wedge-shaped partial view of organs, as seen by ultrasound, is not usually welcomed so enthusiastically by the medical community at large.

But the less cumbersome diagnostic modality of ultrasound is very well suited for assessing the premature and high-risk neonates in the neonatal intensive care unit. In addition, the clear separation of organs often seen in CT scans of adults is largely due to the presence of body fat, which is lacking in premature infants. Body MR imaging is subjected to serious image degradation caused by respiratory, peristaltic, and other body motions, which are difficult to control in small infants. Ultrasound, then, is the modality best adapted for detecting abdominal pathology in the newborn nursery. This chapter is dedicated to a review of the abdominal disease processes most frequently encountered in the premature infant.

When utilizing ultrasound to examine the abdomen of the neonate in the intensive care unit, it is useful to remember that one's hands as well as the transducer should be clean. It is also important to pay special attention to the placement of the transducer and its cable. Careless manipulation of these may result in the dislodging of the multiple catheters, lines, and life supports systems being used on the patient. Since a large amount of cold gel on very small neonates may lower the body temperature, lukewarm contact gel should be used as sparingly as possible. Once the examination is finished, the remainder of the gel should be wiped off. If the neonate is not in an incubator and the examination is expected to be time consuming, then the body temperature should be maintained by using a heat lamp. Remember to place the heat lamp facing opposite to the ultrasound unit in order to keep unwanted light reflection on the screen to a minimum.

The pathologic processes that one encounters in the abdomen during the neonatal period can be grouped as follows:

1. *Congenital anomalies:* A good rule of thumb is that if one congenital anomaly is present others may be also. Thoroughly examine the abdomen.
2. *Normal variations:* Lack of familiarity with the appearance of immature organs may raise confusion. The classic example of this is the kidney, which in the neonate presents a different echogenic pattern as well as a different shape.
3. *Iatrogenic disorders:* These are usually seen in neonates who weigh less than 1,500 g. Examples of this include vascular injuries, biliary calculi, and nephrocalcinosis.

THE DIAPHRAGM

Ultrasound shows the diaphragm as a curved, echogenic structure whose concavity faces the abdomen. The diaphragm is better studied by using sagittal and transverse sections in order to visualize either spontaneous respiration or respiration induced by mechanical ventilation.[1] Supradiaphragmatic processes can then be clearly visualized. Effusions are usually seen as anechoic collections. A large fluid accumulation may lead to inversion of the diaphragm. Pulmonary consolidations or intrathoracic masses may also be visualized through the diaphragm.

Diaphragmatic Paralysis

Diaphragmatic paralysis is not infrequently seen in neonates who have undergone surgery for closure of the ductus arteriosus or repair of an aortic coarctation. These lesions usually involve the left phrenic nerve, with subsequent paralysis of the ipsilateral hemidiaphragm. This paralysis is easily evaluated by placing the transducer immediately below the xiphoid and obtaining transverse images. These transverse images will allow the inspection of both diaphragms during respiration. The injured side will remain low and fixed with minimal movement during inspiration and expiration. Newborns with brachial plexus paralysis generally will not show alterations of diaphragmatic movement on the involved side (Fig. 8-1). Focal segmental diaphragmatic eventrations or relaxations can be seen as segmental "humps" or elevations along the diaphragmatic surface.

Diaphragmatic Hernia

The diaphragmatic hernia is better studied by using longitudinal ultrasound sections. These hernias are seen as interrupted segments of the diaphragmatic hyperechogenicity. Those of the posterior portion, or Bochdalek's hernias, are easily identified. The thoracic cavity may contain multiple intestinal loops that can be easily recognized by the use of real-time ultrasound and by visualizing the movement of the fluid within the bowel. It is important to realize that during the first few hours of life the herniated bowel will contain mostly fluid and very little if any gas (Fig. 8-2). In addition, an overlying hypoplastic lung is identified. The kidney and the adrenal gland are usually displaced superiorly. Occasionally, one may encounter a defect in the central portion of the diaphragm. The liver, gallbladder, spleen, pancreas, and mesentery may herniate through this defect.

LIVER, GALLBLADDER, AND BILIARY SYSTEM

It is possible to detect slush within the gallbladder in the newborn. This material is brightly echogenic because the gallbladder is mostly collapsed in the newborn. This slush tends to remain in the same vesi-

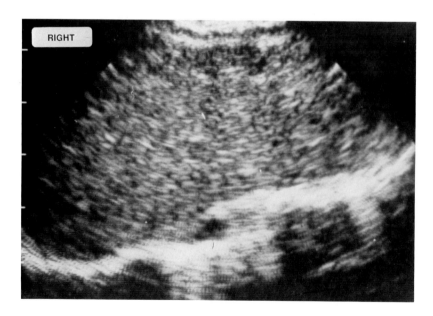

Fig. 8-1. Right hemidiaphragmatic paralysis evidencing no ascent during expiration (axial scan).

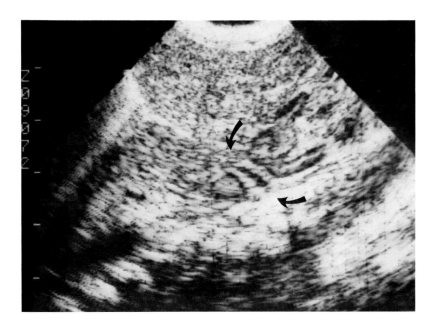

Fig. 8-2. Diaphragmatic hernia with defect in the diaphragm and displacement of loops of bowel (arrows) to the chest (left sagittal plane scan).

cular area. Biliary slush can be detected in utero or during the first days of life. Gallbladder calculi may develop in utero.[2] These may appear as semilunar hyperechogenic structures generally measuring less than 1 cm. Often the intra- or extrahepatic biliary system is not distended (Fig. 8-3). Not infrequently, the calculi are spontaneously passed into the bowel during the first weeks of life.[3]

In biliary atresia the gallbladder cannot be found even after prolonged periods of fasting. This differs from neonatal hepatitis, in which a small gallbladder can be visualized after fasting.[4-7] The hepatic parenchyma as well as the intra- and extrahepatic biliary systems may be normal in both of the above processes.

Multiple processes may lead to edema of the gallbladder wall, a condition that remains unexplained in a large percentage of cases. The most common cause

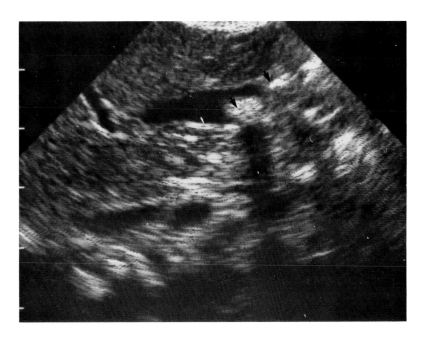

Fig. 8-3. Congenital gallstones (arrows) of irregular contour and homogeneous echogenicity with acoustic shadowing.

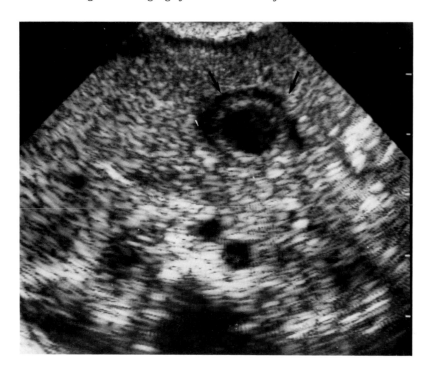

Fig. 8-4. Edema (arrow) of the gall-bladder wall.

is blood group incompatibility, which is usually accompanied by hypoproteinemia and ascites.[7,8] Multiple infections, which usually occur in the low-birth-weight neonate, can also lead to edema of the gallbladder wall (Fig. 8-4). The ultrasound appearance of the edema of the gallbladder wall is that of two densely echogenic lines separated by a less echogenic area.

Early ultrasound examination of neonates treated with total parenteral nutrition or of neonates who have undergone long periods of fasting will demonstrate a mildly edematous gallbladder that can be dis-

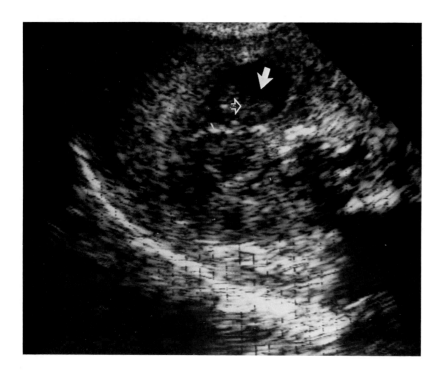

Fig. 8-5. Intravesicular biliary sludge (open arrow), more echogenic than the normal supernatant bile (arrow).

tended but usually contains bile of normal echogenicity.[9] Subsequently, a dense and more echogenic biliary sludge can be seen on top of the normal bile at the sloping end of the gallbladder (Fig. 8-5). In the more chronic stages, this type of abnormal bile may become even more hyperechogenic and may aggregate so as to form small hyperechogenic nodules devoid of posterior acoustic shadowing; further aggregates of these nodules can then progress to frank calculi formation.[10]

Throughout the different stages of biliary calculi formation, the abnormal material can be spontaneously passed into the bowel or can be seen filling the entire extrahepatic biliary system (Fig. 8-6). Clinically, spontaneous passing of this abnormal bile can give rise to jaundice and acute abdominal pain. However, ultrasound examination during this phase may demonstrate the extrahepatic system to be of normal dimensions. Ultrasound is the method of choice to document the presence of biliary calculi. It should be remembered that abdominal roentgenograms during the first months of life are not sensitive since the biliary calculi contain very little calcium.

Sclerosis and Atrophy of the Gallbladder

When the gallbladder is faintly visible, does not become distended following a fasting period, and contains posterior acoustic shadowing due to multiple intravesicular calculi, then the possibility of sclerosis and atrophy of the gallbladder should be considered. Sclerosis and atrophy of the gallbladder is usually seen in neonates who harbor multiple infectious processes and/or who are given total parenteral nutrition for prolonged periods of time (Fig. 8-7).

Air in the Gallbladder

Ultrasound can demonstrate multiple small hyperechogenic densities with a dirty posterior shadowing, representing air bubbles within the gallbladder. These bubbles will move freely and constantly (Fig. 8-8). This can spontaneously result from immaturity of the sphincter of Oddi; it may present rarely in "micropremies."[11]

Inspissated Bile

Thick bile may become impacted in the distal common bile duct.[12-14] Normally, the common bile duct will measure less than 1 mm in the premature newborn. However, the size of the duct actually depends upon the birthweight. It is important to differentiate the common bile duct from the portal vein. If the anatomic differentiation between these structures becomes difficult, then Doppler ultrasound will clearly identify the venous structure (Fig. 8-9). A dis-

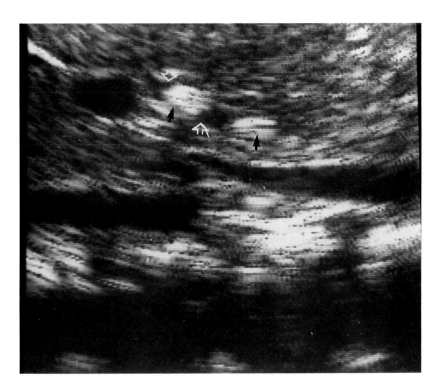

Fig. 8-6. Stones without shadowing (arrows) in a nondilated common bile duct (open arrows).

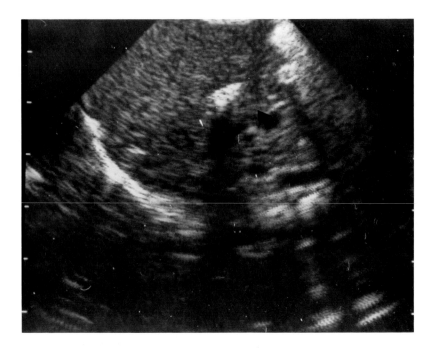

Fig. 8-7. Sclerotic and atrophic, nondistensible gallbladder (arrow), with its walls and contents indiscernible.

tended biliary duct may also show edema of its walls, which will resolve spontaneously once the bile plug has been passed.

Biliary Hydrops

Distension of the gallbladder (biliary hydrops) may be clinically present in those neonates undergoing prolonged periods of fasting and/or parenteral nutrition.[8,15,16] Clinically, biliary hydrops can present as a painless mass in the right upper quadrant. Ultra- sound examination usually demonstrates a remarkably distended gallbladder with thin walls; no calculi or biliary sludge is present. Once oral feeding is started the distended gallbladder drains and returns to normal without sequelae.

Acute Acalculous Cholecystitis

Ultrasound may show a distended gallbladder with well-defined but thickened walls. Calculi or biliary sludge are not present. There is no dilatation of the

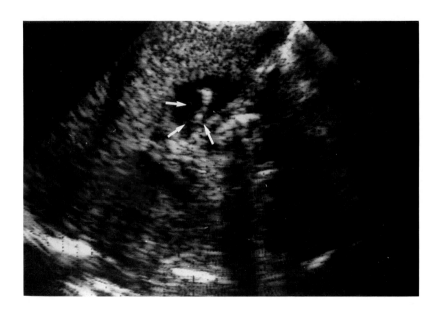

Fig. 8-8. Air within the gallbladder, expressed by small, freely movable bubbles (arrows).

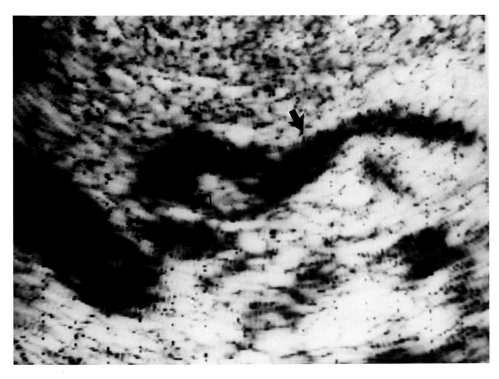

Fig. 8-9. Oblique close-up of the portal region: thickened, retained bile in a dilated common bile duct also containing sludge (open arrow) and interfacing with the splenic vein (arrow).

intrahepatic biliary tree. Placement of the transducer over the distended gallbladder will produce pain. Once the appropriate antibiotic treatment has been established the gallbladder dilatation and the pain will resolve in a matter of days[17] (Fig. 8-10).

Hepatic Masses

Hepatic Hemangioendothelioma

Hepatic hemangioendothelioma can result in hepatomegaly, high-output cardiac failure, and abnormal clotting mechanisms. Ultrasound usually demonstrates a solitary mass. However, when multiple hemangioendotheliomas are present they usually can be found in the periphery of the gland (Fig. 8-11). These tumors have different degrees of echogenicity and at times one may perceive areas of low echogenicity within them, probably representing neoplastic blood vessels. The suprahepatic veins may be displaced or collapsed as a result of compression by the adjacent mass, which can reach a large size. The mass can be large enough to compress the superior aspect of the intra-abdominal aorta (well visualized in midline sagittal sections), and the celiac trunk can have an

abnormally large size, giving rise to a very large hepatic artery.

Before the surgical removal of the mass, it is helpful to perform intra-arterial embolization at different settings.[18,19] This is done in such a manner as to avoid acute hemodynamic decompensation. Once the mass has been surgically removed, ultrasound will show multiple emboli of "echogenic material" in the surgical bed. The liver then returns to its normal size and the suprahepatic veins will be of normal caliber and in their normal position.

Hepatic Hemangiomas

Small and benign angiomas may be seen throughout the liver. Ultrasound shows these masses to be of high echogenicity and to contain a center of relatively low echoes (Fig. 8-12). These masses may spontaneously regress once the fetal circulation is no longer present. At times these masses will remain present for several weeks, and follow-up ultrasound examinations are suggested. When larger angiomas are present within the liver, it is also useful to perform serial ultrasound examinations because the majority

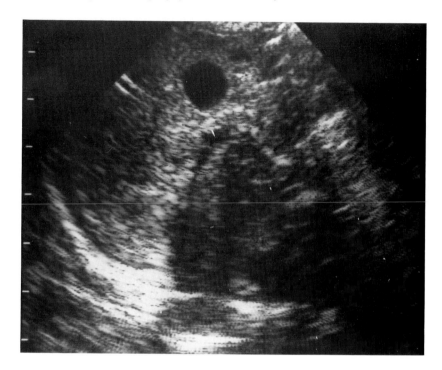

Fig. 8-10. Distended gallbladder in acute acalculous cholecystitis.

of the tumors will diminish in size during the first days or weeks of life.

Hepatic Rhabdomyosarcoma

Hepatic rhabdomyosarcoma is an exceptionally rare neoplasm in the newborn. Ultrasound shows a large mass of variable echogenicity usually causing hepatomegaly. The normal structures within the he-

patic parenchyma are displaced (Fig. 8-13). By the time the tumor is discovered ultrasound may show multiple masses throughout the liver parenchyma.

Intrahepatic Hematomas

Intrahepatic hematomas can be secondary to traumatic deliveries, especially in those neonates with a large birthweight, such as the offspring of diabetic

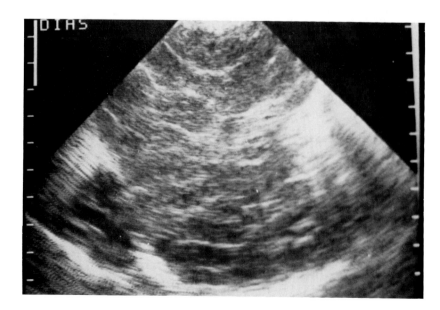

Fig. 8-11. Massive hepatic hemangioma occupying the whole liver, with hyperechogenic septae (sagittal plane scan).

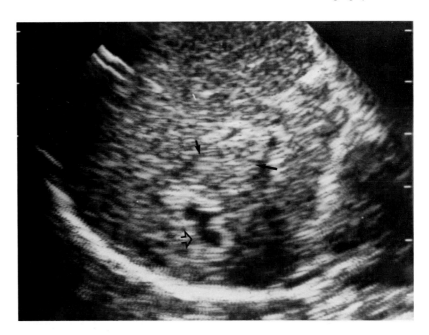

Fig. 8-12. Small intrahepatic hemangioma (arrows) with a feeding vessel located in the periphery of the liver (open arrow).

mothers, or in those newborns with alterations of the clotting mechanisms. Sonographic examination will show hepatomegaly and the presence of focal or diffused areas of hyperechogenicity. Placement of the transducer over the distended liver is usually painful. Serial ultrasound examination will usually show progressive involution of these hemorrhages.[20] As the clots become absorbed, both hepatomegaly and pain lessen. In the chronic stage, ultrasound examination may show calcifications with posterior shadowing at the site where the hematomas were previously documented.

Other findings seen in association with intrahepatic hematoma include a distended gallbladder containing abundant biliary sludge secondary to the lysis of the hematoma. Hemorrhage in other organs such as the adrenal glands can also be present. The presence of multiple large hepatic hematomas in a neonate with no history of traumatic delivery should raise the question of hemophilia (Fig. 8-14).

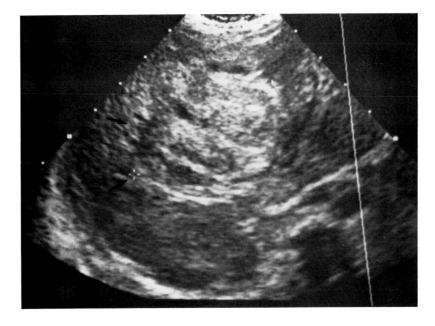

Fig. 8-13. Liver rhabdomyosarcoma with a hyperechoic, heterogeneous mass in relation to the surrounding liver, which is also infiltrated by the spreading tumor (arrows). (Courtesy of Dr. Prieto, Pediatric Radiology Department, Hospital Infantil "La Paz," Madrid, Spain.)

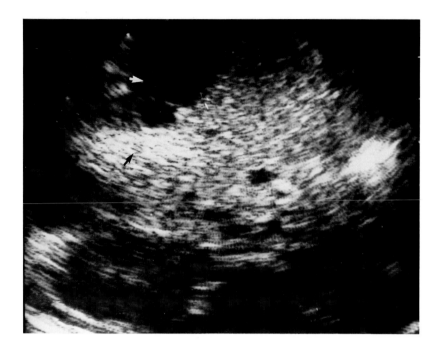

Fig. 8-14. Transverse scan of liver hematoma in a newborn with hemophilia; alternating zones of different echogenicity corresponding to bleeding in different phases of evolution (arrow).

Galactosemia

In the neonate suffering with galactosemia, ultrasound may show diffuse increased echogenicity throughout the liver parenchyma. Hepatomegaly is also present. In chronic stages fatty metamorphosis of the liver may develop, and ultrasound may even detect the formation of regenerating nodules[21] (Fig. 8-15).

Congenital Intrahepatic Calcifications

At times congenital intrahepatic calcifications may be diagnosed in utero or found incidentally during ultrasound of the abdomen done for different reasons. These calcifications tend to be small and hyperechogenic, round, solitary or multiple, and in one or more groups. Ultrasound often detects posterior acoustic shadowing (Fig. 8-16). Although by ultra-

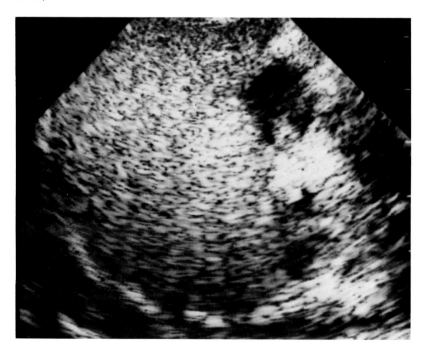

Fig. 8-15. Galactosemia with hepatomegaly and diffuse hyperechogenicity from the first hours of life.

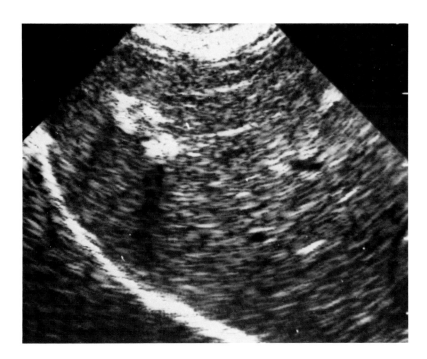

Fig. 8-16. Calcified liver granulomas in newborn with CMV infection acquired in utero.

sound most of these calcifications will show posterior acoustic shadowing, plain films of the abdomen are not sensitive enough for their detection. The cause of such calcifications is not found in the majority of these cases; however, in utero infections such as cytomegalovirus (CMV) may induce them. Other causes for hepatic calcifications include old hematomas or long-standing catheterization of the umbilical vein.[22]

Intrahepatic Gas

Intrahepatic gas is frequently encountered by ultrasound, and necrotizing enterocolitis is the most frequent cause. Ultrasound shows the bubbles of air as areas of hyperechogenicity, usually within the periphery of the liver in its more dependent portion. The gas shows diffuse acoustic shadowing often seen

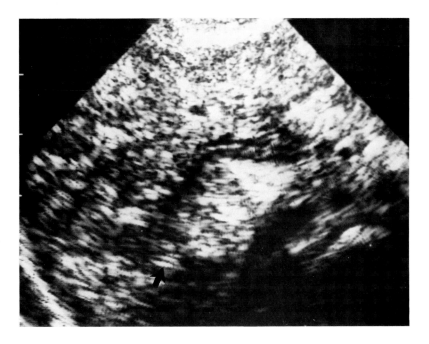

Fig. 8-17. Transverse scan of air bubbles in the liver causing diffuse hyperechogenicity. Air is also present within the lumen of the portal vein, which is difficult to identify (arrow).

in immediate contact with the hyperechogenic diaphragm.[23] At times the gas within the hepatic portal vessels can be so extensive that the liver may demonstrate a diffuse echogenicity (Fig. 8-17). Ultrasound appears to be a more sensitive way of detecting intrahepatic gas than plain radiographs, because the small size of the gas bubbles may be undetected on the abdominal radiographs. The prognosis is directly related to the quantity of gas visualized; the more gas the worse the prognosis will be.

PANCREAS

Pancreatic disease during the neonatal period is very rare. At times one can see increased pancreatic echogenicity in some infants of diabetic mothers, but the gland size usually remains normal and in exceptional cases pancreatic cysts may be visualized.

Nesidioblastosis

As a result of nesidioblastosis, or hypertrophy of the B pancreatic cells, the neonate can suffer hypoglycemia. On ultrasound a very large and echogenic pancreatic gland is easily identified (Fig. 8-18). This

pancreatic disease is seen in association with other congenital anomalies such as those present in the Beckwith-Wiedemann syndrome. Other reported patients with this syndrome present a hyperechogenic pancreas but of a normal size and with an absence of hypoglycemia.[24-28] Nesidioblastosis is seen in association with other anomalies such as esophageal atresia and anomalous venous return under the diaphragm into the portal vein. Treatment for the hypertrophy of these B cells of the pancreas is surgical, with partial resection of the gland.

SPLEEN

The abnormal location of the spleen may produce an abdominal mass on palpation that is confirmed by abdominal ultrasound.[29] Traumatic delivery may produce splenic hematomas, which can show an intrasplenic mass or masses of increased echogenicity. These masses are small and asymptomatic and they resolve on follow-up examinations. Infants suffering from CMV infections will present with splenomegaly, which may reach the iliac crest and present a prominent and tortuous splenic vein.

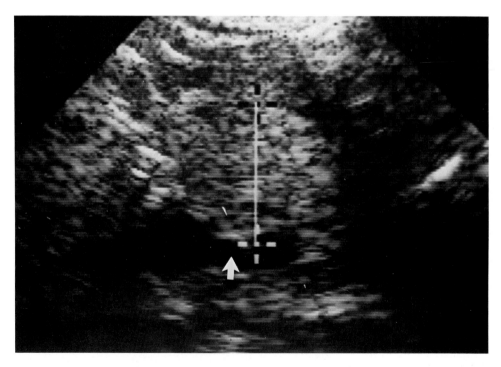

Fig. 8-18. Nesidioblastosis with enlargement and hyperechogenicity of the pancreatic body (transverse mid-abdominal scan).

KIDNEYS, URETERS, AND BLADDER

"Micropremies" usually have kidneys with scalloped contours, the so-called fetal lobulations. At this stage of immature life the kidneys have an increased cortical parenchymal echogenicity. In contrast with the decreased echoes seen at the renal pyramids, the apices of these pyramids will show a small echogenic nodule, which represents the flow through the arcuate artery.[30]

Renal Agenesis

In instances of congenital absence of the kidney, the usual sagittal ultrasound section of the abdominal flank will present a clearer appearance of the psoas muscle. In addition, the adrenal gland will appear elongated, flattened, and larger, losing its typical triangular shape and measuring up to 6.0 cm in length or even in transverse diameter (Fig. 8-19). This abnormally large adrenal gland is an indirect sign of renal agenesis. In this situation we would scan the rest of the abdomen and retroperitoneum, including the lower abdominal region and pelvis.[31] At times the

kidney may be ectopic and placed in the lower abdomen, or its absence may be seen in association with uterine abnormalities.

Those infants born with bilateral renal agenesis will present with pulmonary hypoplasia air leak, pneumothorax, and death. In certain diagnosed cases of unilateral renal agenesis the "absent kidney" may in fact be very small, hypoplastic, and ectopic, and because the intestinal loops fill in the renal fossa it may be overlooked during the ultrasound examination. A follow-up intravenous pyelogram (IVP) during late infancy may demonstrate some function in this small kidney. This dysplastic, poorly functioning, ectopic kidney may have a ureter ending abnormally at the seminal gland, and it can consequently produce obstruction. It may be visualized on the IVP as an ectopic, urine-concentrating mass, usually in the pelvic region.

Renal Hypoplasia

Severe renal hypoplasia or dysplasia may be observed in its normal location at the renal fossa, displaying an abnormal renal parenchyma of an unusually small size. This small organ will have cystic cavities

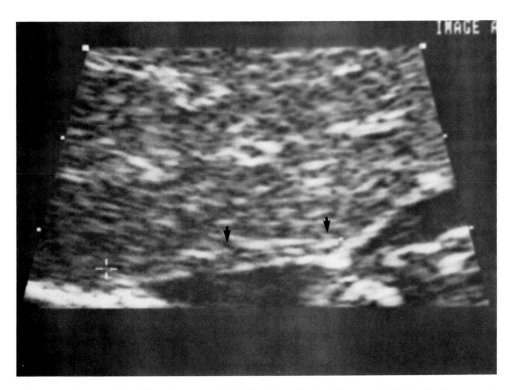

Fig. 8-19. Renal agenesis with a large, unfolded adrenal gland (arrows) (right flank coronal scan).

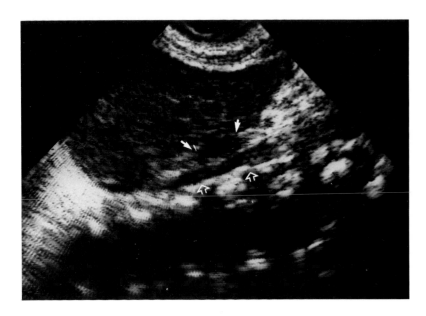

Fig. 8-20. Right flank coronal scan of renal hypoplasia with a small cystic remnant (arrows) in front of the inferior vena cava (open arrows).

within it.[31] The adjacent adrenal gland will have a more normal configuration and size (Fig. 8-20).

Pyelocalyceal Ectasia

Moderate distension of the renal pelvis and calices would be noted on physical examination; this anomaly may resolve later in infancy and ultrasound follow-ups are then recommended. If it does not resolve in the first few months of life, ureteropelvic junction stenosis with or without partial obstruction should be considered.[32] Those cases of hydronephrosis or pye-localiceal ectasia diagnosed in utero should be re-examined several days postpartum. The reason for this waiting period is the newborn delay in the physiologic formation of urine during the first 2 to 3 days of life.

Ureteropelvic Junction Stenosis with Obstruction

Under ultrasound examination the renal parenchyma is diminished in ureteropelvic junction stenosis but the corticomedullary differentiation is preserved. The calices will be dilated as well as the renal

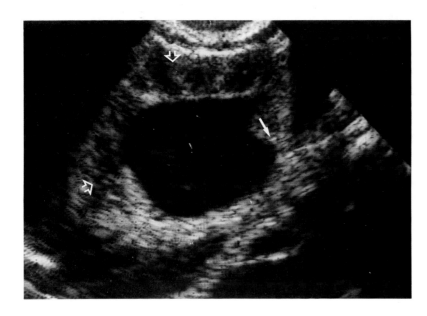

Fig. 8-21. Right flank coronal scan or ureteropelvic junction stenosis (arrow), with enlargement of the pelvis and decreased cortical thickness (open arrows).

pelvis, which usually acquires a round shape with no echoes within it (Fig. 8-21). The renal pelvis stays within the kidney in mild cases or it becomes extrarenal if the abnormality is more severe. The nondilated ureter is absent from the ultrasound field of view. The bladder should be scanned to rule out the presence of distal dilation of the ureters. Ureteral reflux may be detected during micturation with transient dilatation of the pyelocaliceal system.

Multicystic Kidney

A multicystic kidney will be larger than average (0.2 to 2 cm in axial diameter) and it will contain large and uneven cystic and echo-free cavities on ultrasound. No communication is demonstrated between these different-sized cavities, which otherwise present strong posterior wall acoustic enhancement. The renal pelvis is small when present, and difficult to differentiate from the other cystic cavities. The renal parenchyma is sparse and irregular in distribution and without corticomedullary differentiation (Fig. 8-22). The contralateral kidney may be normal or it may present mild hydronephrosis, which usually is idiopathic and disappears with time. There is a higher

incidence of other renal congenital anomalies in the "contralateral normal" kidney.[33]

Polycystic Renal Disease

Both dominant (DPC) and recessive (RPC) polycystic diseases can be seen at birth and/or be diagnosed earlier by obstetric ultrasound. Both may show large, bilateral echogenic kidneys with loss of the normal corticomedullaly differentiation (Fig. 8-23). The pathologic defects in RPC disease are enlargement of the collecting tubule and cellular hyperplasia. RPC disease is usually lethal after birth, but there are several gradations of severity, according to the number of renal tubules involved. Biliary ductal hyperplasia and portal fibrosis are present and they are inversely proportional to those changes in the kidneys.[34]

DPC disease is characterized by formation of cysts in the renal tubular space. The varying severity in the genetic expression of DPC disease may manifest itself with small intrarenal cysts and a macroscopic morphology similar to the kidneys of neonates with RPC disease or with the more characteristic clinical and diagnostic picture of large intrarenal cysts. The small

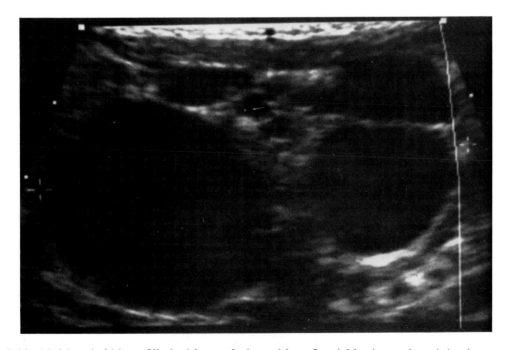

Fig. 8-22. Multicystic kidney filled with anechoic cavities of variable size and a minimal amount of interspersed renal parenchyma (left flank coronal scan).

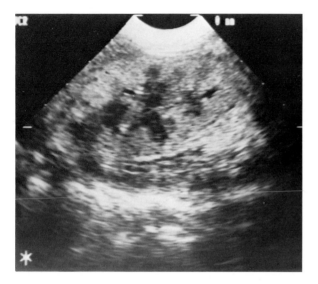

Fig. 8-23. Sagittal scan through the right kidney of an asymptomatic newborn with dominant polycystic renal disease. A grandmother, the father, and two brothers suffered from the same disorder. The ultrasound findings (large, echogenic kidney with loss of the normal corticomedullary differentiation) are similar, in this case, to those of the more typical conditions of recessive polycystic renal disease.

cysts may remain unchanged until later in adulthood or enlarge and create obvious symptoms at any time.[35]

Glomerulocystic renal disease (GCD), a nongenetic disorder with small cortical macroscopic cysts, also presents at birth. The cysts can regress with time but on ultrasound they can look very similar to RPC or DPC disease.[36]

Simple Renal Cysts

A simple renal cyst is a single cystic cavity of variable size localized at the renal cortical periphery. During the neonatal period it may be confused with hypoechoic renal pyramids.[37] The cyst should have a thin, capsular rim and posterior wall acoustic enhancement (Fig. 8-24).

Ectopic Ureterocele

The complete duplication of the pyelocaliceal system is visualized on ultrasound as an echo-free round mass that corresponds to the urine-filled renal pelvis of the upper moiety. This duplicated upper segment has a thin parenchyma with no corticomedullary differentiation (Fig. 8-25A). Its echo-free renal pelvis will be in continuation with a dilated ureter on its way down toward the pelvis, until it ends inside the bladder through a cystic intravesical mass or ureterocele. This cystic structure will have a fine and well-outlined wall (Fig. 8-25B). The lower moiety of the duplicated pyelocaliceal system maintains a more normal renal morphology, although its upper limits can be com-

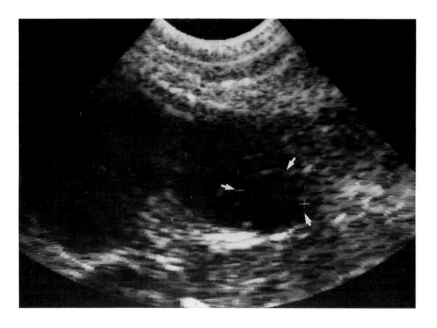

Fig. 8-24. Simple renal cyst (arrows) with a thin capsule at the lower pole (axial scan). (Courtesy of Dr. Del Hoyo, Pediatric Radiology Department, Hospital Infantil "La Paz," Madrid, Spain.)

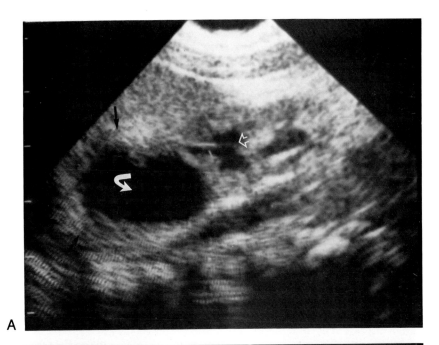

A

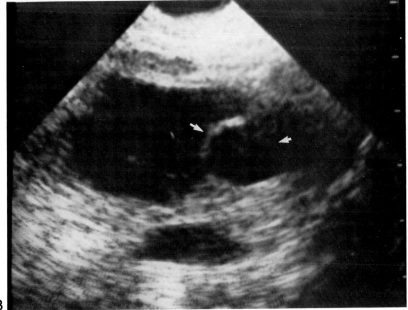

B

Fig. 8-25. **(A)** Sagittal scan of hydronephrosis secondary to ureterocele (curved arrow), showing thinned renal parenchyma (arrow) and slight dilatation of lower pole calices (open arrow). **(B)** Transverse lower abdominal scan of ureterocele within the bladder (arrows).

pressed by the dilated upper moiety. The lower pyelocaliceal system may show dilatation if the ureterocele of the upper system is large enough to compress the ureter of the lower moiety at its vesical entrance. The entrance of the ureter of the lower system is always above the ureterocele.

The contralateral kidney may present similar duplication abnormalties with or without ureterocele, or it could be a completely normal nonduplicated kidney.

There is a higher incidence of renal duplication in girls and the ureterocele may be ectopically present in the urethra or the vagina.[38,39]

Prune-Belly Syndrome

In prune-belly syndrome the kidneys are usually dysplastic or hydronephrotic with good renal parenchyma. The dilatation of the pyelocaliceal systems and

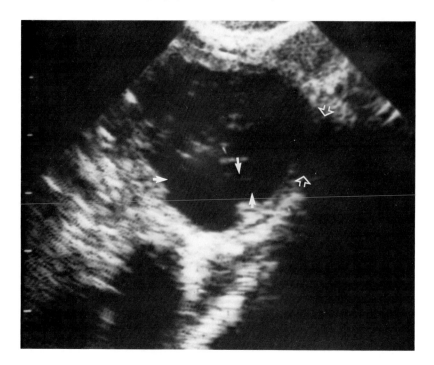

Fig. 8-26. Sagittal plane of the pelvis in a neonate with prune-belly syndrome showing dilated and tortuous distal ureter abutting the bladder wall (arrows). The bladder outlet is also dilated (open arrows).

ureters can reach enormous proportions, and the ureters become very tortuous along their entire pathway.[40] On real-time ultrasound it is possible to visualize the jet effect at the ureterovesical junction if any associated stenosis is present at this level. The vesical wall may be thickened and the neck of the bladder dilated or enlarged, as in cases with posterior urethral valves (Fig. 8-26).

Horseshoe Kidney

The detection of small kidneys on the lateral flank areas should prompt the scanning of the lower midline abdomen. Fusion of the lower renal poles with a mass of lower echogenicity than the kidney may be found. This mass corresponds to renal pyramids lying over the lower lumbar spine, the aorta, and the infe-

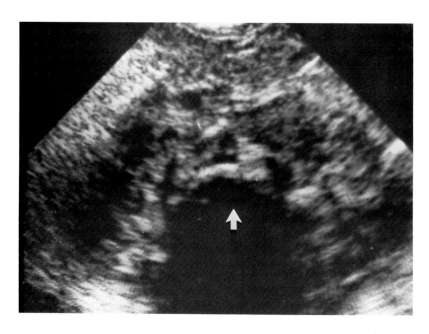

Fig. 8-27. Horseshoe kidney in a transverse section showing renal parenchyma traversing from one to the other renal fossa in front of the spine (arrow), aorta, and vena cava.

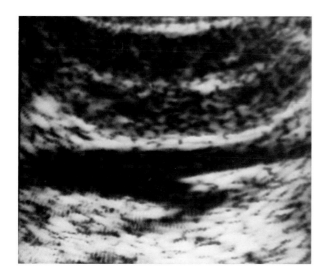

Fig. 8-28. Normal-appearing pelvic kidney at the level of the common iliac arteries on coronal scan.

rior vena cava. The pyelocaliceal systems are not usually dilated if the newborn is asymptomatic (Fig. 8-27). To best visualize this low prevertebral horseshoe kidney, pressure should be applied over the periumbilical region, thus displacing the superimposed bowel loops with the ultrasound transducer.

Pelvic Kidney

The pelvic inlet is the most common place for localization of an ectopic kidney outside the renal fossa. After gentle compression on the lower abdomen to

spread and separate the bowel loops, this ectopic pelvic kidney will appear under the transducer as a mass on top of or behind the bladder or even parellel to the iliac vessels. Its echographic characteristics are those of a normal kidney, although its size may be smaller (Fig. 8-28).

Renal Rupture

Renal rupture may be seen in the newborn with posterior urethral valves.[41] The kidney will contain an echo-free subcapsular area corresponding to the leaked urine, or it may have increased echogenicity when the subcapsular content represents blood outside the renal parenchyma. In cases of severe fracture, the kidney will be seen as a deformed, large mass filled with free echoes, and multiple cysts filled with urine and/or blood and irregularly distributed. Multiple septae will cross this deformed mass, usually outlined by the renal capsule (Fig. 8-29).

Air in the Pyelocaliceal System

Infants born with a distal urinary obstruction may have undergone a decompressive ureterostomy or ureterocalicostomy. On ultrasound examination one may see decreasing size of the previously dilated system and at the same time may observe air bubbles within it coming up from the ureterocalicostomy, seen as movable echogenic material with posterior reverberation shadows. These images are mostly localized at the most dilated upper caliceal group or at the dilated pelvis with hydronephrosis (Fig. 8-30).

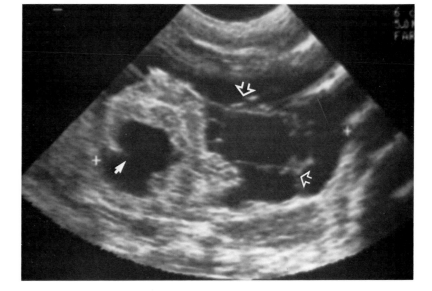

Fig. 8-29. Fractured kidney with disappearance of normal renal echotexture, dilated pelvis (arrow), and subcapsular extravasation of urine (open arrows). (Courtesy of Dr. Gutierrez, Pediatric Radiology Department, Hospital Infantil "La Paz," Madrid, Spain.)

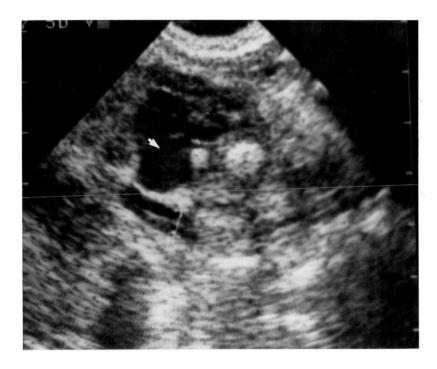

Fig. 8-30. Sagittal scan showing air in a distended pyelocaliceal system; notice small bubbles surrounded by urine (arrow).

Renal Parenchymal Disease: Transient Acute Tubular Disease or Tubular Blockade

The benign course of and rapid recovery from transient acute tubular disease are commonly seen in normal newborns; the condition is due to decreased fluid intake during the first few days of life with precipitation of proteins within the distal collecting tubuli. This phenomenon leads to transitory renal insufficiency and produces increased echogenicity of the renal pyramids in contraposition with the rest of the renal cortical parenchyma (Fig. 8-31). It should not be confused with acute tubular necrosis (ATN),

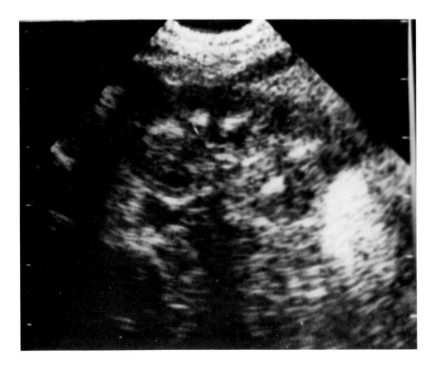

Fig. 8-31. Tubular blockage in a newborn; increased echoes in the renal pyramids with normal cortex.

since no anoxic episodes can be documented. If an IVP is made in search of the cause of anuria, a delay in the renal concentration and excretion of the contrast media will be observed that may last 2 or 3 days after the injection of contrast. Proper hydration of the neonate would correct those abnormalities in the IVP or the abnormally increased echoes in the renal pyramids seen by ultrasound. There are usually no clinical complications. In some infants these abnormally increased intrarenal echogenicities may persist for years and may even cause posterior acoustic shadowing, which makes transient acute tubular disease more difficult to differentiate from nephrocalcinosis.[42]

Renal Vein Thrombosis

Renal vein thrombosis is usually seen in infants suffering from adrenal hemorrhage or in infants of diabetic mothers. The easy palpation of a prominent kidney in one or both flanks should raise the suspicion of renal vein thrombosis, even though hematuria may not yet be present. On real-time ultrasound one or both kidneys are enlarged and the cortical echogenicity is decreased in contraposition with the rest of the renal parenchyma (Fig. 8-32); the normal anatomic

parenchymal landmarks will be lost.[43] Early medical treatment may avoid renal parenchymal atrophy and further growth of the thrombus toward the inferior vena cava. Patency of the inferior vena cava must be checked during the first ultrasound examination and in later follow-ups.

Renal Ischemia

In renal ischemia the kidneys present a generalized increased echogenicity, without corticomedullary differentiation and with normal size and shape. These findings can be seen in premature infants and infants of low birthweight suffering from hypoxia during delivery, or in infants immediately after cardiac surgery (Fig. 8-33).

Nephrocalcinosis

Increased echogenicity in the renal pyramids can be observed in nephrocalcinosis; these echoes correspond to calcium deposits, which are usually caused by long treatment with furosemide for bronchopulmonary dysplasia (Fig. 8-34). In more severe stages of this pulmonary disorder these increased echoes can produce posterior acoustic shadowing. The microcal-

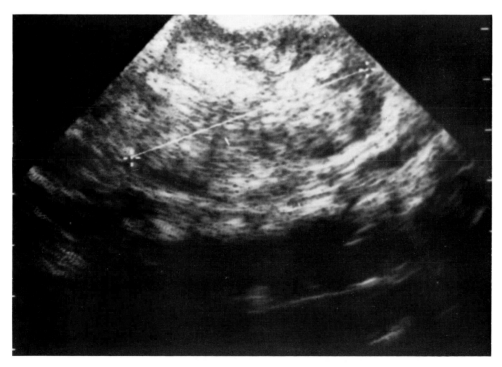

Fig. 8-32. Renal vein thrombosis with enlarged kidneys and increased echogenicity at the medullary portion of the parenchyma.

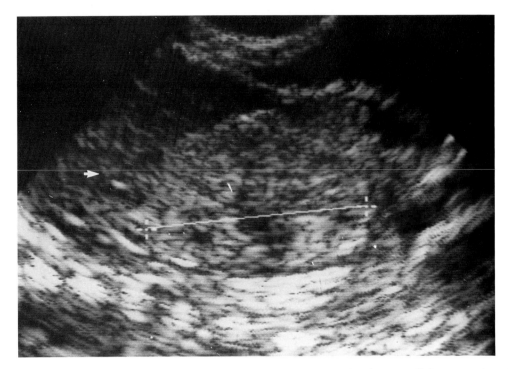

Fig. 8-33. Renal ischemia: a small kidney but of proportionate size in a small-for-gestational-age newborn. The echogenicity is higher than that of the liver (arrow) and lacks corticomedullary differentiation (sagittal scan).

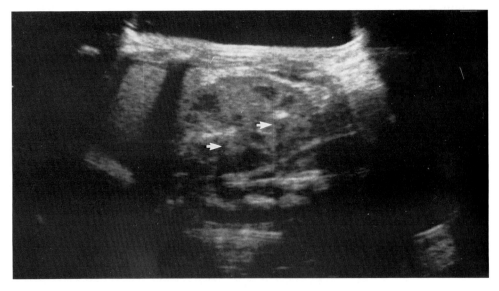

Fig. 8-34. Nephrocalcinosis secondary to diuretic treatment with minimal posterior acoustic shadowing (arrows) (sagittal scan).

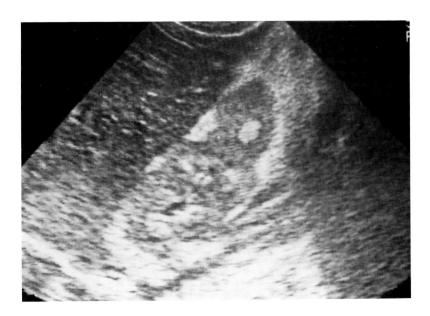

Fig. 8-35. Nephrocalcinosis secondary to vitamin A and D intoxication in the newborn period (sagittal scan).

cifications usually disappear after cessation of treatment but in those infants requiring protracted treatment, large calculi can form inside the kidneys and obstruct the pyelocaliceal systems.[44] These calculi may be excreted later, as seen in older infants after long treatment with diuretics; these infants presented with bouts of abdominal pain and microscopic hematuria. Follow-up ultrasound scans demonstrated the disappearance of these echogenic intrarenal acoustic shadows and improvement of the caliceal ectasia. No treatment is required when the caliceal group dilatation is moderate.

Congenital nephrocalcinosis has also been observed by ultrasound in the first day of life; the mothers of these infants were on a diet high in vitamins and minerals during pregnancy. Nephrocalcinosis can also be present after the acute phase of neonatal renal vein thrombosis subsides; the affected kidney usually becomes smaller. Congenital nephrocalcinosis is also seen in association with congenital ictiosis and thrombosis of the inferior vena cava and after resolution, in some newborns, of an episode of ATN; it may disappear slowly but spontaneously or it may persist during the first years of life. Neonatal

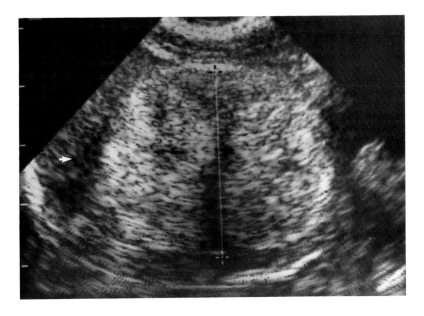

Fig. 8-36. Globular kidney with more echogenicity than the liver parenchyma (arrow) in an infant with sialicosis (right sagittal scan).

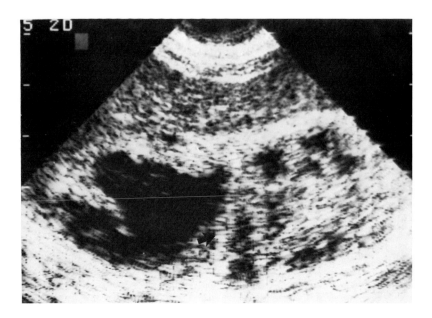

Fig. 8-37. In utero adrenal hemorrhage with hypoechoic characteristics compressing the upper renal pole and separated by a thin interphase (arrow) (sagittal scan).

vitamin A and D intoxication can also produce nephrocalcinosis and increased echogenicity of the renal parenchyma. This hyperechoic cortex will contrast with the normal hypoechoic renal pyramids and the normal echoes of the liver and spleen; these findings are reversible after discontinuing the administration of vitamins (Fig. 8-35).

Sialicosis

Sialicosis is caused by massive renal excretion of sialic acid, which is also present in high concentrations in blood. The infant presents with ascites, hepatomegaly, and prominent round kidneys of increased echogenicity with absence of the corticomedullary differentiation on ultrasound (Fig. 8-36).

ADRENAL GLAND

Adrenal Hemorrhage

The sagittal ultrasound plane will reveal the masses of increased echogenicity at the adrenal gland, displacing inferiorly the adjacent kidney with a compressed upper pole, in adrenal hemorrhage. The

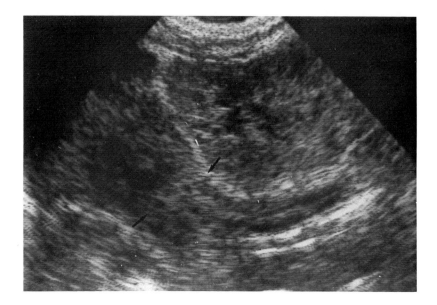

Fig. 8-38. Recent adrenal hemorrhage with widening of the gland cranially (arrow) and preservation of part of the normal gland (coronal scan) (sagittal scan).

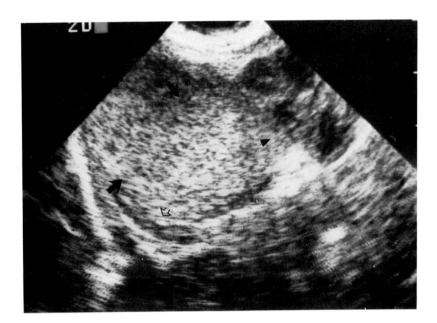

Fig. 8-39. Neuroblastoma (arrows) displacing the adrenal gland superiorly (open arrow) and the kidney inferiorly (arrowhead). Notice the high echogenicity and lack of separation from the kidney (sagittal scan).

mass or masses become less echogenic with time and end up as small residual calcified speckles after several weeks or months.[45] At times the adrenal hemorrhage may have occurred before delivery. An immediate postnatal abdominal ultrasound can show an echo-free or cystic-appearing adrenal gland; it will compress and displace inferiorly and anteriorly the adjacent kidney as an expression of its antenatal origin[46] (Fig. 8-37).

At delivery, adrenal hemorrhage presents with increase echogenicity as described above (Fig. 8-38). In either case the intra-adrenal hemorrhage will alter the normal parenchyma of the gland. In cases of bilateral or large adrenal hemorrhages a syndrome of acute adrenal insufficiency tends to develop, with a very poor prognosis. Adrenal hemorrhage can be seen also in association with neonatal jaundice or thrombosis of the renal vein.[47] Adrenal hemorrhage and congenital neuroblastoma have a similar ultrasound pattern; the neuroblastoma can also bleed and

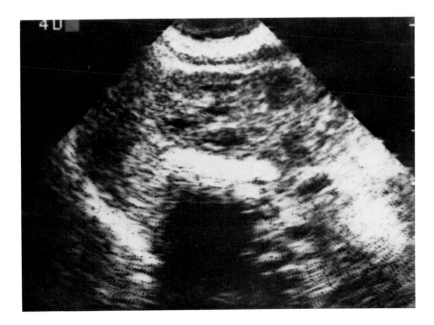

Fig. 8-40. In utero calcified neuroblastoma containing few echoes and minimal mass effect (sagittal scan).

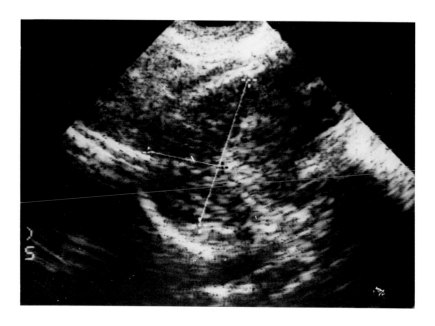

Fig. 8-41. Congenital adrenal hyperplasia secondary to 21-hydroxylase deficiency. The gland appears enlarged and disorganized on this right flank coronal scan.

become either echogenic or a mixed mass of echogenic and hypoechoic texture. Further tests are then necessary for the differential diagnosis.

Congenital Neuroblastoma

Congenital neuroblastoma can be seen on ultrasound as a round, homogeneous mass with increased or decreased echogenicity, depending on the amount of tumor necrosis. The mass is in contact with the adrenal gland, which may have a normal appearance but is displaced from the adjacent kidney by the tumoral growth. This tumor usually displaces the kidney inferiorly and anteriorly.[46] Metastatic disease is not common when the mass is discovered immediately after birth (Fig. 8-39). Congenital neuroblastoma can be diagnosed by obstetric ultrasound as a calcified mass above the kidney (Fig. 8-40). Under these circumstances, because of the presence of associated intra-adrenal hemorrhage, its differential diagnosis with simple hemorrhage becomes almost impossible.[45,48,49] Congenital neuroblastoma can be detected

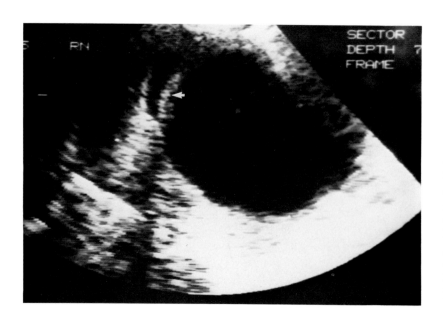

Fig. 8-42. Pyloric duplication in a newborn with an anechoic mass demonstrating posterior acoustic enhancement, and causing displacement of the gallbladder (arrow) (oblique right upper quadrant scan). (Courtesy of Dr. De Pablo, Pediatric Radiology Department, Hospital Infantil "La Paz," Madrid, Spain.)

by palpation during the physical exam as a mass above the kidney or, if smaller in size, may only be detected during a routine neonatal abdominal ultrasound. Extra-adrenal neuroblastomas can also be diagnosed through abdominal ultrasound as echogenic round masses, with sharp boundaries and, at times, with intraparenchymal cystic structures.

Adrenal Hyperplasia

Adrenal hyperplasia can be caused by 21-hydroxylase deficiency. The adrenals will be enlarged with an abnormal parenchyma and no recognition of the normal echogenic central hilar texture can be made.[50] The enlarged gland is completely replaced by a hypoechoic texture, criss-crossed by small septae (Fig. 8-41). The size and configuration of the adrenal gland will return to normal after adequate treatment. Neonatal physiologic adrenal hyperplasia, on the contrary, maintains its normal anatomic texture and configuration and it decreases its enlarged size after the third or fourth week of life.

GASTROINTESTINAL DISEASES DIAGNOSED BY ABDOMINAL ULTRASOUND

Hypertrophic Pyloric Stenosis of the Low-Birthweight Infant

Hypertrophic pyloric stenosis is seen in infants of less than 1,500 g with ultrasound characteristics similar to those seen in the classic muscular hypertrophy of the term newborn of several weeks of age. Increased length of the pyloric channel can be seen along with increased thickness of its muscular layer; the measurements of the abnormal pyloric length and thickness are usually below the range seen in the older infant. A fluid-filled distended stomach with multiple gastric peristaltic contractions can also be seen.

Duodenal Duplication

A variable size, echo-free mass will be seen on ultrasound in duodenal duplication, with sharp contours and, at times, posterior wall acoustic enhancement (Fig. 8-42). The mass may vary in size from 1.0 to several centimeters. When small in size this mass will be surrounded by echogenic air bubbles in the duodenal lumen following the jet phenomenon of the gastric emptying mechanism.[51]

Jejunal Atresia

In jejunal atresia enlargement of the jejunum with dilatation of the proximal bowel loops can be seen on ultrasound as a result of the large amount of fluid-filled intestine (Fig. 8-43). The walls of these loops are well visualized and they end in a round cavity or loop that is usually larger than the others and represents the most proximal loop from the atresia.[52] The diagnosis of proximal or distal jejunal atresia will depend on the number of fluid-filled dilated bowel loops identified.

Meconium Ileus

Meconium can be seen on ultrasound at the ileocecal valve and along the colonic frame as intraluminal masses of increased echogenicity but with central decreased echoes (Fig. 8-44). These masses are usually close to each other or minimally separated; normal meconium, in contrast, has less echogenicity. The bowel loops proximal to these abnormally echogenic masses are distended and filled with fluid.[53] The abnormal meconium echogenicity is caused by a certain degree of intrameconial calcification that is not seen on the abdominal radiograph. Meconium ileus is often seen in association with cystic fibrosis of the pancreas.

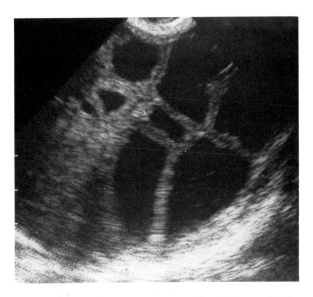

Fig. 8-43. Mid-abdominal scan of an infant with jejunal atresia showing several dilated, fluid-containing loops of bowel. (Courtesy of Dr. Berrocal, Pediatric Radiology Department, Hospital Infantil "La Paz," Madrid, Spain.)

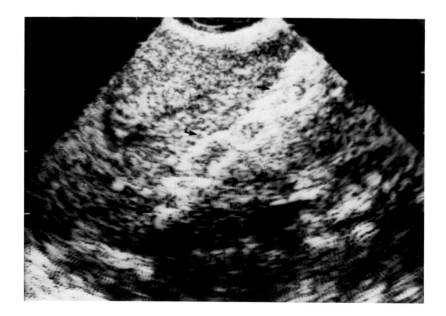

Fig. 8-44. Meconium ileus: small rounded images of abnormal calcified meconium following the course of the colon (arrows) (sagittal mid-abdominal scan).

Meconium Cyst

The newborn infant with a meconium cyst presents with abdominal distension. The abdominal radiograph shows a paucity of intraintestinal air and ultrasound examination can demonstrate large cystic cavities with intracavitary echogenicities representing trapped bowel loops (Fig. 8-45); these bright echogenic loops retain peristaltic motion (snow storm) but no intraluminal air.[54] The cyst walls are poorly defined and sometimes this cyst may rupture during delivery because of its large size; its content may be seen spilling over the peritoneum. It is usually seen in association with cystic fibrosis of the pancreas.

Matted Bowel Loops Caused by Perforation with Peritonitis in Necrotizing Enterocolitis

The abdominal radiograph of perforation-induced matted bowel loops demonstrates a mass defect in the mid-abdomen and an abnormal bowel gas pattern. On ultrasound an abdominal mass of variable size is

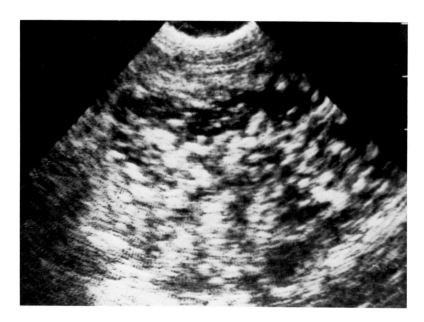

Fig. 8-45. Meconium cyst: cavity full of echoes that shifted continuously on real-time examination (mid-abdominal sagittal scan).

identified (Fig. 8-46) with round contours and low peripheral echogenicity due to the presence of edema.[55] The center of the mass has increased echogenicity and air bubbles within the echogenic fluid-filled cavities (representing bowel loops trapped into the inflammatory process). The identified loops will not be displaced under the pressure exerted by the ultrasound transducer, and pain will be elicited with this maneuver (Fig. 8-46A). The matted mass of bowel loops may have the appearance of a dysplastic kidney but with air bubbles within it (Fig. 8-46B).

Nonspecific Enteritis

Dilated loops of thickened bowel that contain fluid in continuous motion may be seen in newborns with rotavirus infections (Fig. 8-47). The loops are not as dilated as in atresias.

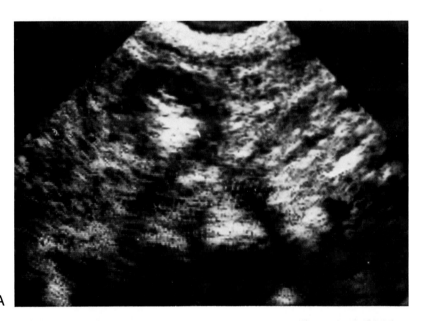

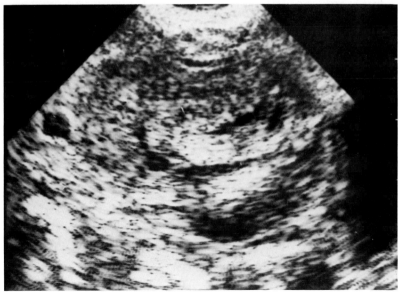

Fig. 8-46. **(A)** Matted bowel loops secondary to necrotizing enterocolitis in a segment of descending colon with wall edema. **(B)** Notice the involvement of several loops (mid-abdominal axial scans).

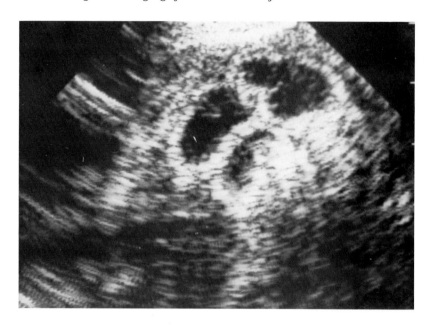

Fig. 8-47. Rotavirus enteritis, with fluid-filled distended loops of small bowel (fluid abdominal axial scan).

OTHER ABDOMINAL MASSES OF EXTRA-ABDOMINAL ORIGIN

Sacrococcygeal Teratoma

Sacrococcygeal teratoma presents with masses of variable size and echogenicity, ranging from echo free to hyperechoic, and with acoustic shadowing if it contains calcium (bone). These teratomas can involve the prerectal space or expand beyond it into the abdominal cavity (Fig. 8-48), displacing intestinal loops.[56] Since the teratoma is in contact with the spine, the cord should be scanned to rule out an intradural origin of the mass.

Infradiaphragmatic Pulmonary Sequestration

Infradiaphragmatic pulmonary sequestration is rare and may present as a highly echogenic mass with several fluid cavities within, displacing the left kidney anteriorly and inferiorly and in contact with the adre-

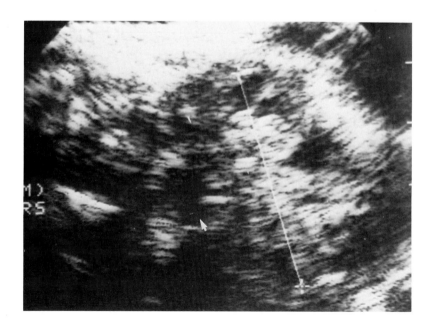

Fig. 8-48. Lower abdominal scan of sacrococcygeal teratoma showing a mass of variable echogenicity in the true pelvis extending to the distal aorta (arrow).

nal gland.[57] The aortic feeding artery is difficult to identify because of its small caliber and length (Fig. 8-49). Differential diagnosis with neuroblastoma should be considered if the feeding artery is not identified. MR imaging is then recommended.

VESSELS

Catheter Position

Ultrasound complements the anteroposterior and lateral radiographs of the chest and abdomen when looking for the exact position of the intraluminal lines or catheters. Using ultrasound it is possible to locate which vessels contain catheters (usually the umbilical vessels) and where the tips of the catheters lie. An umbilical artery catheter can be followed from the bifurcation of the common iliac arteries to its passage along the renal arteries (superior to inferior), the celiac trunk, and superior mesenteric artery or to the diaphragm. A venous line can be followed up to the ductus venosus and beyond until reaching the level of the right atrium.

Aorta

The abdominal aorta can be identified with the newborn in the supine position by placing the ultrasound transducer in a longitudinal orientation over the left flank and angling it superiorly, until the transducer almost touches the bedding. In this way, the

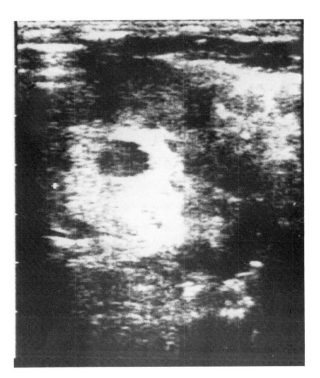

Fig. 8-49. Extralobar pulmonary sequestration in the vicinity of the upper abdominal aorta on left flank coronal scan. Highly echogenic mass with cystic cavity. (Courtesy of Dr. Gonzalez, Madrid, Spain.)

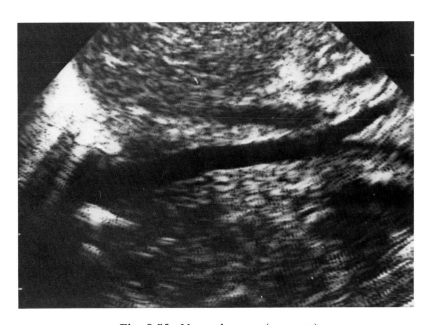

Fig. 8-50. Normal aorta. (see text.)

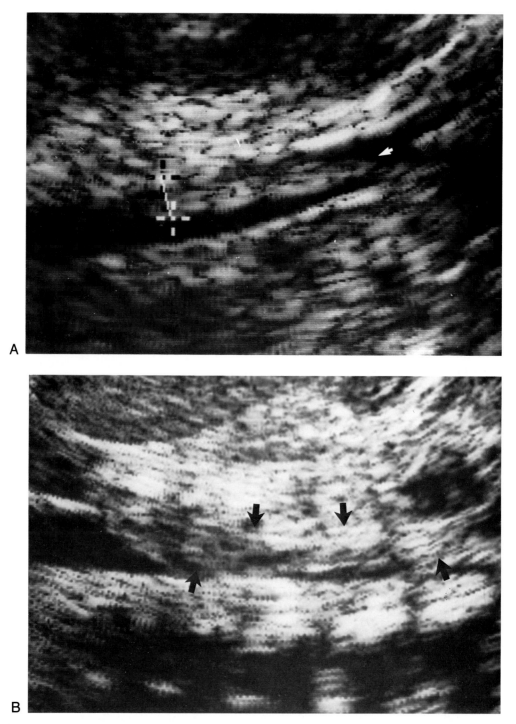

Fig. 8-51. **(A)** Thrombus in the aorta extending to the right common iliac artery (arrow). **(B)** Complete occlusion of the lumen of the aorta in another premature infant by a large thrombus extension (arrows).

gastrointestinal gas located anteriorly is avoided. The infradiaphragmatic aorta can be seen in its full length as a linear structure of mildly echogenic parallel walls and hypoechoic lumen. Its caliber diminishes slightly until it bifurcates at the level of the common iliacs (the left common iliac will be nearest to the transducer if the left-sided approach is utilized). The internal and external iliac arteries can also be identified, measuring about 1 mm in diameter (Fig. 8-50). Frequently, two parallel structures can be seen on each side of the aorta, containing some echoes, that correspond to the diaphragmatic pillars.

Thrombosis of the Aorta

Thrombosis of the aorta happens with relative frequency if the umbilical arteries have been catheterized for too long in the newborn period. Its incidence in necropsies reaches 10 percent but ultrasonographic studies show it occurs more often. The thrombus is identified as an echogenic filiform structure adherent to one of the walls of the vessel, usually above the renal arteries; it may extend inferiorly as a freely movable clot to obstruct completely the ipsilateral catheterized iliac artery. The contralateral artery is usually patent (Fig. 8-51A). Occasionally, the thrombus may extend to the origin of the superior mesenteric artery. Rarely, at the tip of the catheter a freely floating echogenic thrombus can be seen; removal of the catheter should then be performed, aspirating with caution to avoid dislodgement of the thrombus.

Thrombosis of the aorta should be suspected in the presence of hypertension of unknown cause, when there is difficulty in placing the catheter (possible vessel wall injury), and when the catheter appears obstructed (no backflow). The thrombi usually disappear spontaneously within a week of catheter removal. Sometimes a slightly echogenic foci may remain at the site of origin of the thrombus. Exceptionally, thrombosis may totally involve the lumen of the aorta; this is seen as an echogenic mass filling the lumen of the vessel, with no flow distally (Fig. 8-51B). These cases can be lethal if not treated promptly.[58]

Aortic Calcification

Rarely, aortic calcification is seen on ultrasound as a highly echogenic wall of the aorta also involving its branches, such as the superior mesenteric and iliacs arteries (Fig. 8-52). The hypechoic lumen cannot be

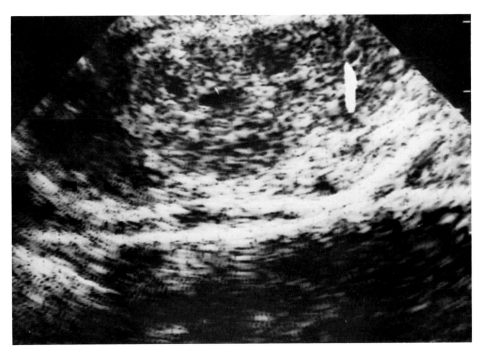

Fig. 8-52. Aortic and iliac wall calcifications with obscuration of the lumen of the aorta and stenosis at the level of the bifurcation.

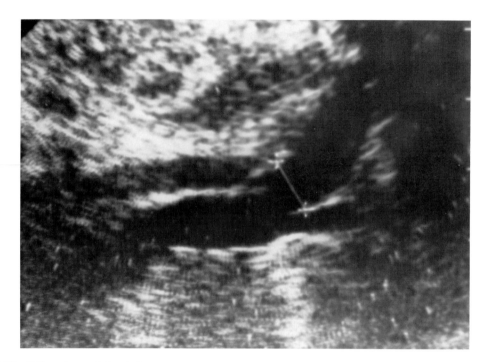

Fig. 8-53. Dilatation of the left iliac vein in relation to the right one in angioma of the left lower extremity.

seen. Aortic calcification is associated with periarticular calcifications as well as calcium deposits on peripheral arteries in Conradi's syndrome. The radiograph shows faint parallel calcifications near the vertebral column that are better appreciated in arteries of the limbs.

Inferior Vena Cava

The full length of the inferior vena cava (IVC) can be identified by scanning in longitudinal sections from the liver area or from the right flank. The iliac veins can be seen as of larger caliber than the arteries. The iliac vein nearest to the transducer will correspond to the ipsilateral iliac vein.

Dilatation of the Left Iliac Vein

Dilatation of the left iliac vein, in which the diameter of the vessel is much greater than that of the contralateral vein, may be seen in cases of hemangiomas of the ipsilateral limb. The iliac artery is not enlarged. Treatment can be achieved by selective arterial embolization of the feeding vessel (Fig. 8-53).

Thrombosis of the IVC

Thrombosis of the IVC is not frequent but is seen in association with renal vein thrombosis. Ultrasound will show echogenic masses within the lumen of the vein with a less echogenic central portion and posterior acoustic shadowing. The lumen of the vessel may be completely occluded and dilated. In the newborn depicted in Figure 8-54A nephrocalcinosis and cutaneous lesions of congenital dominant ichthyosiform erythrodermia were associated. Plain radiographs will show an ovoid calcification superimposed on the liver.[59] Exceptionally, if the venous thrombus is freely movable it may be seen as a rounded, moderately echogenic structure that shifts toward the heart (Fig. 8-54B).

Dilated IVC

A dilated IVC can be seen in the hemodynamic changes of heart failure. The suprahepatic veins may also be dilated. Possible causes include myocardiopathies, intracardiac tumors, and thrombus. The most frequent cause in the newborn is rhabdomyoma asso-

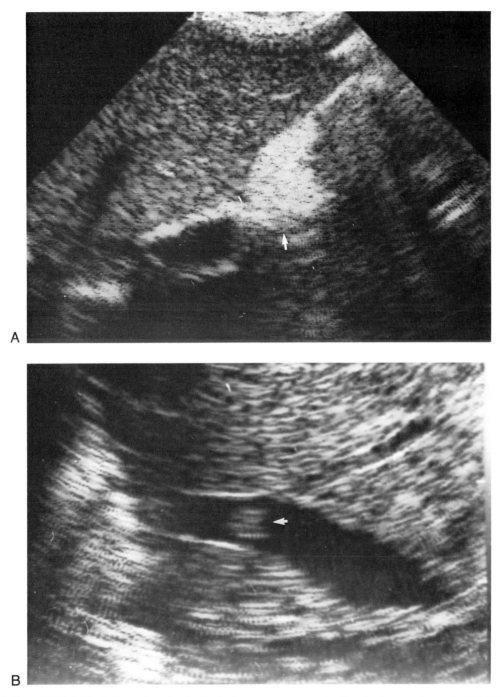

Fig. 8-54. **(A)** Calcified thrombus in the inferior vena cava occluding its lumen (arrow). **(B)** Thromboembolus that ascends freely toward the heart (arrow) (sagittal scans).

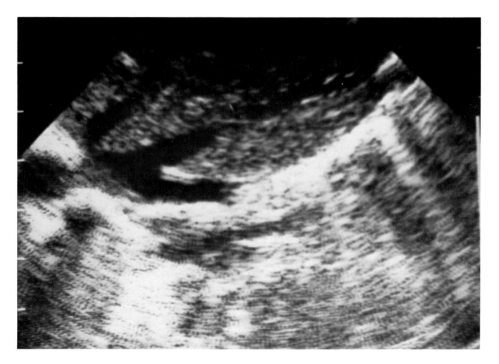

Fig. 8-55. Sagittal right upper quadrant scan showing dilated suprahepatic veins in a newborn with right atrial myxoma.

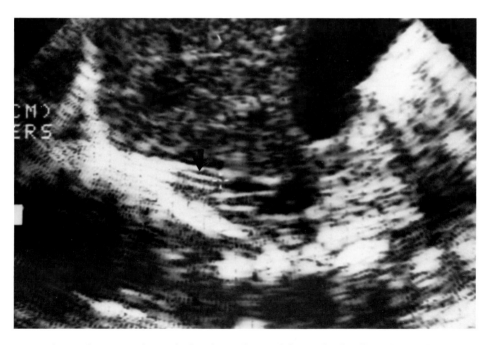

Fig. 8-56. Catheter fragment (arrow) that has migrated from the basilic vein in the left arm to the inferior vena cava (sagittal scan).

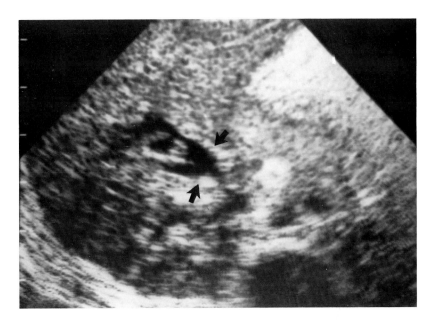

Fig. 8-57. Portal venous thrombosis due to *Candida albicans* mycetoma; notice dilatation of the lumen of the portal vein (arrows) (oblique scan, right upper quadrant).

ciated with phakomatosis and right atrial myxomata (Fig. 8-55). Hepatomegaly is also a frequently detectable ultrasonographic finding.

Fragmented Catheter

A catheter fragment may migrate from its insertion point in the arm veins to the right atrium and descend into the IVC. In this latter position it may be seen by abdominal ultrasound as a double parallel echogenic line (Fig. 8-56).

Thrombosis of the Portal Vein

Thrombosis of the portal vein is revealed on ultrasound as irregular enlargement of its caliber. A heterogeneous mass of irregular borders may be seen (Fig. 8-57) corresponding to a fungus ball due to *Candida albicans*. Other fungus balls may be present in vascular structures of main organs, such as the kidneys of a patient suffering from renal candidiasis.[60,61]

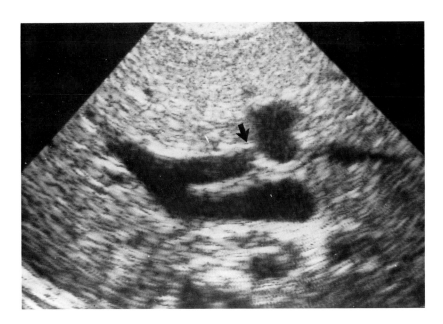

Fig. 8-58. Total anomalous pulmonary venous return below the diaphragm with drainage to the left portal vein (arrow) (oblique scan, right upper quadrant).

Total Anomalous Pulmonary Venous Return below the Diaphragm Draining to the Portal Vein

Within the liver parenchyma and between the dilated left portal vein and the aorta, an aberrant vessel can be identified parallel to the aorta in total anomalous pulmonary venous return below the diaphragm. The vessel descends on the left from the chest and terminates to the right of the spine by joining the main portal vein or its left branch and forming an angle.[62,63] The diameter of the portal vein is markedly enlarged throughout its length,[64] whereas the splenic vein is not dilated and the aorta is smaller in caliber than usual (Fig. 8-58). Doppler analysis facilitates identification of these abnormal vessels.[63]

REFERENCES

1. Shkolnick A, Foley MJ, Riggs TW, Devine S: New application of real time ultrasound in pediatrics. Radiographics 2:422, 1982
2. Wagner LD, Weinberg B, Morrissey WJ et al: Cholelithiasis in a six week old asymptomatic neonate. JCU 17:692, 1989
3. Keller MS, Markle BM, Laffey PA et al: Spontaneous resolution of cholelithiasis in infants. Radiology 157:345, 1985
4. Balistreri WF, Bove KE: Hepatobiliary consequences of parenteral alimentation. Prog Liver Dis 9:567, 1990
5. Ikeda S, Sera Y, Akagi M: Serial ultrasonic examination to differentiate biliary atresia from neonatal hepatitis. Special reference to changes in size of the gallbladder. Eur J Pediatr 148:396, 1989
6. Narula MK, Sachdev HP, Dubey AP et al: Sonographic evaluation of gall bladder in acute viral hepatitis. Indian Pediatr 26:636, 1989
7. Carrol IBA, Oppenheimer DA, Muller HH: High frequency real time ultrasound of the neonatal biliary system. Radiology 145:437, 1982
8. Shlaer WJ, Leopold GR, Scheible FW: Sonography of the thickened gallbladder wall: a nonspecific finding. AJR 136:337, 1981
9. Peevy KJ, Wiseman JH: Gallbladder distension in septic neonates. Arch Dis Child 57:75, 1982
10. Matos C, Avni EF, Van Gansbeke D: Total parenteral nutrition (TPN) and gallbladder diseases in neonates. Sonographic assessment. J Ultrasound Med 6:243, 1987
11. Kirks DR, Baden M: Incompetence of the sphincter of Oddi associated with duodenal stenosis. J Pediatr 83:838, 1973
12. Brown DM: Bile plug syndrome: successful management with a mucolytic agent. Pediatr Surg 25:351, 1990
13. Pfeiffer WR, Robinson LH, Bairasa VJ: Sonographic features of bile plug syndrome. J Ultrasound Med 5:335, 1986
14. Davies C, Daneman A, Stringer DA: Inspissated bile in a neonate with cystic fibrosis. J Ultrasound Med 5:335, 1986
15. Kumari S, Lee WJ, Baron MG: Hydrops of the gallbladder in a child: diagnosis by ultrasound. Pediatrics 63:295, 1979
16. Schrumpf JD, Handmaker H: Hydrops of gallbladder in a premature neonate. Am J Dis Child 136:172, 1982
17. Mukamel E, Zer M, Avidor J et al: Acute acalculous cholecystitis in an infant: a case report. J Pediatr Surg 16:521, 1981
18. Johnson DH, Vinson AM, Wirth FH et al: Management of hepatic hemangioendotheliomas of infancy by transarterial embolization: a report of two cases. Pediatrics 73:546, 1983
19. Stanley P, Grinnel VS, Stanton RE et al: Therapeutic embolization of infantile hepatic hemangioma with polyvinyl alcohol. AJR 141:1047, 1983
20. Zorzi C, Perale R, Benini X, and Angonese I: Diagnostic value of ultrasonography in neonatal liver ruepute. Pediatr Radiol 16:425, 1986
21. Scatariage JC, Scott WW, Donovan PJ et al: Fatty infiltration of the liver: ultrasonographic and computed tomographic correlation. J Ultrasound Med 3:9, 1984
22. Richter E, Globl H, Holthusen W, Lassric MA: Intrahepatic calcifications in infants and children following umbilical vein catheterization. Ann Radiol 27:117, 1984
23. Lindley S, Mollitt DL, Seibert JJ, Golladay ES: Portal vein ultrasonography in the early diagnosis of necrotizing enterocolitis. J Pediatr Surg 21:530, 1986
24. Jacobs DG, Haka Ikse K, Wesson DE et al: Growth and development in patients operated on for islet cell dysplasia. J Pediatr Surg 21:1184, 1986
25. De Morais CF, Lopes EA, Bisi H et al: Nesidioblastosis associated with congenital malformations of the heart. Morphological and immunohistochemical study of 5 necropsy cases. Pathol Res Pract 181:175,1986
26. Synn AY, Mulvihill SJ, Fonkalsrud EW: Surgical disorders of the pancreas in infancy and childhood. Am J Surg 156:201, 1988
27. Goossens A, Gepts W, Saudubray JM et al: Diffuse and focal nesidioblastosis. A clinicopathological study of 24 patients with persistent neonatal hyperinsulinemic hypoglycemia. Am J Surg Pathol 13:766, 1989
28. Walsh E, Cramer B, Pushpanathan C: Pancreatic

echogenicity in premature and newborn infants. Pediatr Radiol 20:323, 1990
29. Seviatan H, Harrell RS, Perret RS: Ectopic spleen: a sonographic diagnosis. Pediatr Radiol 12:152, 1982
30. Hriack H, Slovis TL, Callen PW, Romanski RN: Neonatal kidneys: sonographic-anatomic correlation. Radiology 147:699, 1983
31. Silverman PM, Carroll BA, Moskowitz PS: Adrenal sonography in renal agenesis and dysplasia. AJR 134:600, 1980
32. Chopra A, Telle RL: Hydronephrosis in children: narrowing the differential diagnosis with ultrasound. JCU 8:473, 1980
33. Pedicelli G, Equier S, Bowen A, Boisvert J: Multicystic dysplastic kidneys: spontaneous regression demonstrated with US. Radiology 161:23, 1986
34. Lieberman E, Salinas-Madrigal L, Gwinn JL et al: Clinical, pathological and radiological correlations and comparison with congenital hepatic fibrosis. Medicine 50:277, 1971
35. Fellows RA, Leonidas JC, Beatty EC: Radiologic features of "adult type" polycystic kidney disease in the neonate. Pediatr Radiol 4:87, 1976
36. Fredericks BJ, De Campo M, Chow CU et al: Glomerulocystic renal disease: ultrasound appearance. Pediatr Radiol 19:184, 1989
37. Steinhardt GF, Slovis TL, Perimutter AD: Simple renal cysts in infants. Radiology 155:349, 1985
38. Cremin BJ: A review of the ultrasonographic appearances of posterior urethral valves and ureteroceles. Pediatr Radiol 16:357, 1986
39. Nussbaum AN, Dorst JP, Jeffs RD, Sanders RD: Ectopic ureter and ureterocele: their varied sonographci manifestations. Radiology 159:227, 1986
40. Garris J, Kangarloo H, Sarti D et al: The ultrasound spectrum of prune-belly syndromes. JCU 8:117, 1980
41. Macpherson RI, Gordon L, Bradford BF: Neonatal urinomas: imaging considerations. Pediatr Radiol 14:396, 1984
42. Avni EF, Sphel-Robberecht M, Lebrun D et al: Transient acute tubular disease in the newborn: characteristic ultrasound pattern. Ann Radiol 26:175, 1983
43. Metreweli C, Pearson R: Echogenic diagnosis of neonatal renal venous thrombosis. Pediatr Radiol 14:105, 1984
44. Gilsanz V, Fernal W, Reid BS et al: Nephrolithiasis in premature infants. Radiology 154:107, 1984
45. Wu CC: Sonographic spectrum of neonatal adrenal hemorrhage: report of a case simulating solid tumor. JCU 17:45, 1989
46. Gotoh T, Adachi Y, Nounaka O et al: Adrenal hemorrhage in the newborn with evidence of bleeding in utero. J Urol 141:1145, 1989
47. Brill PW, Jagannath A, Winchester P et al: Adrenal hemorrhage and renal vein thrombosis in the newborn: MR imaging. Radiology 170:95, 1989
48. Nunez R, Cabanez Andres JA, Blesa Sanchez E: Congenital suprarenal hemorrhagic pseudocyst and neuroblastoma in situ. An Esp Pediatr 30:237, 1989
49. Eklof O, Mortensson W, Sandstedt B: Suprarenal hematoma versus neuroblastoma complicated by hemorrhage. A diagnostic dilemma in the newborn. Acta Radiol [Diagn] (Stockh) 27:3, 1986
50. Menzel D, Hauffa BP: Changes in size and sonographic characteristics of the adrenal glands during the first year of life and the sonographic diagnosis of adrenal hyperplasia in infants with 21-hydroxylase deficiency. JCU 18:619, 1990
51. Fried AM, Pulmano CM, Mostowycz x: Duodenal duplication cyst: sonographic and angiographic features. AJR 128:863, 1977
52. Manning C, Strauss A, Gyepes MT: Jejunal atresia with apple peel deformity: a report of eight survivors. J Perinatol 9:281, 1989
53. Pan EY, Chen LY, Yang JZ et al: Radiographic diagnosis of meconium peritonitis: a report of 200 cases including six fetal cases. Pediatr Radiol 13:199, 1983
54. Lawrence PW, Chrispin A: Sonographic appearances in two neonates with generalized meconium peritonitis. The "snowstorm" sign. Br J Radiol 57:340, 1984
55. Kodroff MB, Hartenberg MA, Goldschmidt RA: Ultrasonographic diagnosis of gangrenous bowel in neonatal necrotizing enterocolitis. Pediatr Radiol 14:168, 1984
56. Moazan F, Talbert JL: Congenital anorectal malformation: harbingers of sacroccocygeal teratomas. Ann Surg 120:856, 1985
57. John PR, Beasley SW, Mayne V: Pulmonary sequestration and related congenital disorders: a clinicoradiological review of 41 cases. Pediatr Radiol 20:4, 1989
58. Golberg REA, Cohen AM, Bryan PJ, Olsen M, Martin RJ: Neonatal aortic thrombosis treated with intra-arterial urokinase therapy. J Can Assoc Radiol 40:50, 1989
59. Uglietta JP, Woodruff WW, Effmann EL, Carroll BA: Duplex Doppler ultrasound evaluation of calcified inferior vena cava thrombosis. Pediatr Radiol 19:250, 1989
60. Verdeguer A, Fernandez JM, Esquembre C et al: Hepatosplenic candidiasis in children with acute leukemia. Cancer 665:874, 1990
61. Currie JL: Ultrasound appearances of systemic candidiasis in the neonate. Radiogr Today 55:20, 1989
62. Van Hare GF, Schmidt KG, Cassidy SC et al: Color Doppler flow mapping in the ultrasound diagnosis

of total anomalous pulmonary venous connection. J Am Soc Echocardiogr 1:341, 1988

63. Copper MJ, Teitel DF, Silverman NH, Enderlein MA: Study of the infradiaphragmatic total annomalous pulmonary venous connection with cross-sec-

tional pulsed Doppler echocardiography. Circulation 70:412, 1984

64. Patriquin HB, Perreault G, Grignon A et al: Normal portal venous diameter in children. Pediatr Radiol 20:451, 1990

Musculoskeletal Abnormalities of the High-Risk Newborn

Rodrigo Dominguez

9

The high-risk neonate has an increased incidence of musculoskeletal structural defects, whose etiology can be attributed to chromosomal or other hereditary genetic factors as well as exposure to known teratogenic or other sporadic unknown agents. Such infants may present at delivery with a single primary defect or have a multiple malformation syndrome. A dysmorphology evaluation of an affected newborn is then very appropriate. Because the musculoskeletal system is most commonly involved with single primary defects,[1] radiologic evaluation is an integral part of the clinical work-up, and the pediatric radiologist should be consulted for the selection of the most appropriate imaging modality to optimally display the defect.

DETERMINATION OF SKELETAL MATURATION

Conventional radiology not only displays osseous anomalies but also depicts the status of ossification or dysmaturity of the skeleton. Standards of ossification in the normal or at-risk neonate have been published.[2] It should be remembered that premature infants can show failure of ossification of the pubic bones, and that the distal femoral epiphysis can appear on the roentgenogram of a premature infant of 36 weeks' gestational age and that of the proximal tibia in premature infants of 38 weeks' gestational age; the proximal humeral head appears on roentgenograms of premature infants of 37 weeks' gestational age. Females have advanced ossification when compared with male infants.

Ultrasound can also be used to determine the maturation of the skeleton by assessing the size of the echogenic ossification centers of the distal femur, proximal tibia, and calcaneal bone and their relations with gestational age, body weight, and height.[3] These centers are not yet ossified at this early age, and consequently, they are not visible on conventional roentgenograms.

An unusually wide spinal canal is commonly observed on the anteroposterior projection of the premature infant chest at the cervicothoracic area (Fig. 9-1). This finding should not be interpreted as abnormal or as an expression of possible myelodysplasia. In an analogy with the lumbosacral area, it probably represents normal selective delay in the ossification of the posterior vertebral elements secondary to the bulk of the spinal nerves that exit at these levels. The lack of complete ossification of the posterior elements facilitates an accurate evaluation of the cord size and the position of the filum terminale by ultrasound (Fig. 9-2), particularly when a dimple in the skin at the end of the spine raises the question of occult dysraphism.[4]

CONGENITAL POSTURAL DEFORMITIES

The various forms of talipes and congenital hip dislocations are the most frequently observed congenital postural deformities. Most children with these problems are otherwise normal.[1]

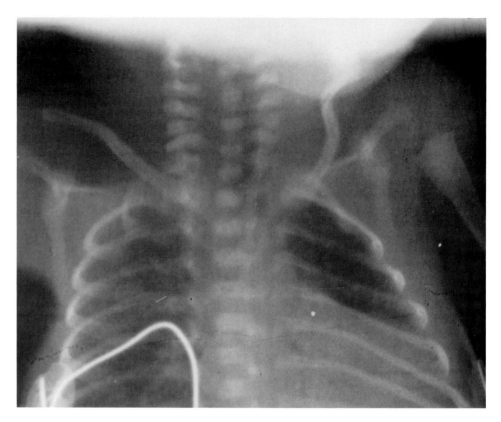

Fig. 9-1. Anteroposterior radiograph of the chest in a premature infant. Notice the unusually wide nonossified portion of the spinal cord at the cervicothoracic region. This is a normal finding in premature and newborn infants. A delayed ossification of the posterior arches produced by the exit of the proportionally larger and bulkier cervical nerve plexus from this anatomic area toward the shoulders and arms.

Talipes

In an infant with talipes a radiographic evaluation of clubfoot is indicated, including a lateral projection with simulated weight bearing, so that the anatomic misalignment of the foot can be evaluated for early treatment when the foot still retains its flexibility (Fig. 9-3).

Congenital Hip Dislocation

Congenital hip dislocation (CHD) requires an early diagnosis to avoid permanent disabilities resulting from nontreatment or sequelae associated with late treatment. The diagnosis of CHD is primarily clinical and especially difficult during prematurity since the acetabular roof is so small and incompletely developed and the joint capsule so extremely lax. Roentgenograms and ultrasound examinations provide static and dynamic confirmation of the clinical suspicion when the physical findings are equivocal.[5]

The usefulness of the frontal radiograph of the neonatal pelvis is limited by both inherent and technical considerations. Lack of ossification of the femoral head and the absence of a well-defined acetabular margin make readiographic recognition of hip dysplasia a limited task. Even mild rotation of the patient or inaccurate positioning of the legs can alter the relation of the radiographic landmarks or formular lines, which classically have been used to help localize the unossified femoral head. In addition, dislocated hips may be relocated during positioning for the radiographic examination (Fig. 9-4A). The frontal radiograph is more valuable during early infancy when the acetabular rim becomes better defined.

High-resolution coronal and transverse ultrasound examinations performed with a linear transducer can solve most of these radiographic limitations, because the echogenic acetabular edge and femoral head are easily outlined and at the same time can be manipulated not only to rule out dysplasia with dislocation

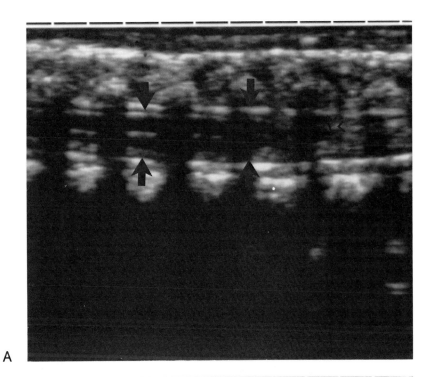

A

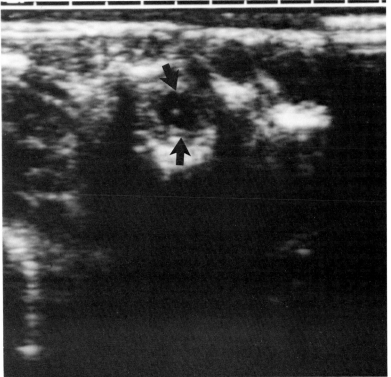

B

Fig. 9-2. Ultrasound scans of the spinal cord in a premature infant in the sagittal **(A)** and axial **(B)** planes. The cord (arrows) is normal in size and sonolucent and the central canal is echogenic. By counting the lumbar vertebral bodies one can assess the level of the filum terminale (open arrowhead).

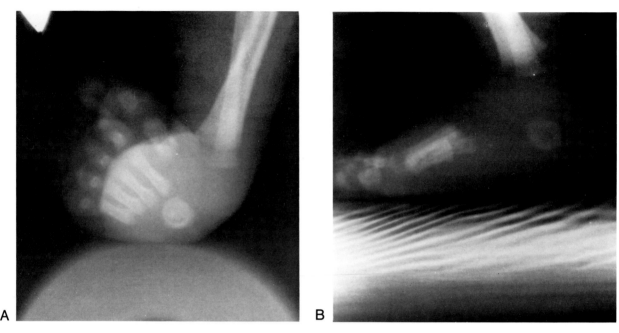

Fig. 9-3. Radiographic evaluation of a congenital talipes equinovarus (**A & B**). Notice the flexibility of this clubfoot at this early age, with adoption of a normal profile when it is forced into the proper position on the simulated weight-bearing lateral projection. (**B**).

but to determine the degree of articular congruency and instability in less deformed hips, which usually presents clinically with a click. This dynamic ultrasound examination requires moderate skills and a cooperative effort between the radiologist, the neonatologist, and/or the pediatric orthopaedic surgeon for the best evaluation of the ultrasound clinical findings. The modified Barlow and Ortolani maneuvers are performed while the hip is imaged; the relationship of the femoral head to the acetabulum is observed during these maneuvers.

Static coronal ultrasound of the hip allows an easier anatomic definition of normalcy, acetabular insufficiency, and/or dysplasia by better visualization of the bony acetabulum, its rim, position of the cartilaginous labrum, and the shape of the cartilaginous roof and gives a more accurate estimate of the acetabular coverage on the femoral head, following downward the vertical line formed by the iliac bone in this ultrasound plane (Fig. 9-4B). Ultrasound examination of the hips is a complimentary study to a carefully performed physical examination; it is more valuable when performed in premature infants at risk of CHD, and performed at 2 to 4 weeks of the full term period following corrected gestational age.

BONE DYSPLASIAS

The main body of these entities are the so-called chondrodysplasias or inherited disorders of the bone, caused by genetic mutations that interfere with the normal linear growth and development of the skeleton. Multiple malformations syndromes involving primarily the musculoskeletal system constitute also part of the bone dysplasias. These abnormalities likewise affect the morphology of the skeleton and stunt its growth. Many dysplasias have an unknown pathogenesis and their classification has been very conflictive over the years, especially because of the presence of many rare, unclassified cases. Various other diseases—metabolic, chromosomal, or inflammatory—have also been studied under bone dysplasias.

A uniform international nomenclature[6] was established by the European Society of Pediatric Radiology in 1969. This classification has been updated on several occasions and is based upon clinical, anatomic, and radiographic criteria. It has helped in bringing some order into this confusing area. A condensed classification based upon the international nomenclature adopted by the European Society of Pediatric Radiology[7] is offered in Table 9-1.

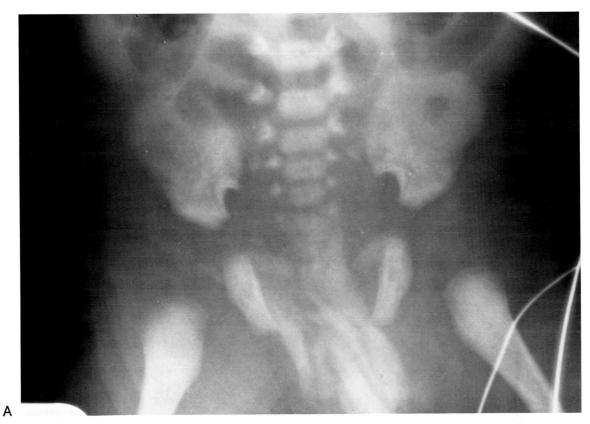

A

Fig. 9-4. (A) Anteroposterior projection of the pelvis, including the hips. Notice the lack of "sclerotic" outlining of the acetabulae at this early age and the complete lack of ossification of the hips. Acetabular dysplasia evaluation is at best inaccurate. **(B)** Coronal ultrasound scann of the right hip in the same premature infant. This exam shows clearly the echogenic labrum of the acetabulum (arrow) and the exact and proper localization and shape of the hip under it.

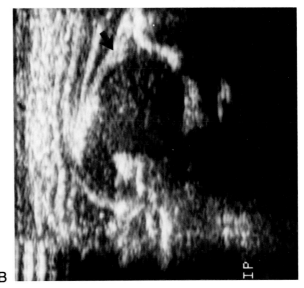

B

TABLE 9-1.   Skeletal Dysplasias (Condensed Classification)[a]

Skeletal Dysplasias resulting in short stature
  Disproportionate   Skeletal dysplasia
  Proportionate   Constitutional delay in growth
                                                        Genetic short stature
                                                        Idiopathic hypopituitarism
                                                        Emotional deprivation
                                                        African pygmies
                                                        Cornelia de Lange's syndrome
                                                        Progeria
                                                        Silver's and Russell's syndromes
                                                        Prader-Willi syndrome
                                                        Hypothyroidism

Bone dysplasias
  Osteochondrodysplasias
    Short extremities
      Acromelia (short hands and feet)   Peripheral dysostosis
      Mesomelia (short forearms and legs)   Nievergelt's syndrome
                                                        Langer syndrome
                                                        Léri-Weill syndrome
      Rhizomelia (short arms and thighs)   Achondroplasia
                                                        Hypochondroplasia
                                                        Multiple epiphyseal dysplasia (rhizomelic type)

      Micromelia
      Lethal dwarfisms at birth   Thanatophoric dwarfism
                                                        Achondrogenesis
                                                        Homozygous achondroplasia
                                                        Ateleosteogenesis
                                                        Severe hypophosphatasia
                                                        Osteogenesis imperfecta congenita
      Short ribs dwarfisms   Ectodermal dysplasia
                                                        Asphyxiating thoracic dysplasia
                                                        Other short ribs–polydactyly syndromes

      Pyknodysostosis
      Diastrophic dwarfism
    Short trunk
      Spondyloepiphyseal dysplasias (SEDs)   Congenita
                                                        Pseudoachondroplasia
                                                        Tarda
      Multiple epiphyseal dysplasias (MEDs)   Tarda
                                                        Conradi-Hünermann syndrome
                                                        Congenita
                                                        Rhizomelic type

      Metatropic dwarfism
      Mucopolysaccharidosis (also considered a
        constitutional disease with known
        pathogenesis)
      Metaphysial dysplasias
  Fibrochondrodysplasias   Enchondromatosis
                                                        Multiple exostosis
                                                        Hemimelic epiphyseal dysplasia
                                                        Fibrodysplasia
  Osteodysplasias   Osteogenesis imperfecta
                                                        Osteopetrosis
                                                        Pyknodysostosis
                                                        Osteopoikilosis
                                                        Melorheostosis
                                                        Osteopathia striata
                                                        Undertubulation and overconstriction dysplasias

continued

TABLE 9-1. *(continued)*   **Skeletal Dysplasias (Condensed Classification)**[a]

Bone dysostosis	
Soft tissues	Fibrodysplasia calcificans progresiva
	Pterygium
	Arthrogryposis
Limbs	Long bone deficiencies or hemimelias
	Congenital bowing or pseudoarthrosis
	Small hands and related anomalies[b]
	Radioulnar synostosis
Craniofacial skeleton	Lacunar skull
	Parietal foramina
	Cranium bifidum
	Craniosynostosis
	Acrocephalosyndactylies
Axial skeleton	Cleidocranial dysostosis
	Sprengel deformity
	Klippel-Feil syndrome
	Caudal regression syndrome
Skeletal growth disturbance in widespread organ	Marfan's syndrome
involvement disorders	Neurofibromatosis
Constitutional diseases with known pathogenesis	
Chromosomal aberrations	Cri du chat (pair #5)
	Trisomy (pair #13)
	Trisomy (pair #18)
	Down's syndrome (pair #21)
	Turner's syndrome (XO)
	Klinefelter syndrome (XYY)
Inborn errors of metabolism	
Calcium/phosphorus	Vitamin D–resistant ricket
	Hypophosphatasia
	Pseudohypoparathyroidism
Carbohydrates	Mucopolysaccharidosis
Lipids	Niemann-Pick disease
	Gaucher's disease
	Eosinophilic granuloma
Amino acids	Homocystinuria

[a] Constitutional bone diseases with changes affecting mainly the morphology of the skeleton and the stature (usually with a decrease in skeletal high). (Some of these entities also are classified under multiple malformation syndromes.)

[b] Brachydactyly, camptodactyly, clinodactyly, polydactyly, syndactyly, synphalangism, adactyly, acheria, ectrodadctyly, brachyphalangy. (Adapted from Jequier et al.,[7] with permission.)

Because of the many problems with classification the role of radiology in the identification of bone dysplasias is very important, and a complete radiographic survey of the skeleton, including a detailed evaluation of the relationship between the trunk and the extremities, should be the standard procedure. The morphology of the distal ends of the long bones, that of the vertebral bodies, the bone density, and combinations of abnormal skeletal features are the clues for the radiographic diagnosis of these dysplasias (Fig. 9-5).

A large number of osseous dysplasias can be recognized at birth, including achondroplasia, asphyxiating thoracic dystrophy (Fig. 9-6), chondrodysplasia punctata, chondroectodermal dysplasia, diastrophic dysplasia, metatropic dysplasia, and spondyloepiphyseal dysplasia congenita. Their identification is of utmost importance in the early evaluation of a premature or high-risk neonate. Some of these entities (the lethal osseous dysplasias) have a poor prognosis: achondrogenesis, rhizomelic chondrodysplasia, homozygous achondroplasia, severe hypophosphatasia,

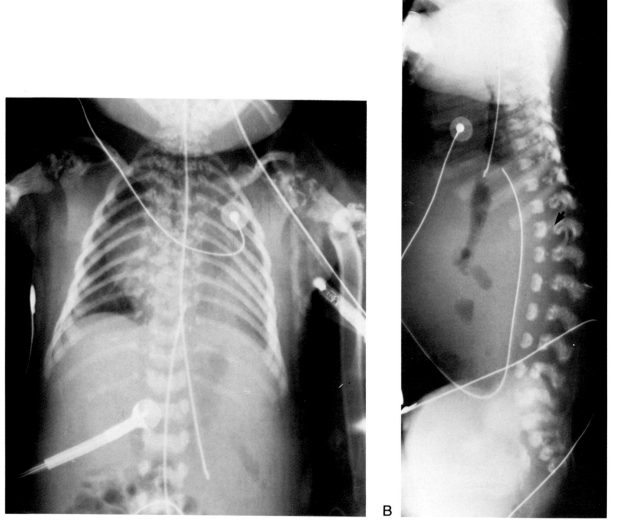

Fig. 9-5. Radiographic skeletal evaluation of a newborn premature infant with a bone dysplasia (chondrodysplasia punctata, rhizamelic type). **(A & B)** Chest and thoracolumbar spine in anteroposterior **(A)** and lateral **(B)** projections; note the abnormal calcifications at the epiphysis and other secondary ossification centers and the presence of coronal clefts at the vertebral bodies (arrow). *(Figure continues.)*

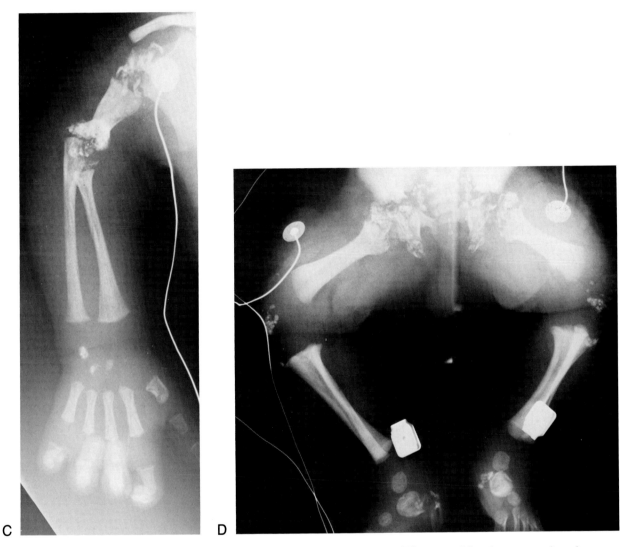

C   D

Fig. 9-5 *(Continued)*. **(C & D)** Views of the upper **(C)** and lower **(D)** extremities demonstrating the marked symmetric shortening of the humeri and femora and the abnormal epiphyseal calcifications and wide and coarse metaphyseal ends of the long bones.

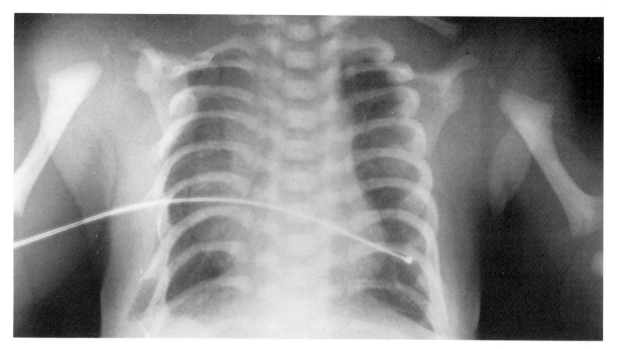

Fig. 9-6. Anteroposterior projection of the chest of a newborn with asphyxiating thoracic dystrophy, or Jeune's syndrome. The shortening of the humeri is moderate; the ribs are also shortened and have wide flaring of their anterior margins.

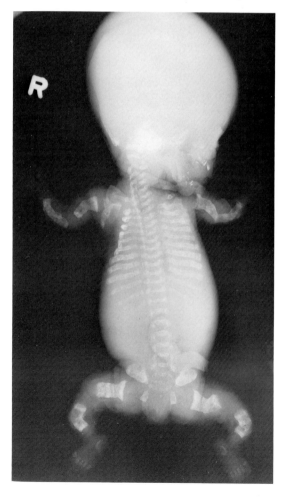

Fig. 9-7. Lethal neonatal short-limbed osseous dysplasia (severe osteogenic imperfecta). This stillborn "babygram" shows the obvious shortening of the extremities and the delayed ossification and osteopenic quality of the skeleton. Multiple deformities of the long bones due to in utero fractures can also be seen.

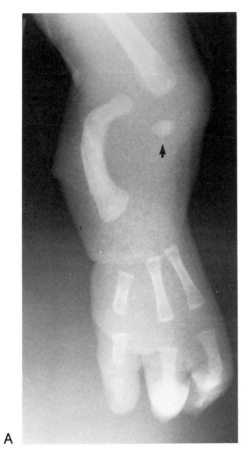 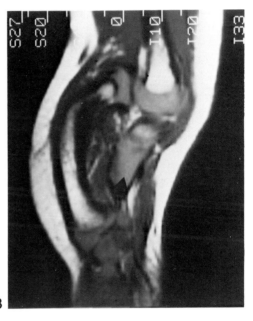

Fig. 9-8. (A) Roentgenogram of an upper extremity dysostosis (longitudinal ulnar hemimelia or deficiency) in a newborn. The ossified proximal ulna (arrow) only is noted, accompanied by a short, curved, and dysplastic radius. **(B)** T_1-weighted MR image of this same extremity showing the cartilaginous anlage of the hypoplastic ulna (arrow), much longer than what it is notice on the roentgenogram. This examination is quite useful to the orthopaedic surgeon in planning reconstructive surgery.

severe osteogenesis imperfecta (Fig. 9-7), and thanatophoric dysplasia. Polydactylies, syndactylies, and other limb dysostoses and/or deficiencies require a baseline radiographic or even magnetic resonance (MR) imaging evaluation when corrective surgery is being considered (Fig. 9-8).

Advances in biotechnology and genetic engineering are leading to new revolutionary insights into the classical approach to bone dysplasias. The capability of studying and even experimentally modifying the genes molecular structures of the chondrocytes, is changing the understanding of the chondrodysplasias pathophysiology. The longer survival of these patients by preventive orthopaedic treatments, coupled with a better prospective of their natural history, have recently shattered the previous, long and descriptive

classifications into essentially eight groups or families. Each group encompasses many of the known syndromes, but they are now seen from common pathogenetic roots, similar natural history, and clinical or radiologic features (that may manifest in a mild, moderate, or severe form within the spectrum). In such a manner the Achondroplasia family would encompass other entities such as hypochondroplasia and tanathophoric dwarfism and so on.

The eight groups are:

1. Achondroplasia
2. Spondyloepiphyseal dysplasia
3. Chondrodysplasia punctata
4. Short ribs polydactylies
5. Metatropic dysplasias

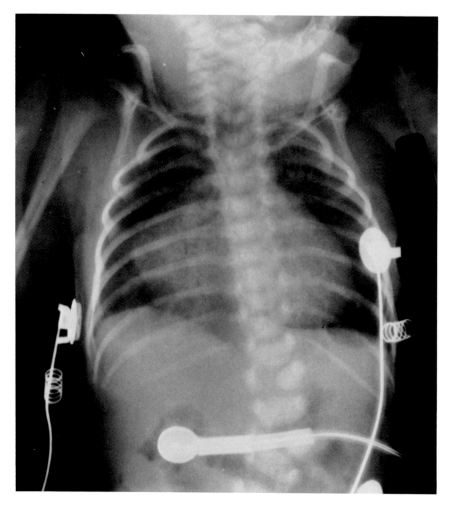

Fig. 9-9. Chest roentgenogram of a premature infant with trisomy 18. Notice the long, arched, and gracile clavicles, cardiomegaly secondary to a complex congenital heart disease, and lumbar vertebrae with segmental anomalies.

6. Metaphyseal dysplasias
7. Brachyolmia (universal platyspondilies)
8. Achromelic dysplasias

Syndromes of chromosomal abnormalities and nonimmune hydrops also benefit from a radiographic survey of the whole skeleton, because certain specific osseous dysmorphologic features can be of help for the syndrome identification: gracile, and clavicles, and dislocation of peripheral joints (trisomies of the chromosomal pairs 18 and 13) (Fig. 9-9), radioulnar synostosis (Klinefelter's syndrome), delayed bone ossification (Turner's syndrome), and so on. The combination of the skeletal anomalies seen

on the roentgenograms and other associated clinical findings may allow the diagnosis of syndromes of unknown etiology, such as VATER syndrome (hemivertebrae, radial dysplasia, tracheoesophageal fistula, and anal atresia) (Fig. 9-10), or syndromes secondary to teratogenic exposure, such as neurocristopathies (craniocerebral anomalies, cleft palate, branchial arch defects, and abnormal skin pigmentation).[8]

MR imaging studies of the musculoskeletal system are also an ideal method for the confirmation and evaluation of muscular dysostoses, such as Larsen's syndrome, arthrogryposis (Fig. 9-11), or amyotonia congenita.

Traumatic deliveries with head, shoulder, or arm

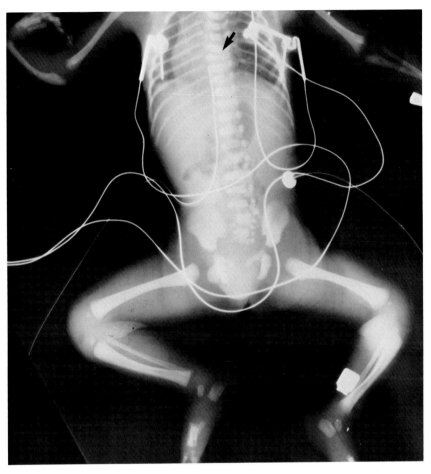

Fig. 9-10. "Babygram" of a newborn with VATER syndrome. The examination helped the diagnosis by outlining the vertebral segmental anomalies (arrow) and the right radial dysostosis.

presentations may result in iatrogenic or spontaneous clavicular fracture or brachial plexus injury and frequently require radiologic documentation. Other traumatic lesions of the skull as a result of birth injury have already been reviewed in Chapter 4.

BONE INFECTIONS

A tailored skeletal survey (anteroposterior views of the long bones) is often requested in the neonatal intensive care unit for those sick neonates whose mothers suffer from or are positive for syphilis or other viral venereal diseases, such as TORCH (toxoplasmosis, rubella, cytomegal ovirus, and herpes simplex). These skeletal infections are acquired by the neonate in utero and are manifested on the roent-

genograms by lucent and irregular metaphyses and/ or diaphyses (in cases of advanced syphilitic involvement) (Fig. 9-12). In many instances of TORCH normo- or microcephalic newborns exhibit periventricular intracraneal calcifications on skull radiographs and/or brain ultrasound studies. These echogenic foci can even be visualized on obstetric ultrasound before delivery, and they may lack acoustic shadowing.[9]

Bacterial osteomyelitis and septic arthritis are usually hematogenous in early life and may be asymptomatic. Both frequently occur concurrently because of the proximity of the joint to the bone and the common blood supply for both epiphysis and metaphysis across the physis. This anomalous dissemination only happens during infancy. Articular fullness and soft tissue swelling and demineralization of the metaphy-

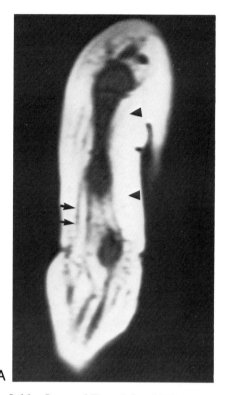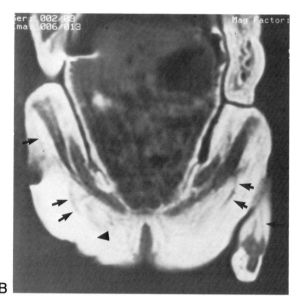

A   B

Fig. 9-11. Coronal T_1-weighted MR images of the right arm **(A)** and lower abdomen and thighs **(B)** of an infant with arthogryposis. The images outline clearly the muscular aplasia (thin strips of low signal intensity; arrows) and secondary fat replacement (large areas of increased signal intensity; arrowheads).

sis may be seen on the roentgenogram in early stages of the osseous infection. They represent the effect of the inflammatory exudate or pus in the joint and limiting bones. Periosteal elevation and bony destruction with, at times, disappearance of the epiphyseal ossification center (vanishing epiphysis) are seen later in the roentgenograms (Fig. 9-13). Ultrasound examination of the affected joint, to assess the presence of fluid and placement of percutaneous drainage, may be all that is diagnostically needed, and it can be very helpful and simple. Technetium-99m methylene diphosphonate (MDP) bone scanning is more sensitive than roentgenograms for early diagnosis of osteomylitis.

Periosteal elevation — a radiographic sign of irritation, destruction, and new buildup of the periostium and a common finding in the high-risk neonate — is usually secondary to either osteomyelitis, healing fractures following treatment for rickets, or the administration of prostaglandin E for closure of the ductus arteriosus.[10]

RICKETS OF THE PREMATURE INFANT

Osteopenia and rickets are increasingly recognized as important problems in immature infants, who may end with chronic lung disease or bronchopulmonary dysplasia (Fig. 9-14). It may be noted that nutritional rickets itself is sometimes associated with diffuse lung disease.[11] Furthermore, preterm infants have been described[12] in whom lung disease appears secondary to the skeletal process. The relationship, if any, of these observations to the chronicity of the lung changes is uncertain.

A variety of causative factors have been implicated, including malabsorption of calcium and phosphorus and dietary deficiencies of calcium, phosphorus, and vitamin D.[11,13-15] Infants with chronic lung disease commonly require extended parenteral nutrition, leading to demineralization and rickets. This mechanism seems to involve inadequate phosphate intake, together with cholestasis secondary to the parenteral

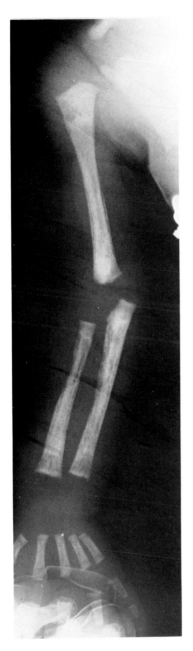

Fig. 9-12. Upper extremity roentgenogram of a premature infant with congenital syphilis. Notice the severe involvement of the metaphyseal ends of the long bones, periostitis at the humeral diaphysis, and lytic destruction of the radial and ulnar diaphyses. This severe osseous involvement also produces a "bone-within-bone" appearance.

protein hydrolysate, causing decreased bile acids in the enterohepatic circulation and a resultant diminished gut absorption of calcium and vitamin D. A negative calcium balance seems to occur also in infants requiring long-term furosemide (used in treatment of cor pulmonale).[16]

Radiographically the earliest findings of rickets seem to be focal demineralization at the growing ends of long bones and in the scapulae and iliac bones, and a "bone-within-bone" appearance of the vertebrae. The process begins at 14 to 30 days and reaches a maximum at 40 days. Between about 50 and 80 days, the demineralization progresses along the diaphyses of the bones and becomes generalized. After these manifestations some patients undergo a gradual return to normal bone density, whereas others, at 60 to 100 days, develop rickets, which subsequently heals after appropriate treatment.[17]

Because the chest is the most frequently radiographed area on these patients, it is reasonable to get as much information as possible regarding skeletal abnormalities from the chest film. The early demineralization of the growing ends of long bones is readily perceived in the proximal humerus.[18]

Rib fractures may be the first suggestion of rickets noted on the chest film.[19] Flaring of the anterior rib ends is an even more reliable sign of rickets. The most commonly fractured bones secondary to rickets are the ribs because the brunt of the chest physiotherapy, necessary in bronchopulmonary dysplasia, is physically directed against the rib cage. Other roentgenographic changes of rickets, such as cupping and then fraying, irregularities, and splaying of the metaphyses, are much better appreciated on a single frontal view of a wrist or knee. These areas are also best for monitoring responses to therapy and healing.

THORACIC CAGE DEFORMITY SECONDARY TO BRONCHOPULMONARY DYSPLASIA

In severe cases of bronchopulmonary dysplasia the chest on the frontal roentgenogram assumes a somewhat rounded shape that usually reflects hyperinflation.[20] In other similar cases associated with severe bone disease, however, this rounded shape becomes unusually pronounced, or there is marked lateral splaying of the inferior ribs.[21] If a lateral view is exposed, the chest is seen to be quite flattened along its

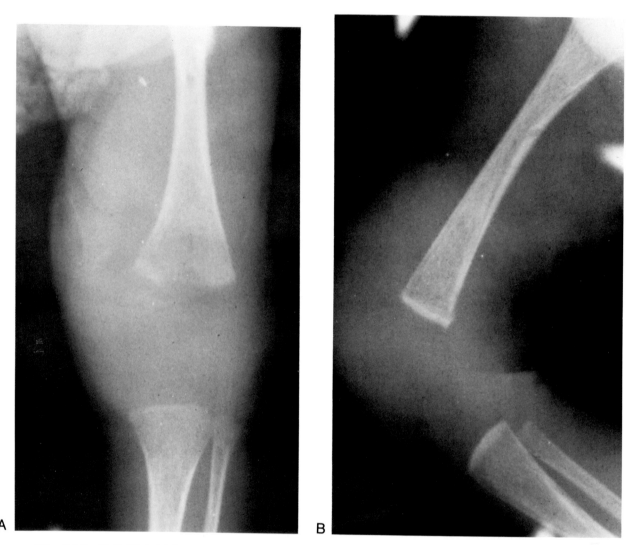

A   B

Fig. 9-13. (A & B) Initial roentgenographic evaluation of a two-week-old, 36 weeks' gestation, premature infant with neonatal sepsis and septic arthritis with accompanying osteomyelitis at the left knee. Only fullness of the joint space and metaphyseal osteopenia are visualized at this time. *(Figure continues.)*

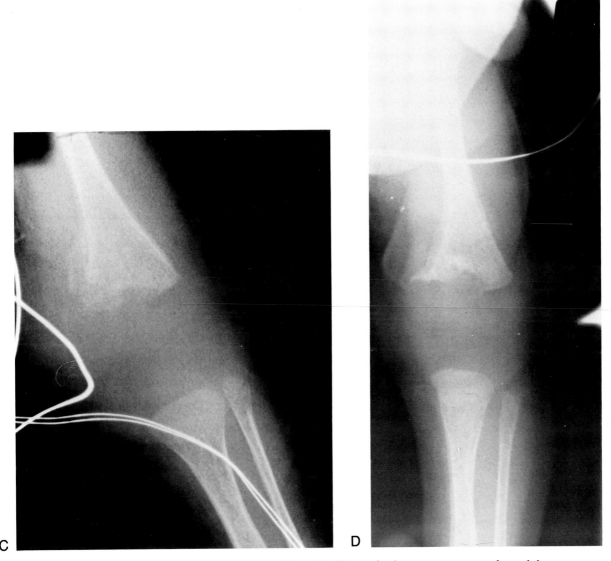

Fig. 9-13 *(Continued).* **(C & D)** Follow-ups at 3 **(C)** and 8 **(D)** weeks demonstrate metaphyseal destruction and periosteal new bone formation; notice the absence of the distal femoral ossification center **(D)** (destroyed by the infection), which should have appeared at this age.

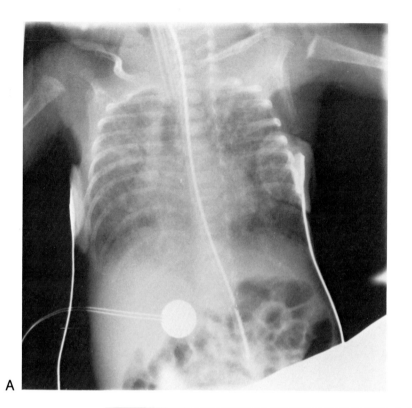

A

Fig. 9-14. (A) Chest roentgenogram of a 56-day-old premature infant with moderate bronchopulmonary dysplasia, enphysematous lungs bases, assisted ventilation, and early osteopenia of the skeleton. (B) On a roentgenogram taken 23 days later the chronic lung changes and the diffuse skeletal osteopenia have become much more evident. The fragile bones have suffered pathologic fractures such as the one seen on the left proximal humerus; notice also flaring of the distal ribs, another sign of neonatal rickets. *(Figure continues.)*

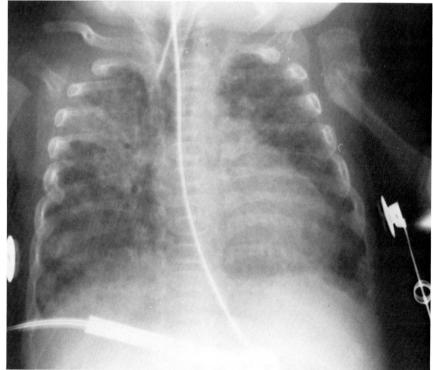

B

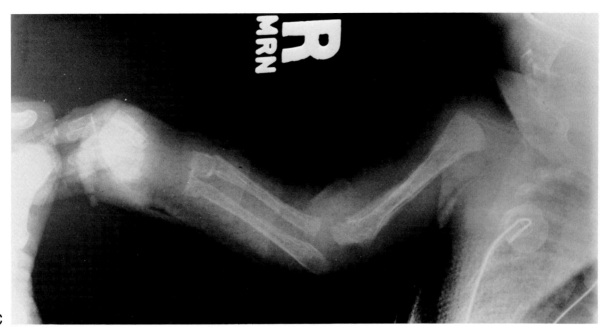

C

Fig. 9-14 *(Continued)*. **(C)** Right upper extremity roentgenogram demonstrating cupping of the distal radial and ulnar metaphyses, severe osteopenia, pathologic fractures, periosteal elevation, and bone remodeling.

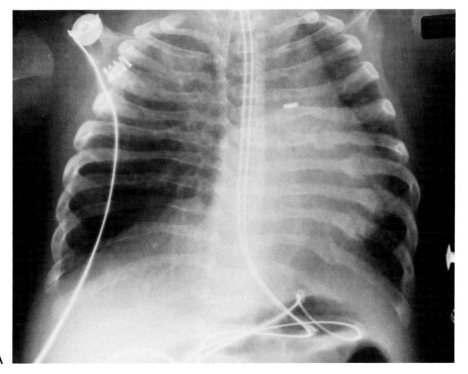

A

Fig. 9-15. **(A)** Anteroposterior chest roentgenogram. *(Figure continues.)*

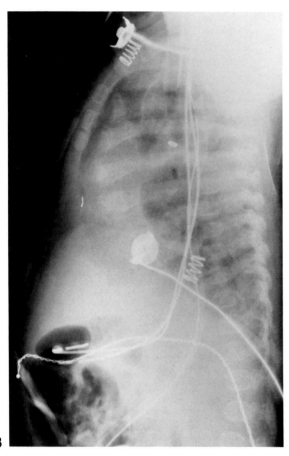

B

Fig. 9-15 *(Continued).* Anteroposterior **(A)** and **(B)** lateral chest roentgenograms of a 90-day-old premature infant with severe bronchopulmonary dysplasia, neonatal rickets (notice osteopenia and several rib fractures), and a rounded shape of the thoracic cavity and lateral splaying of the inferior ribs. The lateral projection demonstrates the shortened anteroposterior diameter of the chest.

anteroposterior axis (Fig. 9-15). The etiology of this appearance is uncertain. It might result from abnormally soft, demineralized bones and months of supine or prone positioning in which the gravitational vector is anteroposterior. The condition seems to improve with age.

REFERENCES

1. Behrman RE, Vaughan VC III: Nelson Textbook of Pediatrics, 13th ed. p. 317. WB Saunders, Philadelphia, 1987

2. Kuhns LR, Finnstrom O: New standards of ossification of the newborn. Radiology 119:655, 1976

3. Pastor I: Determination of state of osseous maturation abstracted. p. 94. In: Proceedings of the 25th Congress of the European Society of Pediatric Radiology, Montreux, Switzerland, 1988

4. Glasier CM, Chadduck WM, Leithiser RE et al: Screening spinal ultrasound in newborns with neural tube defects. J Ultrasound Med 9:339, 1990

5. Leonidas JC: A sound way to identify congenital hip dislocation. Contemp Pediatr January, p. 105, 1989

6. Kozlowski K, Maroteaux P, Silverman F et al: Classification des dysplasies osseouses. Table ronde. Ann Radiol 12:965, 1969

7. Jequier A, Kaufmann S, Labrune H et al: International nomenclature of constitutional diseases of bone. Ann Radiol 27:275, 1984

8. Oelberg DG, Dominguez R, Hebert AA: Neurocristopathy syndrome: review of four cases. Pediatr Dermatol 7(2):87, 1990

9. Sudakoff GS, Mitchell DG et al: Frontal periventricular cysts on the first day of life: a one-year clinical follow-up and its significance. J Ultrasound Med 10:25, 1991

10. Ringel RE, Brenner JI, Haney PJ et al: Prostaglandin-induced periostitis: a complication of long term PGE1 infusion in an infant with congenital heart disease. Radiology 142:657, 1982

11. Khajavi A, Amirhakimi GH: The rachitic lung. Pulmonary findings in 30 infants and children with malnutritional rickets. Clin Pediatr 16:36, 1977

12. Glasgow JFT, Thomas PS: Rachitic respiratory distress in small preterm infants. Arch Dis Child 52:268, 1977

13. Toomey F, Hoag R, Batton D, Vain N: Rickets associated with cholestasis and parenteral nutrition in premature infants. Radiology 142:85, 1982

14. Gefter WB, Epstein DM, Anday EK, Dalinka MK: Rickets presenting as multiple fractures in premature infants on hyperalimentation. Radiology 142:371, 1982

15. Warshaw BL, Anand SK, Kerian A, Lieberman E: The effect of chronic furosemide administration on urinary calcium excretion and calcium balance in growing rats. Pediatr Res 14:1118, 1980

16. Venkataraman PS, Han BK, Tsang RC, Daugherty CC: Secondary hyperparathyroidism and bone disease in infants receiving longterm furosemide therapy. Am J Dis Child 137:1157, 1983

17. Masel JP, Tudehope D, Cartwright D, Cleghorn G: Osteopenia and rickets in the extremely low birth weight infant. A survey of the incidence and a radiological classification. Australas Radiol 2:1041, 1982

18. Poznanski AK, Kuhns LR, Guire KE: New standards of cortical mass in the humerus of neonates: a means

of evaluating bone loss in the premature infant. Radiology 134:639, 1980

19. Geggel RL, Pereira GR, Spackman TJ: Fractured ribs: unusual presentation of rickets in premature infants. J Pediatr 93:680, 1978

20. Mortensson W, Lindroth M: The course of bronchopulmonary dysplasia. A radiographic follow-up. Acta Radiol [Diagn] (Stockh) 27:19, 1986

21. Edwards DK: (Comment by Northway WH, Jr.) The radiology of bronchopulmonary dysplasia and its complications. p. 185. In Merritt TA, Northway WH, Boynton BR (eds): Contemporary Issues In Fetal and Neonatal Medicine, Vol. 4, Bronchopulmonary Dysplasia.

Retinopathy of Prematurity

A. Aguirre Vila-Coro

10

Retinopathy of prematurity (ROP) is an embryologic vascular proliferative disease intimately associated with immaturity of the retinal vascularization of premature infants exposed to high ambient oxygen concentration. Air is hyperoxic as compared to maternal uterine blood, and often premature infants receive further oxygen supplementation.

INCIDENCE

In 1954, the relationship between exposure to oxygen and ROP was confirmed.[1] In the following years, rigid limitation of exposure to oxygen resulted in a drastic decrease in incidence of ROP and in a dramatically higher mortality and morbidity due to brain damage. It is estimated that in the decade 1950 to 1960, for every case of blindness spared, 16 premature babies died as a result of rigid controls in administration of oxygen.[2,3] In recent years oxygen has been administered on the basis of need as assessed by arterial, percutaneous, and pulse oximetry. Increased use of oxygen and high technology equipment and procedures in neonatal intensive care units allow survival of many more infants, although some of them develop advanced stages of ROP. In the United States, approximately 500 children became blind as a result of ROP every year before cryotherapy was proven to reduce the risk of blindness.[4] The incidence of ROP correlates with prematurity and exposure to oxygen, with a reported incidence of up to 72 percent in infants with birthweight below 1,200 g and 66 percent in infants born before 32 weeks of gestation.[5]

Infants with a birthweight less than 750 or those at 27 weeks' gestation or less are at high risk of developing severe ROP.[5]

ETIOLOGY

Prematurity and hyperoxia are the main risk factors in the development of ROP. Continuous transcutaneous oxygen monitoring has not been shown to be more effective in reducing the incidence of ROP as compared with standard intermittent arterial blood sampling, supporting the hypothesis of multifactorial etiology in the development of ROP. Risk factors associated with ROP include poor prenatal care, ventilator hours, treatment with xanthines, low birthweight and gestational age, maternal bleeding, multiple births, and exposure to bright light.[5-7] Hyperoxia induces a vasoconstriction of the retinal vessels, which probably has a protective effect regulating the amount of oxygen delivered to the retina. Dilation of the retinal vessels in response to acidemia and hypercapnia may reverse the protective vasoconstriction, and could explain the observation that in extremely premature babies ROP may be more closely associated with acidemia and hypercapnia than with the degree of hyperoxemia.[8] Retinopathy of prematurity or similar disease processes have been reported in full-term infants who have not received supplemental oxygen. These include patients with cyanotic heart disease, incontinentia pigmenti, familial exudative vitreoretinopathy, and severe central nervous system abnormalities such as anencephaly.[9-13]

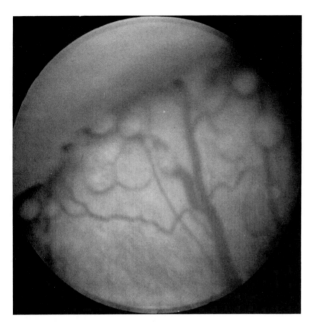

Fig. 10-1. Ophthalmoscopic appearance of retinopathy of prematurity (ROP) stage 1. Notice the sharp demarcation line between the vascularized and avascular retina. Abnormal branching can be seen behind the demarcation line.

PATHOGENESIS

Vascularization of the retina begins around the 16th week of gestation, progressing radially from the optic nerve toward the periphery.[14] Around the 34th to 35th week of gestation, retinal vascularization has reached the ora serrata nasally, but the temporal retina anterior to the equator remains avascular.[15] Complete vascularization of the temporal retina occurs around 1 month following full-term delivery.[16] Sustained hyperoxia causes retinal vasoconstriction and an arrest in the normal development of retinal vessels. The primitive mesenchymal cells (spindle-shaped cells located anteriorly in the developing retina) stop their maturation into endothelial cells and undergo hyperplasia. Extensive gap junctions develop between adjacent spindle cells. These gap junctions may represent a secondary phenomenon commonly observed in vitro when cells reach confluence and stop to proliferate, indicating that the stimulus to grow has stopped.[17] Behind this vanguard of spindle cells there is a rearguard of proliferating endothelial cells and newly formed capillaries.[18] The demarcation line between the anterior avascular retina with hyperplastic spindle cells and the posterior vascularized retina becomes ophthalmoscopically visible as a whitish sharp line (Fig. 10-1).

As the disease progresses the rearguard endothelium proliferates, with formation of vascular channels and capillaries whose walls are permeable to fluorescein. Ophthalmoscopically this proliferation becomes recognizable as a ridge, a visible elevation of the retinal surface (Fig. 10-2). The ridge is white initially, then pink. Close behind the ridge, isolated tufts of capillaries on the surface of the retina may occur. Later fibrovascular tissue develops from the posterior aspect of the ridge, with the formation of shunt vessels along the ridge. Fibrovascular proliferation progresses on the retinal surface at the vitreoretina interface and extends into the vitreous cavity (Fig. 10-3). This fibrovascular tissue contains myofibroblasts, which are fusiform fibroblasts replete with contractile filaments. The abnormal new vessels leak plasma and blood, eliciting more fibroglial cell proliferation. Retinal detachment probably develops as a result of increasing traction and not exudation. The detachments have a concave (tractional) configuration, whereas exudation detachments, like the detachment of the uveal effusion syndrome, have a convex configuration.[19]

The proliferation of fibrovascular tissue into the vitreous causes reorientation of the vitreous collagen, which then directs the proliferating tissue toward the lens. This results in traction on the retina anteriorly and circumferentially. The peripheral avascular retina, thus stretched, causes the formation of the peripheral trough and the narrowing of the anterior funnel in end-stage ROP. Narrowing of the posterior funnel occurs through glial proliferation in the vicinity of the optic disc and the hyaloid vessels.[19] The retinal detachment may progress from partial (Fig. 10-4) to total (Figs. 10-5 and 10-6). A totally detached retina may fold and rest behind the lens, to which it may become attached, constituting retrolental fibroplasia. Eventually the fibrovascular tissue anterior to the detachment increases its collagen content and loses cells, becoming whiter on ophthalmoscopy. Progressive vascular incompetence may manifest as increasing dilation and tortuosity of the peripheral retinal vessels, engorgement of the iris vessels, rigidity of the pupil, and vitreous haze. Dilation and tortuosity of the retinal vessels sometimes is permanent, persisting following regression of ROP. This may reflect endothelial cell hyperplasia in response to angiogenic stimulation.

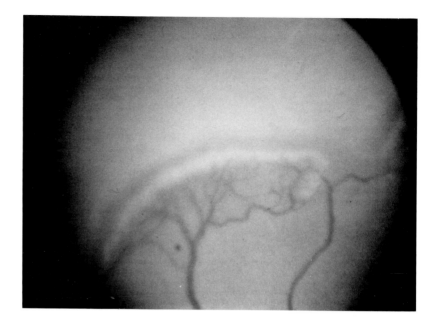

Fig. 10-2. Ophthalmoscopic appearance of ROP stage 2. Notice the elevated tridimensional ridge with tufts of new vessels behind the ridge. Some retinal vessels leave the plane of the retina to enter the elevated ridge.

The iris may show dilation of stromal vessels and neovascularization during the acute phase of the disease, sometimes resulting in rigidity of the pupil, which is unable to dilate. Posterior synechiae, persistence of the pupillary membrane with patent blood vessels, and migration of the iris pigment epithelium onto the anterior surface of the iris (ectropion uveae) may occur. Total retinal detachment with retrolental fibroplasia may cause shallowing of the anterior chamber and secondary glaucoma. A cyclitic membrane may develop if the pars plicata is caught up in the retrolental fibrotic tissue.

CLASSIFICATION

An international classification of ROP developed by an ad hoc committee sorts the disease in terms of location, stage, involvement of the posterior retinal vessels, and regression.[20,21] To specify location, the

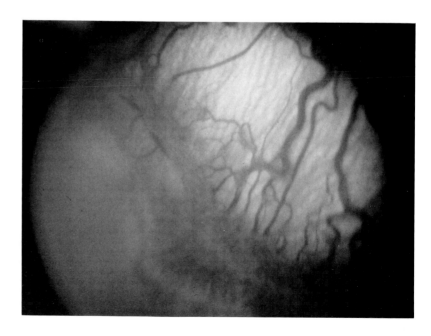

Fig. 10-3. Ophthalmoscopic appearance of ROP stage 3, severe. Notice massive proliferation of extraretinal fibrovascular tissue originated behind the ridge, becoming out of focus as it enters into the vitreous.

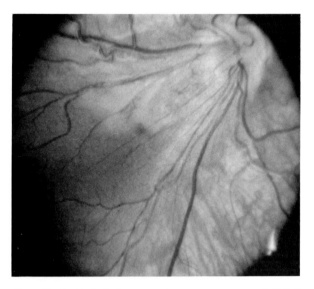

Fig. 10-4. Ophthalmoscopic appearance of ROP stage 4b. Notice the tractional retinal detachment, including the fovea.

retina is divided into three concentric zones defined by two circumferences around the optic disc:

Zone I extends from the disc to twice the distance from the disc to the center of the macula.

Zone II extends from the anterior edge of Zone I to

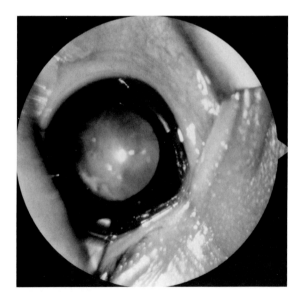

Fig. 10-5. Ophthalmoscopic appearance of ROP stage 5. The retina, totally detached, is visible as a vascularized white mass behind the lens.

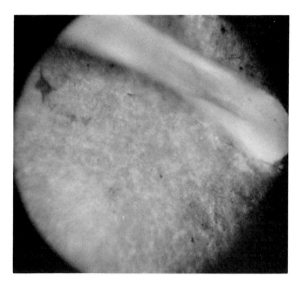

Fig. 10-6. Ophthalmoscopic appearance of regressed ROP. A total retinal detachment (funnel shaped narrow posteriorly and narrow anteriorly) extends temporally. The naked choroid is directly visible.

the most nasal point of the ora serrata and to approximately the temporal equator.

Zone III represents the crescent of retina anterior to Zone II.

Extent of involvement is specified by hours of the clock (Fig. 10-7).

Stages

Various stages describe the severity of the retinal changes (Table 10-1).

Normal Immature Retina

Normal immature retina corresponds to the ophthalmoloscopic recognition in the preterm infant of a vascularized posterior retina and an avascular anterior retina without a sharp or clear-cut limit between them. The fundus seen through the translucent avascular retina appears pale gray, as opposed to the more posterior orange fundus seen through transparent vascularized retina. The avascular retina extends 360° behind the ora serrata, more posteriorly in infants of lower gestational age. Intraretinal hemorrhages related to birth trauma are commonly found

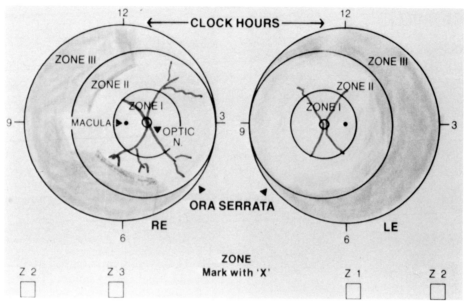

Fig. 10-7. Schematic charting of the ophthalmoscopic appearance of ROP: stage 1 at 9:00 to 12:00 in Zone II, stage 2 at 5:00 to 8:00 O.D., immature retina in anterior Zone II O.S.

in neonates and resolve spontaneously over a period of several weeks.

Stage 1: Demarcation Line

Stage 1 occurs when a thin, white, unidimensional line can be recognized as sharply separating the avascular retina anteriorly from the vascularized retina posteriorly. Abnormal arcading or branching vessels can be recognized behind the demarcation line (Fig. 10-1).

TABLE 10-1. Stages of Retinopathy of Prematurity

Stage No.	Characteristic	
1	Demarcation line	
2	Ridge	
3	Ridge with extraretinal fibrovascular proliferation	
4	Subtotal retinal detachment	
5	Total retinal detachment	
	Funnel:	
	Anterior part	Posterior part
	Open	Open
	Narrow	Narrow
	Open	Narrow
	Narrow	Open

(From International Committee for the Classification of Retinopathy of Prematurity,[21] with permission.)

Stage 2: Ridge

In stage 2 the demarcation line has become tridimensional and extends out of the plane of the retina; it has a white-pink color. Retinal vessels may leave the plane of the retina to enter the elevated ridge and tufts of new vessels on the retinal surface may occur behind the ridge (Fig. 10-2).

Stage 3: Ridge with Extraretinal Fibrovascular Proliferation

Fibrovascular proliferative tissue is found behind the ridge with or without connection with the posterior aspect of the ridge in Stage 3. The finding of fibrovascular proliferation into the vitreous, perpendicular to the retinal plane, also indicates stage 3 (Fig. 10-3). Stage 3 is subdivided into mild, moderate, or severe according to whether fibrovascular proliferative tissue is found in limited, significant, or massive amounts, respectively.

Stage 4: Subtotal Retinal Detachment

Unequivocal detachment of the retina defines stage 4. While the detachment may have exudative features, traction detachment is the main cause of visual loss and blindness in ROP. Stage 4 is subdivided

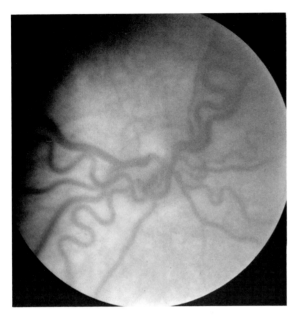

Fig. 10-8. Ophthalmoscopic appearance of "plus" disease. Notice enlargement of the veins and tortuosity of the arterioles in the posterior retina.

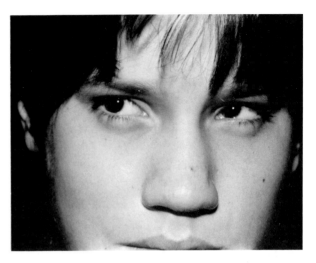

Fig. 10-9. Child with regressed ROP in both eyes looking straight at the camera. The left eye (blind) has sensory esotropia and is turned in; the right eye has a macula markedly dragged temporally, causing a false exotropia due to a very large positive angle kappa.

into two groups depending on the location of the detachment.

Stage 4a: Extrafoveal Retinal Detachment

Extrafoveal retinal detachment is a concave peripheral traction detachment that does not involve the macula. It may be circumferential (360°) or segmental and it is usually located in Zone III or anterior Zone II.

Stage 4b: Retinal Detachment Including the Fovea

This segmental detachment usually extends in the form of a fold from the disc through Zone I to involve Zones II and III (Fig. 10-4).

Stage 5: Total Retinal Detachment (Funnel Shaped)

Total retinal detachment is always funnel shaped in ROP (Figs. 10-5 and 10-6). Subdivision of stage 5 depends on the configuration of the funnel. When the funnel is open anteriorly and posteriorly, the detachment has a concave configuration and extends to the optic disc. Another configuration occurs when the funnel is narrow in both its anterior and posterior aspects and the detached retina is located just behind the lens. A less common type exhibits a funnel open

anteriorly and narrowed posteriorly. The least common type is one in which the funnel is narrow anteriorly and open posteriorly.

"Plus" Disease

"Plus" disease is typified by enlargement of the veins and tortuosity of the arterioles in the posterior retina (Fig. 10-8). It represents a poor prognostic sign probably because it reflects increased proliferative activity.

Regressed ROP

Regression occurs in the vast majority (over 90 percent) of patients with ROP and may occur at any stage, leaving various retinal and vascular changes. The more severe the original disease, the more serious the changes left behind will be when the acute process regresses (Table 10-2)[21] (Fig. 10-9).

DIAGNOSIS

Screening

Neonatal intensive care units should establish a screening program for detection of ROP among premature infants. The most commonly accepted

TABLE 10-2. Regressed Retinopathy of Prematurity

Peripheral Changes

Vascular
1. Failure to vascularize peripheral retina
2. Abnormal, nondichotomous branching of retinal vessels
3. Vascular arcades with circumferential interconnection
4. Telangiectatic vessels

Retinal
1. Pigmentary changes
2. Vitreoretinal interface changes
3. Thin retina
4. Peripheral folds
5. Vitreous membranes with or without attachment to retina
6. Latticelike degeneration
7. Retinal breaks
8. Traction/rhegmatogenous retinal detachment

Posterior Changes

Vascular
1. Vascular tortuosity
2. Straightening of blood vessels in temporal arcade
3. Decrease in angle of insertion of major temporal arcade

Retinal
1. Pigmentary changes
2. Distortion and ectopia of macula
3. Stretching and folding of retina in macular region leading to periphery
4. Vitreoretinal interface changes
5. Vitreous membrane
6. Dragging of retina over disc
7. Traction/rhegmatogenous retinal detachment

(From International Committee for the Classification of Retinopathy of Prematurity,[21] with permission.)

current criteria for surgical treatment of ROP to prevent retinal detachment imply the presence of "plus" disease: enlargement of the veins and tortuous arterioles in the posterior retina.[4] Diagnosis of "plus" disease can be made by any pediatrician with minimal experience in the use of the direct ophthalmoscope. A more appropriate screening can be done by an ophthalmologist skilled in the detection of ROP, by examining the peripheral retinas of all infants who weighed less than a locally established birthweight criterion, usually between 1,300 and 2,000 g. If a single screening is made, it should be done at age 7 to 9 weeks.[22] High-risk infants with birthweights less than 1,250 g should be examined initially at 4 to 6 weeks of age. Examination of critically ill infants in the first weeks of life is not indicated. Affected infants

are followed periodically at intervals based upon the risk factors and the severity of the changes noted.

Ophthalmoscopy

Binocular indirect ophthalmoscopy is the technique of choice to visualize the peripheral retina. A Sauer lid speculum (Storz Ophthalmic Instruments, 3368 Tree Court Industrial Blvd., St. Louis, MO 63122) and an assistant to restrain the patient's head and arms are invaluable. Manual rotation of the patient's head allows reflexive doll's head eye movement to rotate the eye to visualize the peripheral retina. A small paper clip is very useful to rotate the eye and perform scleral depression. Topical anesthesia should be used to minimize the pain caused by the lid speculum, as well as the eye rotations and scleral depressions performed with the paper clip, especially if there is contact with the cornea.[23] Bradicardia and other reflex responses[24] of the premature infant produced by examination of the fundus are probably decreased by the use of topical anesthesia.

Pupillary dilation can be obtained with one drop or a solution containing 1% phenylephrine and 0.2% cyclopentolate 30 minutes before the examination. Darkly pigmented infants usually need repeat dropping 5 minutes after the initial drop. The systemic side effects of the drops[25] can be decreased by using small-sized drops with a micropipette and, in older infants with patent lacrimal passages, by applying pressure to the lacrimal puncta for 2 minutes after the eye has been dropped.

Particular care should be taken in avoiding injury to the corneal epithelium during the examination. Some *Pseudomonas* species, frequent contaminents of instruments used in neonatal intensive care units, can rapidly cause perforation of the cornea and endophthalmitis if the corneal epithelium is violated.

Immature fundi show a gray discoloration in the periphery (seen through a translucent avascular retina) as opposed to the more central orange fundus (seen through a transparent vascularized retina); there is a gradual transition between the peripheral gray and central orange areas, without clear-cut demarcation lankmarks. Stage 1 shows a sharp demarcation line between the vascularized and nonvascularized retina. This line may be discontinuous or continuous and may involve only the temporal periphery or the entire circumference of the retina (Fig. 10-1). Stage 2 shows a distinct neovascular ridge originated by enlargement of the demarcation line (Fig.

10-2); stage 3 shows extraretinal proliferation from the posterior aspect of the ridge (Fig. 10-3). Stage 4 shows partial retinal detachment, either extrafoveal (stage 4a) or including the fovea (stage 4b) (Fig. 10-4). Stage 5, total retinal detachment, is seen ophthalmoscopically as a whitish opaque mass behind the lens during the acute phase of ROP (Fig. 10-5). Details of the detachment may become more clearly visible upon regression of the acute phase (Fig. 10-6).

Ultrasonography

Ultrasonography is useful in patients with ROP for two different purposes: (1) to aid in the diagnosis of ROP as part of the differential diagnosis in patients presenting with leukocoria without known history of ROP, and (2) to evaluate the intraocular status of a patient with known ROP to assist in monitoring retinal detachment (e.g., for sequential or perioperative evaluation). Ultrasonography is especially valuable in the evaluation of patients with leukocoria because it allows appreciation of areas inaccessible to ophthalmoscopy.

A series of typical changes are often found along the entire globe and orbit in eyes with stage 4 or 5 ROP, which help the ultrasonographer to differentiate ROP from other causes of leukocoria, such as retinoblastoma:

1. Increased thickness of the cornea and choroid
2. Decreased depth of the anterior chamber
3. Anomalies of the lens
   a. Malposition: anterior or posterior displacement
   b. Intralenticular echoes: cataract
   c. Lens unrecognizable
   d. Abnormalities in the shape of the lens with loss of the normal biconcave appearance
4. Anomalies of the vitreous
   a. Low-amplitude anterior echoes: retrolental fibrovascular tissue (RLF)
   b. Higher amplitude echoes—membrane patterns: retinal detachment (RD) or retinal folds
   c. Complex (low- and high-amplitude) echo patterns due to RLF and RD
5. Anomalies of the orbit: acoustic shadowing of the orbital fat echo complex

Increased thickness of the cornea and choroid often represent prephthisical changes seen in eyes with profound hypotony. Corneal thickening may also be seen in secondary glaucoma as a result of

anterior displacement of the lens. Decreased depth of the anterior chamber is a frequent finding in eyes with stage 5 ROP, often associated with anterior displacement of the lens and secondary angle-closure glaucoma. Malposition of the crystalline lens with anterior displacement is seen in cases of florid retrolental fibroplasia, in which the lens is being pushed forward by a large retrolental mass. Posterior displacement of the lens is due to posterior traction by retracting fibrovascular tissue attached to the posterior aspect of the lens. Internal echoes within the crystalline lens are due to formation of cataract. Inability to clearly discern the lens echoes occurs in cases of marked internal disorganization of the eye with abundant retrolental tissue acoustically similar to the lens. The high-amplitude membrane echo patterns in the vitreous cavity may be due to total or partial retinal detachment or to retinal folds. Complex echo patterns in the vitreous cavity are usually due to the combined presence of fibroproliferative tissue and total retinal detachment. The orbit may show a pattern of decreased echoes suggestive of atrophy of the orbital fat with acoustic shadowing of the orbital fat echo complex. Shadowing of the orbital fat is an ultrasonographic feature often seen in retinoblastoma. Shadowing in retinoblastoma is due to the effects of mass, density, and calcification of the tumor[26]; in ROP, the acoustically dense and complex intraocular fibrovascular changes cause sufficient attenuation of sound to create shadowing of the orbital fat.[27]

While none of the above echographic characteristics is pathognomonic of ROP, taken together they suggest ROP to the clinician confronted with a case of leukocoria of unknown origin. For example, retinoblastoma, an important entity usually presenting as leukocoria, shows foreign body–type echoes in the vitreous as a result of intraocular calcification; the cornea, anterior chamber, and lens are usually normal. Cataract is seen extremely rarely and the tumor can often be distinctly visualized ultrasonographically.[26]

In patients with known ROP the use of current high-resolution B scans allows precise imaging of intraocular structures through safe, noninvasive techniques to assist in diagnosing the stage and severity of ROP as well as in perioperative evaluation.[27] Ultrasonographic examination is a valuable tool in stages 3, 4, and 5 of ROP to rule out, recognize, and classify retinal detachment. Ophthalmoscopy is often insufficient to clearly recognize and delimit shallow retinal

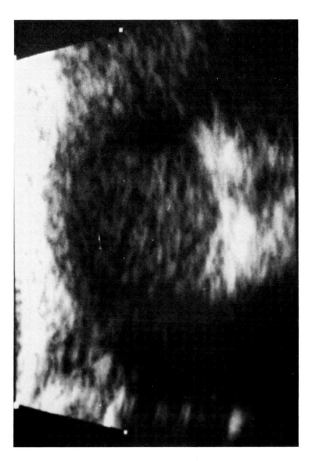

Fig. 10-10. Ultrasonographic appearance of ROP stage 5. Notice massive hemorrhage occupying the whole vitreous cavity. (Courtesy of C. Prieto, M.D., and I. Pastor Abascal, M.D.)

detachments with exudation. Even experienced observers may encounter considerable difficulty in recognizing the type and severity of retinal detachment. The pupil often dilates poorly as a result of persistent pupillary membrane, posterior synechiae, or iris hyperemia during the active phases of the disease. Excessive administration of dilating drops may cause potentially lethal cardiopulmonary, central nervous system, and gastrointestinal side effects in these fragile infants.[25] The media often lose transparency because of retrolental fibrovascular membranes or vitreous hemorrhages.[27,29]

B scan ultrasonography is valuable to determine the presence, configuration, and extension of retinal detachment, facilitating judgment of the type and severity of the detachment and in determining the location and size of the peripheral trough in funnel-

shaped detachments in stage 5.[19] Its use is also indicated in stage 3, 4, and 5 of ROP. In stage 3 it facilitates postoperative monitoring following ablation of the avascular retina by cryosurgery or laser. In stages 4 and 5, sequential ultrasonographic examinations may show the progression of the detachment as a result of increased traction.[19,30] In stages 4 and 5 it allows one to monitor perioperatively, before and after repairing retinal detachment by scleral buckle or by vitrectomy. After surgery for stages 3, 4, and 5 ROP, ophthalmoscopy may become especially difficult because of postoperative periocular edema preventing adequate exposure of the eye.

Subretinal blood and exudate may be identifiable by ultrasonographic examination. Subretinal and choroidal hemorrhages are recognized by a high and diffuse reflectivity in the appropriate areas. Vitreous pathology, such as the shape, extension, and location of fibrovascular proliferation into the vitreous or a vitreous hemorrhage, can be best observed by setting the ultrasonograph at a high gain (Fig. 10-10). The presence and degree of subretinal or choroidal exudate or hemorrhage can easily be defined by ultrasonography. While the subretinal echoes of subretinal hemorrhage are easily recognized, it may be difficult to differentiate between subretinal blood and exudate with current instruments.[21] New devices currently being developed will probably allow better imaging of intraocular pathology.[31]

Ultrasound is important in diagnosing subretinal hemorrhage because this hemorrhage carries such a poor prognosis in retinal detachment from ROP that some authorities elect not to operate such eyes.[19] Hemorrhagic choroidal detachment can be diagnosed by ultrasonography and can assist in the surgical planning by determining where to place sclerotomies to externally drain the hemorrhage. Comparing the preoperative ultrasonographic appearance with the operative findings in the various substages of stages 4 and 5, the ultrasonographic picture appears to correlate well with the operative findings, with a 90 percent correlation in some studies when hyaloid vessels were present.[32] Such high correlation is only possible when ultrasonography is performed by an experienced examiner with a clear understanding of its dynamic nature, the way the detachment develops, and the multiplicity of presentations in stages 4 and 5 of ROP. Standard horizontal and vertical optic nerve views would not accurately disclose a funnel dragged in an oblique superolateral direction, but customizing the views can be done in such a fashion as to refect

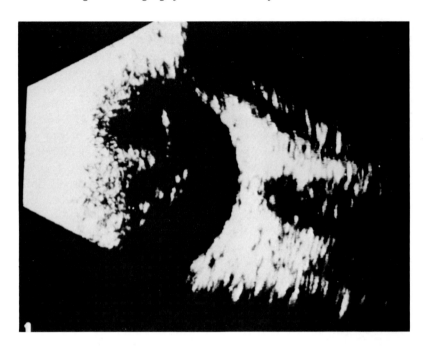

Fig. 10-11. Ultrasonographic appearance of ROP stage 4a. Notice early peripheral retinal detachment (concave) caused by traction by the fibrovascular tissue proliferated from the ridge. (From E. de Juan,[19] with permission.)

the pathology in full detail. Several studies have shown that the configuration of the detachment has strong prognostic significance regarding reattachment.[28,30,32–35] The rate of success decreases as the funnel of detached retina narrows.[30,32,34,35] The importance in diagnosing by ultrasonography the subtypes of stage 5 ROP with open posterior funnel is related to the fact that these are more easily operated upon and have a better prognosis for reattachment as compared with eyes with stage 5 ROP with narrow

posterior funnels, in which the retina often cannot be reattached surgically. Ultrasonography can thus be used to temporally monitor the morphology of the detachment and operate while the funnel is still wide in cases in which progressive narrowing can be demonstrated on repeated B scans.

Besides the morphology of the retinal detachment, other significant prognostic indicators of bad surgical result in stage 5 ROP are immature iris or pupil, vascularized epiretinal membranes, retinal folds,

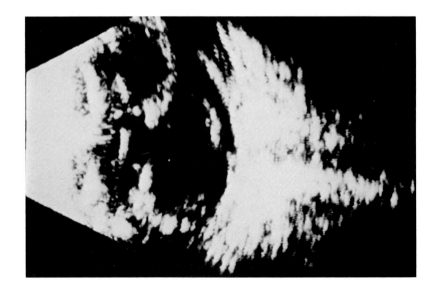

Fig. 10-12. Ultrasonographic appearance of ROP stage 5. Same eye as in Figure 10-11, 8 days later. Notice the funnel configuration, open anterior and narrow posterior (From E. de Juan,[19] with permission.)

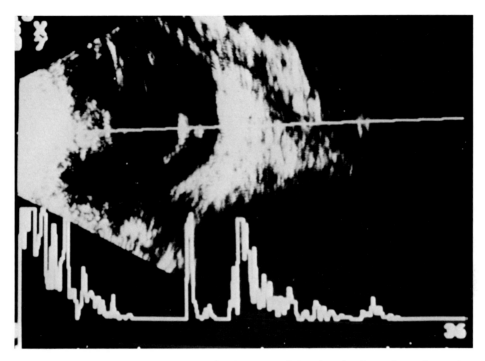

Fig. 10-13. Ultrasonographic appearance of ROP stage 5. Notice the funnel configuration, narrow anterior and narrow posterior. (From E. de Juan,[19] with permission.)

tractional retinoschisis, persistent hyaloid system, and subretinal blood or organization.[32] All of those factors can be assessed with reasonable accuracy by ultrasonography with the exception of some of the membrane morphology. In the latter case, however, ultrasonography provides some indirect clues regarding the extension of preretinal membranes behind the retrolental mass: ultrasonographic recognition of multiple folds, retinal dragging, and closed funnels correlate highly with the presence of prere-

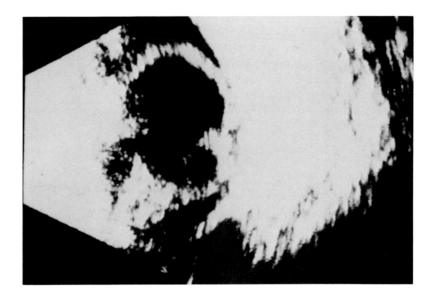

Fig. 10-14. Ultrasonographic appearance of ROP stage 5. Notice the funnel configuration, narrow anterior and open posterior (From E. de Juan,[19] with permission.)

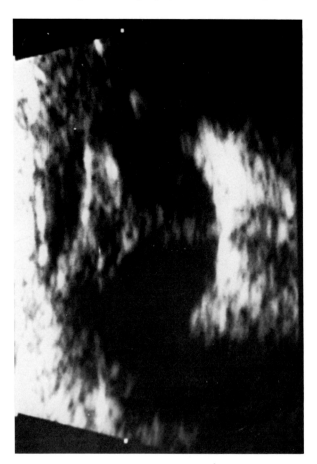

Fig. 10-15. Ultrasonographic appearance of ROP stage 5. Notice the funnel configuration, narrow posterior and open anterior. (Courtesy of C. Prieto, M.D., and I. Pastor Abascal, M.D.)

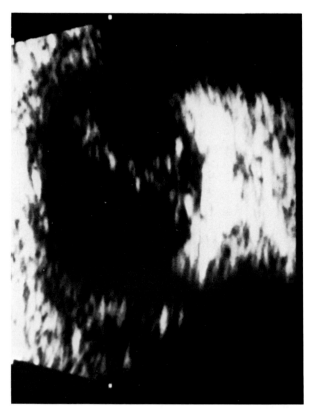

Fig. 10-16. Ultrasonographic appearance of ROP stage 5. Notice the configuration of the funnel, obliquely directed, narrow anterior and open posterior. (Courtesy of C. Prieto, M.D., and I. Pastor Abascal, M.D.)

tinal membranes.[32] Some experts, however, dispute the practical prognostic value of ultrasonography in stage 5 ROP and do not include it as part of the routine preoperative evaluation in these patients (S.T. Charles, personal communication, 1991). Figures 10-11 through 10-16 show the ultrasonographic appearance of Stage 4 and various subdivisions of stage 5 ROP.

Computed Tomography and Magnetic Resonance Imaging

The current level of resolution in computed tomography (CT) and magnetic resonance (MR) imaging is probably insufficient for their clinical use in sequential or perioperative evaluation of ROP. Both CT and MR imaging, however, are invaluable in the differential diagnosis of leukocoria. Diffuse retinoblastoma may be misdiagnosed on clinical or ultrasonic examination as an inflammatory process. CT is superior to MR imaging in identifying the intratumoral calcifications typical of retinoblastoma. The pineal gland must be examined by CT or MR imaging to rule out the so-called trilateral retinoblastoma (i.e., pinealoma associated with retinoblastoma of both eyes). Persistent hyperplastic primary vitreous (PHPV), another fairly common cause of leukocoria, may be seen on CT scan as retrolental dense images often extending from the posterior pole to the lens (Fig. 10-17). Eyes with Stage 5 ROP show disorganization and increased density of the intraocular content. The retinal detachment may be visible, as well as anomalies in the density of the lens (secondary cataract) or in the position of the lens (anterior or posterior displacement) (Fig. 10-18).

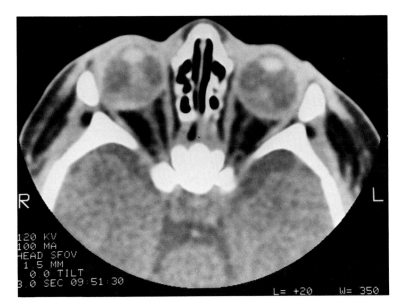

Fig. 10-17. Computed tomography scan of persistent hyperplastic primary vitreous. Observe the bilateral dense structure anterior to the retina. In the right eye it can be seen extending up to the lens. (Courtesy of J.W. Yeakley, M.D., University of Texas Medical School, Houston.)

TREATMENT

Prophylaxis

Since ROP is essentially a developmental vasculopathy of the prematurely born infant, it is obvious that adequate prenatal care decreasing the incidence of premature babies is the most important prophylaxis. Administration of adrenocorticosteroids to the pregnant mother shortly before delivery causes maturation of the fetal lungs and decreases the incidence of respiratory distress syndrome. By decreasing the likelihood of need for supplementary oxygen it is likely that this will be associated with decreased risk for ROP. Knowledge of the premature delivery is in most cases unfortunately not early enough to allow time for lung maturation, but it certainly seems an appropriate prophylactic measure whenever possible. Widespread use of exogenous surfactant will similarly decrease the morbidity of borderline premature infants but, like prenatal adenocorticoster-

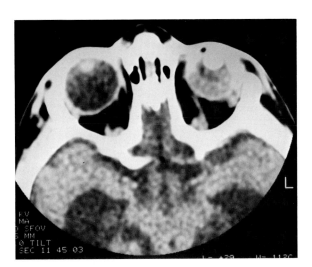

Fig. 10-18. Computed tomography scan of ROP stage 5, left eye. Notice disorganization of the intraocular content due to total retinal detachment and fibrovascular tissue in the vitreous cavity. (Courtesy of J.W. Yeakley, M.D., University of Texas Medical School, Houston.)

TABLE 10-3. Guidelines for Re-Examination of Infants with ROP Based on Appearance of the Fundus

	Re-examine in:
Zone III findings	
Immature retinas	4–6 weeks
Stage 1 or 2	2 weeks
Stage 2+ or 3	1 week
Zone II findings	
Stage 1	2 weeks
Stage 2	1 week
Prethreshold disease	
Any stage Zone I	3–7 days
Stage 2+ Zone II	
Stage 3	
Stage 3+ less than 5 clock hours	

oids, it also will increase viability of infants too premature for survival at the present time.

Administration of vitamin E supplements to the premature infant has been proposed to prevent or ameliorate ROP because these infants are known to carry low serum levels of vitamin E, because vitamin E acts as scavenger of free radicals, and because studies show beneficial effects of vitamin E in oxygen-induced retinopathy in some full-term newborn animals. Clinical use of vitamin E for ROP has resulted in conflicting reports regarding efficacy, dosage, mode of administration, and safety. A recent study by the U.S. Institute of Medicine found no conclusive evidence of benefit from vitamin E administration for ROP.[36]

Stages 1 through 3

No treatment is indicated for the initial stages of ROP. Repeat ophthalmoscopic examinations are timed based on the appearance of the fundus and the risk factors. The guidelines described in Table 10-3 are modified based on associated risk factors. The current recommendation of the Cryotherapy for Retinopathy of Prematurity Cooperative Group is to treat eyes with "threshold disease," defined as five or more continuous or eight cummulative 30° sectors (clock hours) of stage 3 ROP in Zone I or II in the presence of "plus" disease.[4] Treatment for threshold disease consists in ablation of the avascular peripheral retina up to the anterior edge of the ridge. The risk for blindness in threshold disease is about 50 percent, and cryoablation has proven to be effective in reducing by one-half the risk of unfavorable outcome (retinal fold, retinal detachment, or retrolental tissue) in eyes with threshold disease receiving treatment.[4] About 25 percent of eyes receiving treatment for threshold disease will still evolve to unfavorable outcome, but in most treated eyes ROP regresses. Following cryoablation the signs of "plus" disease usually disappear within 24 hours. Within 2 weeks the ridge regresses and normal retinal vessels grow across the ridge.

Systemic complications of cryoablation include bradycardia, cyanosis, hypoxemia, and respiratory depression.[4] Respiratory arrest and cardiorespiratory arrest have been reported, probably caused by excessive use of local anesthetics.[37] Local complications include vitreous, retinal, or preretinal hemor-

rhages and hematomas or lacerations of the conjunctiva.[4] Late complications of cryoablation are not well defined. Rhegmatogenous retinal detachment has been reported 1 to 4 years following cryoablation, and this author has seen three cases of severe anisometropic myopia in the treated eye in patients with bilateral symmetric disease in which ROP regressed in both eyes following cryoablation of one eye. Some authors have performed cryoablation of the fibrovascular ridge and adjacent areas[38,39] but its benefits are controversial[40]; serious side effects such as triggering proliferative vitreoretinopathy or optic nerve atrophy appear to be more likely than with cryoablation of the retina anterior to the shunt.[38] Laser photocoagulation has been used for many years in Japan and it appears a desirable alternative for eyes with clear media.[41]

Stages 4 and 5

Stage 4

Treatment of stage 4 is controversial. Some authorities recommend no treatment (S.T. Charles personal communication, 1990) while others recommend scleral buckling and/or vitrectomy.[42-44] Some patients with non-rhegmatogenous retinal detachment will improve spontaneously, and there is no good evidence that visual results are better in eyes treated with scleral buckling as compared with no surgery. Most published series include numbers too small for hard conclusions.[42-44] Scleral buckling, however, remains an accepted procedure as part of the treatment of rhegmatogenous retinal detachment in children with stages 4 and 5 ROP[45,46] or in late-onset retinal detachment in regressed ROP.[47]

Stage 5

Treatment of stage 5 is usually recommended months to years following resolution of the active acute phase of ROP.[48] The techniques currently used —vitrectomy with delamination, peeling of membranes, and internal tamponade—may be done through open-sky[49,50] or closed-eye[28,33,51,52] approaches. Closed-eye technique appears to achieve slightly better results[28,33,49-52] but the global results are disappointing. Anatomic reattachment occurs in less than 50 percent of patients in most series[28,33,35,49,52]; visual success depends on visual criteria and varies between 10 and 80 percent of those with anatomic success.[28,33,48-50,52] A consecutive series of 580 eyes undergoing closed-eye vitrectomy during 1977 to 1985 recorded an anatomic success rate of 46 percent and visual success rates 10 percent less than anatomic success.[52]

A recent report using data collected by investigators of the Multicenter Trial of Cryotherapy for Retinopathy of Prematurity showed that vitreous surgery has little effect on visual outcome in retinal detachment due to ROP even when the retina was anatomically reattached.[53] Of 129 eyes with stage 5 ROP, 58 eyes did not undergo retinal detachment surgery. Ten percent of those showed partial spontaneous rattachment (without recovery of vision). Of the 71 eyes operated for repair of total retinal detachment (closed-eye or open-sky vitrectomy), the anatomic success rate was 28 percent. Only two eyes (one infant) showed any evidence of pattern vision.[53] In any case, following reattachment of the retina it is imperative to fully correct all factors predisposing to amblyopia and to wait, since it may take months or years to clinically see visual improvement.[50]

REFERENCES

1. Kinsey VE: Retrolental fibroplasia. Cooperative study of retrolental fibroplasia and the use of oxygen. Arch Ophthalmol 56:481, 1956
2. McDonald AD: Neurological and ophthalmic disorders in children of very low birth weight. Br Med J 1:895, 1962
3. Cross KW: Cost of preventing retrolental fibroplasia? Lancet 2:954, 1973
4. Cryotherapy for Retinopathy of Prematurity Cooperative Group: Multicenter trial of cryotherapy for retinopathy of prematurity. Preliminary results. Arch Ophthalmol 106:471, 1988
5. Charles JB, Ganthier R, Apphia AP: Incidence and characteristics of retinopathy of prematurity in a low-income inner-city population. Ophthalmology 98:14, 1991
6. Hammer ME, Mullen PW, Ferguson JG et al: Logistic analysis of risk factors in acute retinopathy of prematurity. Am J Ophthalmol 102:1, 1986
7. Glass P, Avery GB, Subramanian KN et al: Effect of bright light in the hospital nursery on the incidence of retinopathy of prematurity. N Engl J Med 313:401, 1985
8. Garner A: The pathology of retinopathy of prematurity. p. 19. In Silverman WA, Flynn JT (eds): Retinopathy of Prematurity. Blackwell Scientific Publishers, Boston, 1985
9. Bruckner HL: Retrolental fibroplasia: associated with intrauterine anoxia? Arch Ophthalmol 80:504, 1968
10. Stefan FH, Ehalt H: Non-oxygen induced retinitis proliferans and retinal detachment in full-term infants. Br J Ophthalmol 54:490, 1974
11. Rosenfeld SI, Smith ME: Ocular findings in incontinentia pigmenti. Ophthalmology 92:543, 1985
12. Brookhurst RJ, Albert DM, Zakow ZN: Pathologic findings in familial exudative vitreoretinopathy. Arch Ophthalmol 99:2143, 1981
13. Addison DJ, Font RL, Manschot W: Proliferative retinopathy in anencephalic babies. Am J Ophthalmol 74:967, 1972
14. Flower RW: Perinatal retinal vascular physiology. p. 97. In Silvermann WA, Flynn JT (eds): Retinopathy of Prematurity. Blackwell Scientific Publications, Boston, 1986
15. Ashton N: Retinal angiogenesis in the human embryo. Br Med Bull 26:103, 1970
16. Payne JW: Retinopathy of prematurity. p. 909. In Avey ME, Taeusch HW (eds): Schaffer's Diseases of the Newborn, 5th Ed. WB Saunders, Philadelphia, 1984
17. Yee AG, Revel RP: Loss and reappearance of gap-junctions in regenerating liver. J Cell Biol 78:554, 1978
18. Foos RY: Acute retrolental fibroplasia. Graefes Arch Clin Exp Ophthalmol 195:87, 1975
19. de Juan E Jr, Shields S, Machemer R: The role of ultrasound in the management of retinopathy of prematurity. Ophthalmology 95:884, 1988
20. Committee for the Classification of Retinopathy of Prematurity: an international classification of retinopathy of prematurity. Arch Ophthalmol 102:1130, 1984
21. International Committee for the Classification of Retinopathy of Prematurity: An international classification of retinopathy of prematurity II; the classification of retinal detachment. Arch Ophthalmol 105:906, 1987
22. Palmer EA: Optimal timing of examination for acute retrolental fibroplasia. Ophthalmology 88:662, 1981
23. Anand KJS, Hickey PR: Pain and its effects in the human neonate and fetus. N Engl J Med 317:1321, 1987
24. Clark WN, Hodges R, Noel LP et al: The oculocardiac reflex during ophthalmoscopy in premature infants. Am J Ophthalmol 99:649, 1985

25. Isenberg SJ, Abrams C, Hyman PE: Effects of cyclopentolate eyedrops on gastric secretory function in pre-term infants. Ophthalmology 92:698, 1985

26. Sterns GK, Coleman DF, Ellsworth, RM: The ultrasonic characteristics of retinoblastoma. Am J Ophthalmol 78:606, 1974

27. Shapiro DR, Stone RD: Ultrasonic characteristics of retinopathy of prematurity presenting with leukokoria. Arch Ophthalmol 103:1690, 1985

28. Chong LP, Machemer R, de Juan E: Vitrectomy for advanced stages of retinopathy of prematurity. Am J Ophthalmol 102:710 1986

29. Palmer EA: Discussion of Tasman W, Brown GC, Schaffer DB et al: Cryotherapy for active retinopathy of prematurity. Ophthalmology 93:585, 1986

30. de Juan E Jr, Machemer R: Retinopathy of prematurity: surgical technique. Retina 7:63, 1987

31. Paulin CJ, Harasiewicz K, Sherar MD, Foster FS: Clinical use of ultrasound biomicroscopy. Ophthalmology 98:287, 1991

32. Jabbour NM, Eller AE, Hiroshe T et al: Stage 5 retinopathy of prematurity. Prognostic value of morphologic findings. Ophthalmology 94:1640, 1987

33. Trese MT: Visual results and prognostic factors for vision following surgery for stage V retinopathy of prematurity. Ophthalmology 93:574, 1986

34. de Juan E Jr, Machemer R, Charles ST et al: Surgery for stage 5 retinopathy of prematurity, letter. Arch Ophthalmol 105:21, 1987

35. Tasman WS: Discussion of Jabbour NM, Eller AE, Hiroshe T et al: Stage 5 retinopathy of prematurity. Prognostic value of morphologic findings. Ophthalmology 94:1646, 1987

36. Vitamin E and Retinopathy of Prematurity. Institute of Medicine Publication 86-02. National Academy Press, Washington, DC, 1986

37. Brown GC, Tasman WS, Naidoff M et al: Systemic complications associated with retinal cryoablation for retinopathy of prematurity. Ophthalmology 97:855, 1991

38. Kingham JD: Acute retrolental fibroplasia II. Treatment by cyrosurgery. Arch Ophthalmol 96:2049, 1978

39. Hindle NW, Leyton J: Prevention of cicatricial retrolental fibroplasia by cryotherapy. Can J Ophthalmol 13:277, 1978

40. Keith CG: Visual outcome and effect of treatment in stage III developing retrolental fibroplasia. Br J Ophthalmol 66:446, 1982

41. Tamai M: Treatment of acute retinopathy of prematurity by cryotherapy and photocoagulation. p. 151. In McPherson AR, Hittner HM, Kretzer FL: Retinopathy of Prematurity. Current Concepts and Controversies. BC Decker, Philadelphia, 1986

42. Baruch E, Bracha R, Godel V, Lazar M: Buckling procedure in infant retrolental fibroplasia. J Ocular Ther Surg 1:65, 1981

43. Tasman W: Management of retinopathy of prematurity. Ophthalmology 92:995, 1985

44. Topilow HW, Ackerman AL, Wang FM: The treatment of advanced retinopathy of prematurity by cryotherapy and scleral buckling surgery. Ophthalmology 92:379, 1985

45. Starzycka M, Ciechanowska A, Gergovich A: Retinal detachment in retrolental fibroplasia. Ophthalmologica 181:261, 1980

46. Tasman W: Retinal detachment in retrolental fibroplasia. Graefes Arch Clin Exp Ophthalmol 195:130, 1975

47. Sneed SR, Pulido JS, Blodi CF et al: Surgical management of late-onset retinal detachments associated with regressed retinopathy of prematurity. Ophthalmology 97:179, 1990.

48. Zilis JD, de Juan E, Machemer R: Advanced retinopathy of prematurity. The anatomic and visual results of vitreous surgery. Ophthalmology 97:821, 1990

49. Hirose T, Schepens CL: Open-sky vitrectomy in retrolental fibroplasia. Paper presented at the American Academy of Ophthalmology Annual Meeting, November 12, 1984

50. Tasman W, Borrone RN, Bolling J: Open sky vitrectomy for total retinal detachment in retinopathy of prematurity. Ophthalmology 94:449, 1987

51. Machemer R: Closed vitrectomy for severe retrolental fibroplasia in infants. Ophthalmology 90:436, 1983

52. Charles ST: Vitrectomy with ciliary body entry for retrolental fibroplasia. p. 225. In McPherson AR, Hittner HM, Kretzer FL (eds): Retinopathy of Prematurity. Current Concepts and Controversies. BC Decker, Philadelphia, 1986

53. Quinn GE, Dobson V, Barr CC et al: Visual acuity in infants after vitrectomy for severe retinopathy of prematurity. Ophthalmology 98:5, 1991

Index

Page numbers followed by f *indicate figures; those followed by* t *indicate tables.*
Page ranges with final f *or* t *indicate a figure or table within the range.*

A

Abdomen
    gasless, 166, 168
    pathologic processes of, 203
    ultrasound of, 203
Abdominal masses, of extra-abdominal
        origin, 232–233f
Abdominal wall defects, 18, 169, 171,
        173f
ABO isoimmune hemolytic anemia, 8
Absent pulmonary valve syndrome,
        144
Acalculous cholecystitis, acute,
        208–210f
Acquired immunodeficiency syn-
        drome. *See* TORCH
        infections, intrauterine
Adaptation, 2
Adenoma sebaceum, 60
ADH (antidiuretic hormone), 4
Adrenal gland disorders, 22, 226–229f
Adrenocorticosteroids, for retinopa-
        thy of prematurity,
        277–278
Adrenoleukodystrophy, 76, 79f
Adult respiratory distress syndrome
        (ARDS), 93f, 94, 109
Aganglionic megacolon
        (Hirschsprung's disease),
        18, 188, 192–194f
Agyria, 61
Air
    in gallbladder, 207, 208f
    in gastrointestinal tract, normal
        passage of, 165, 166f
    in pyelocaliceal system, 221–222f
    in sigmoid colon, 166, 167f
Air leak syndromes, 16
AIUM (American Institute of
        Ultrasound in Medicine),
        33
Alexander's disease, 76, 79f
Alobar holoprosencephaly, 56
Alpha-fetoprotein, 6
American Institute of Ultrasound in
        Medicine (AIUM), 33
Amniocentesis, 6
Amniotic fluid, production of, 3

Anemia, 8, 20
Anencephaly, 51
Annular pancreas, 178
Anomalous coronary arteries, 157
Anorectal anomalies, 193, 196–197f
Antidiuretic hormone (ADH), 4
Antral diaphragm, 174, 178
Aorta
    coarctation of, 152–153f
    normal abdominal, ultrasonogra-
        phy of, 233f, 235
    thrombosis of, 234f, 235
    two-dimensional echocardio-
        graphy, 144
Aortic arch
    anomalies, vascular ring of, 137,
        138f
    laterality of, 122
Aortic calcification, 235–236f
Aortic valve stenosis, 122, 135
Aortopulmonary window, 122
Apnea of prematurity, 17
Apoproteins, 4
Aqueductal stenosis, 53, 58, 59f
Arachnoid cysts, 59
ARDS (adult respiratory distress
        syndrome), 93f, 94, 109
Arnold-Chiari malformation, 13, 53,
        54f–55f
Arteriovenous fistula of vein of Galen,
        59f
Arteriovenous malformations,
        58–59f
Arthrogryposis, 254, 256f
Asphyxia neonatorum, 11, 80f
Astrocytomas, 60
Atresia
    of pulmonary artery, 120
    of small bowel, 178, 182f–184f
Atria-branchia concordance, 127
Atrial localization, 127
Atrial septal defect, 129, 131, 154
Atrial septum, two-dimensional
        echocardiography of, 142
Atrial situs, 127, 140f
Atrioventricular canal defects, 118,
        131
Atrioventricular connection, 139–140,
        141f

Atrioventricular valves, two-dimen-
        sional echocardiography
        of, 142–143
Autoregulation, 66

B

Barium, 26–27
Barotrauma, 94, 95f–96f
Basilar impression, 53
B cells, 5
Beckwith-Weidmann syndrome,
        214
Bernouilli equation, 146–147
Bile, inspissated, 207–209f
Biliary atresia, 38, 39f, 205
Biliary calculi, 207f
Biliary hydrops, 208
Biliary sludge, intravesicular,
        206–207f
Bilirubin, 6
Biological clock, 2
Birth asphyxia, 78, 83f
Birth injuries, 9
Birth trauma, brain pathology from,
        83, 84f
Boerhaave's syndrome, 173
Bone dysplasias. *See* Skeletal dysplasias
Bone infections, 255–259f
Bone scan, radionuclide, 42–44f
Bootshaped heart, 124
Bowel gas, 165, 167f
Bradycardia, 126
Brain
    atrophy, 64, 68f
    characteristics, 49–50
    death, diagnosis of, 37–38
    developing, degenerative diseases
        of, 76–83f
    maturation, patterns of, 71, 74–76f
    pathology, diagnosis of, 50
    secondary acquired injuries, 64,
        66–71f
Brain lesions, of circulatory origin,
        64, 66–67, 70–71f
Brain SPECT, 37–38f
Brain tumors, congenital, 59
Breast milk jaundice, 19

Great arteries, transposition of, 133–134f, 150–151f
Group B streptococcal pneumonitis, 107, 108f
Gut, functional immaturity of, 18

H

Hamartomas, 60
Heart. *See also* Cardiac entries
  fetal-premature, 3–4
  function, M-mode echocardiography of, 145–147f
  position anomalies of, 126–128f
  size and shape, 122–126f
Heart disease, congenital, 14–15. *See also specific congenital diseases*
  classification by degrees of pulmonary arterial vascularity, 118t
  decreased pulmonary arterial markings of, 134–135f
  increased pulmonary arterial markings of, 128–134f
  normal pulmonary arterial markings of, 135–137f
  positional anomalies, bony thorax abnormalities and, 127–128
  right aortic arch in, 123t
Heart rate, fetal, 7
Hemangioendothelioma, hepatic, 209, 210f
Hemangiomas, hepatic, 209–210, 211f
Hematopoietic system, fetal-premature, 5
Hemimelia, longitudinal ulnar, 253f
Hemoglobin, 5
Hemorrhage
  adrenal, 22, 226–228f
  gastrointestinal, 18, 39–41f
  intracranial, 12–13, 67
  intraventricular, 64, 66, 68
  periventricular, 12
  pulmonary, 17, 100f
  subependymal, 64, 67–68, 70f
  subretinal and choroidal, 273f
Hemorrhagic brain lesions, 64, 66–67
Hemostasis, abnormal, 20
Hepatic veins, two-dimensional echocardiography of, 143
Hepatitis B virus infection. *See* TORCH infections, intrauterine
Hepatobiliary tree abnormalities, radionuclide studies of, 38–39f

Hernia, diaphragmatic, 168–171f, 204, 205f
Herpes simplex infections, 83, 84f, 110f–111f. *See also* TORCH infections, intrauterine
Heterotopia, 51, 53f, 61, 62f
High-risk newborns, 49
High-risk pregnancy, fetal surveillance during, 7
Hip dislocation, congenital, 22, 244, 246–247f
Hirschsprung's disease (aganglionic megacolon), 18, 188, 192–194f
Histogenesis, 58
Holoprosencephaly, 56f
Horseshoe kidney, 220–221f
Hyaline membrane, 105
Hyaline membrane disease
  with cardiomegaly, 100f
  clinical similarities with neonatal pneumonitis, 107
  treatment of, 104–106f, 114f
Hydranencephaly, 63
Hydrocephalus
  with aqueductal stenosis, 53
  with arteriovenous fistula of vein of Galen, 59f
  cerebral hemisphere destruction in, 63–64, 66f
  posthemorrhagic, 12
  vs. alobar holoprosencephaly, 56
Hydromyelia, 53
Hydronephrosis, secondary to ureterocele, 218–219f
Hydrops fetalis, 107f
21-Hydroxylase deficiency, secondary congenital adrenal hyperplasia of, 228f, 229
Hyperbilirubinemia, 19
Hyperinsulinism, 21
Hyperplasia, congenital adrenal, 228f, 229
Hypertension, pregnancy-induced, 8–9
Hypertrophy of B pancreatic cells, 214f
Hypertrophic pyloric stenosis, of low-birthweight infant, 229
Hypoglycemia, 21
Hypoplastic left heart syndrome, 122, 134, 153–154
Hypothyroidism, congenital, 21

I

Ileal atresia, 178, 184f
Iliac artery wall calcifications, 235f
Imaging methods, costs of, 49

Immmunoglobulins, 5
Immune system, fetal-premature, 5
Imperforate anus, 18, 196f, 197f
Inborn errors of metabolism, 20–21
Incidence, of prematurity, 49
Indium-111, 36
Infections, 83. *See also* Bone infections; *specific infections*
Inferior vena cava
  abdominal ultrasonography of, 236–239f
  dilated, 236, 238f, 239
  fragmented catheter in, 238f, 239
  thrombosis of, 236, 237f
  two-dimensional echocardiography of, 143
Infradiaphragmatic pulmonary sequestration, 232–233f
Intelligence quotient (IQ), in mental retardation, 14
Intensive care unit, 87
Intestinal fixation and malrotation, abnormal, 180–182, 185f–186f
Intracranial hemorrhages, 12–13, 67. *See also specific types of intracranial hemorrhage*
Intrahepatic calcifications, congenital, 212–213f
Intrahepatic gas, 213–214f
Intrahepatic hematomas, 210–212f
Intrauterine growth retardation (IUGR), 1, 2, 7
Intraventricular hemorrhage, 64, 66, 68
IQ (Intelligence quotient), in mental retardation, 14
Isolated dextrocardia, 127
IUGR (intrauterine growth retardation), 1, 2, 7

J

Jaundice, neonatal, 19
Jejunal atresia, 178, 183f, 229f
Jejunal stenosis, 178, 182f
Jejunoileal atresia, 18
Jeune's syndrome, 252f

K

Kartagener's syndrome, 127
Kawasaki disease, 157
Kerley B lines, 119, 129, 132
Kidney. *See also* Renal entries
  air in pyelocaliceal system, 221–222f

R

Radiation
    acute effects of, 25
    from x-rays, early effects of, 26
Radioiodine, 36
Radioisotopes. *See* Radionuclides;
    specific radionuclides
Radionuclide angiography, 157
Radionuclides, 31, 35–36. *See also*
    Nuclear Medicine
    absorbed radiation doses from,
        29–31t
    dosage, 36–37
Radiopharmaceuticals. *See* Nuclear
    Medicine; Radionuclides
Real-time duplex Doppler ultrasound,
    203
Recessive polycystic renal disease, 217
Renal agenesis, 215f
Renal cysts, simple, 218f
Renal hypoplasia, 215–216f
Renal insufficiency and failure, in
    premature newborn,
        19–20
Renal ischemia, 223, 224f
Renal masses, identification of,
    41–42f
Renal parenchymal disease, 222–223f
Renal rupture, 221f
Renal system, fetal-premature, 4–5
Renal tubular acidosis, 20
Renal vein thrombosis, 223f
Respiration control, fetal-premature, 4
Respiratory distress syndrome, 15, 94,
    96
Retina, normal immature, 268–269
Retinal detachment
    in retinopathy of prematurity,
        268f, 269–270
    rhegmatogenous, 278
    ultrasonography of, 273–274f
Retinopathy of prematurity (ROP)
    classification, 267–269f
    computed tomography of,
        276–277f
    etiology, 265
    incidence, 11–2, 265
    magnetic resonance imaging of, 276
    ophthalmoscopic diagnosis,
        271–272
    pathogenesis, 11–12, 266–268f
    prophylactic treatment, 277–279t
    regressed, 270f, 271t
    screening, diagnostic, 270–271
    stages, 268–270t
    ultrasonography of, 272–276f
Rhabdomyoma, 126
Rhabdomyosarcoma, 126, 210, 211f

Rh immune globulin, 8
Rh isoimmune hemolytic anemia, 8
Rhombencephalon, 55
Rib notching, 127
Rickets, 21, 256–257, 260f
ROP. *See* Retinopathy of prematurity
Rotavirus enteritis, 231, 232f
Rubella. *See* TORCH infections,
    intrauterine
Rubeola. *See* TORCH infections,
    intrauterine

S

Sacrococcygeal teratoma, 232f
Sail sign, 123f
Schizencephaly, 61–62, 63f, 64f
Schwannomas, 60
Scimitar syndrome, 1333
Scintigraphy, gastroesophageal, 174
Scoliosis, idiopathic, 127
Secondary neurulation
    derangements of, 53
    description of, 51, 53
Seizures, 13
Semilobar holoprosencephaly, 56
Semilunar valves, two-dimensional
    echocardiography, 143f
Sepsis neonatorum, in premature
    newborns, 11
Septic arthritis, 258f–259f
Septo-optic dysplasia, 56–57f
SGA (small for gestational age), 1
Shunt, left-to-right, 118
Sialicosis, 225f, 226
Single photon emission computed
    tomography (SPECT),
        45
Situs ambiguus, 127
Situs inversus, 127, 140f
Situs solitus, 127, 140f
Skeletal dysplasias, 22
    classification of, 248f–249t
    group classification, 253–354
    radiographic diagnosis of,
        249–255f
Skeletal system
    abnormalities of, 127–128
    determination of maturation level,
        243, 244f–245f
    maturation, 127
Skull fractures, 83
Small bowel disorders, 178, 180–186f
Small-for-gestational-age (SGA), 1
Small left colon syndrome, 183, 188,
    192f
Sodium, fractional excretion of, at
    birth, 4–5

SPECT (single photon emission com-
    puted tomography), 45
Spina bifida, 13, 53
Spinal canal, wide, 243, 244f
Spleen, abnormal location of, 214
Spontaneous abortion, 8
State screens, neonatal, 20–21
Stenosis, pulmonary, 118
Sternal ossification, premature fusion,
    127
Stomach, disorders of, 174, 178–179f
Stroke, perinatal, 63
Sturge-Weber syndrome, 60f
Subacute necrotizing
    encephalomyelitis, 76,
        78f
Subarachnoid hemorrhage, 12–13
Subdural hematomas, 83
Subdural hemorrhage, 12
Subependymal hemorrhages, 64,
    67–68, 70f
Superior vena cava, two-dimensional
    echocardiography of, 143
Surfactant, pulmonary, respiratory
    distress syndrome and, 15
Syphilis, 109f, 257f. *See also* TORCH
    infections, intrauterine
Syringomyelia, 53
Systemic-to-pulmonary flow rate, 146

T

Tachyarrhythmias, 126
Talipes equinovarus deformities,
    22–23, 244, 246f
TAPVC (total anomalous pulmonary
    venous connection),
        132–133
T cells, 5
Technetium-99m-labeled compounds
    absorbed doses from studies, 31
    IDA hepatobiliary studies, 39
    risks of, 30, 31t
    usage of, 35–36
Telencephalon, 55
Teratoma, sacrococcygeal, 232f
Tetralogy of Fallot
    peripheral pulmonic stenosis and,
        154
    pulmonary artery underdevelop-
        ment and, 120
    pulmonary vascularity and, 118,
        134, 135f
    with scoliosis, 127, 128f
Thoracic cage deformity, secondary
    to bronchopulmonary
        dysplasia, 257, 261–262f
Thoracic dystrophy, 252f